Ever Widening Circles

& Mystical Moments

Jean Shinoda Bolen, MD

International Author & Speaker, Activist, Feminist, Psychiatrist, Jungian Analyst

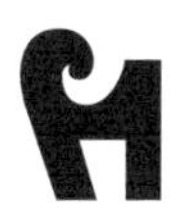

CHIRON PUBLICATIONS • ASHEVILLE, NORTH CAROLINA

Original Cover Artwork by Jean Shinoda Bolen, M.D.
Cover Design and Book Chapter Photomontage Artwork by Lynda Carré
Cover Portrait Photograph by D. Kelly Images
Interior design by Danijela Mijailovic

Published in 2025 by Chiron Publications, P.O. Box 19690, Asheville, N.C. 28815-1690.

Printed primarily in the United States of America.

ISBN 978-1-68503-540-2 paperback
ISBN 978-1-68503-541-9 hardcover
ISBN 978-1-68503-539-6 electronic
ISBN 978-1-68503-537-2 limited edition paperback
ISBN 978-1-68503-538-9 limited edition hardcover

Library of Congress Cataloging-in-Publication Data Pending

BOOKS by JEAN SHINODA BOLEN

The Tao of Psychology

Goddesses in Everywoman

Gods in Everyman

Ring of Power

Crossing to Avalon

Close to the Bone

The Millionth Circle

Goddesses in Older Women

Crones Don't Whine

Urgent Message from Mother

Like a Tree

Moving Toward the Millionth Circle

Artemis

I live my life in widening circles
that reach out across the world
I may not complete this last one
but I give myself to it.

~ Rainer Maria Rilke, *The Book of Hours*
Translation by Joanna Macy and Anita Barrows

There is no linear evolution: there is only a
circumambulation of the self.

~ C. G. Jung, *Memories, Dreams, Reflections*

One sees clearly only with the heart. Anything
essential is invisible to the eyes.

~ Antoine de Saint-Exupéry, *The Little Prince*

Contents

Preface

Every Widening Circles & Mystical Moments

I was a child whose life was dramatically affected by historical events. After Japan bombed Pearl Harbor in Hawaii and the United States entered World War II, all people of Japanese ancestry on the west coast of the United States were to be rounded up and imprisoned behind barbed wire in remote relocation camps. It did not matter that we were American citizens. To avoid this, my family became instead, in the language of the United Nations, "internally displaced refugees" for a short time. I was in kindergarten when we left Los Angeles for central California, while my father went to Sacramento to get papers that would allow us to leave the state. Once we crossed the state boundary, we were free American citizens again. This was the beginning of many moves during the war years in which I went to four elementary schools in a variety of places.

Until I wrote this book, I've said very little about my personal life while speaking and teaching nationally and internationally. My public and professional persona is as an author, an advocate for women's rights, a psychiatrist and a Jungian analyst. I am breaking two major taboos telling personal stories about my family and myself. There is my family of origin, with hundreds of years of Japanese tradition of maintaining appearance, which means that writing about my impaired younger brother is revealing a family secret.

Then there was the Freudian psychoanalytic training in my psychiatric residency which taught me to be a neutral blank screen and to volunteer no personal information. Instead, I listen with compassion, feel with, care about, and want the best outcome for the individuals who work with me (patients, analysands by professional definition).

Dreams reveal, in the language of metaphors and memories, what it is that we have tried to forget, need to forgive, or no longer suppress in order to remember and be ourselves now. I listen with empathy as I hear their experiences and feelings. I respond from my heart and mind with words that can lead to insights as well as healing. Trust grows as bottled-up grief and shame as well as joy comes and is shared with me.

Memoirs are retrospective. In life, significant events may not always seem so until later: "We had the experience but missed the meaning / And approach to the meaning restores the experience in a different form." These are words from T. S. Eliot's *Four Quartets*—and how true they are! This is what I found out when I returned to long ago experiences in this memoir. The poem recalls and reflects upon ineffable personal moments, with references to history and to places, which I found myself also doing.

The second half of the title of my memoir is "and Mystical Moments." Mystical, spiritual, subjective soul experiences are threshold or liminal perceptions, where visible and invisible worlds merge, where ordinary time and eternal time overlap, when "music heard so deeply / That it is not heard at all, but you are the music / While the music lasts" (words from *Four Quartets*, "The Dry Salvages" by T.S. Eliot). In childhood, late adolescence, and as an adult, mystical moments and insights gave me a sense of coming into this world with meaning and purpose about what I could do with my life.

I also pay attention to synchronicity, which was the subject of my first book, *The Tao of Psychology: Synchronicity and the Self.* At the time, "synchronicity" (a word coined by C. G. Jung for "meaningful coincidences") was considered too esoteric a word to be in the title. Many significant, life-changing meetings, and many personally transformative spontaneous events came about through synchronicity, and could not be explained by cause and effect. Such moments, large and small events that can't be explained, are like miracles of significant timing, or opportunities that evoke gratitude and wonder.

Once we know how and what affects us deeply, and remember how we adapted in order to be acceptable (and may still do so), there is still time and timing (as long as we are still here) to know ourselves. There is still time to learn how we can help and why we are still here. How and what can we learn, how can we help, and will we discover that there are reasons to still be here?

In this memoir, I am making "rounds" on my own life, as I share my stories and insights. Maybe you will find some pearls of information here, words that bring back memory, a definition of something of importance that you didn't have words for before, a metaphor that fits, or the clarity of a psychological insight or a Jungian concept expressed in ordinary English.

While young adults often struggle to do or become whatever it is that matters to them, so does accomplishment and position on retirement become an obstacle for elders. It gets in the way of doing and learning something new that could be meaningful or creative. Fear of looking foolish is a major obstacle when a spouse or grown children reflect this back, just as failure at relationships or work is also often an obstacle to a young or midlife adult. It takes insight and time, as well as courage, intention, choice, and synchronicity to choose to do what is meaningful personally and to make a commitment to follow through.

My personal insights and commentary are meant to illuminate the lives of those who read my memoir and find themselves remembering their own childhood and years since. There are the personality patterns with which we came into the world, that show up in infancy as extraverted energy and movement or introverted quiet, as well as the deeper aspects: archetypes or talents with which we were born. Depending on what gender, what culture, what family we were born into, they are aspects in us that were either valued and developed or ridiculed and suppressed.

As I looked back on the path my life has taken, I see that my personal journey resembles a series of circles that resemble a widening spiral. What was inwardly meaningful and touched my soul fit the concept of "circumambulating the self," Jung's description of the journey of individuation, the *Self* being the archetype of meaning (divinity by whatever name, within and outside of us).

Historical events, gender, ethnicity, religion, family circumstances

Indirectly—sometimes directly

Shaped and limited many of the decisions I made.

When I was a child, I had some profound experiences.

That were purely subjective knowing, a deep comfort.

Though few and far-between.

As I grew older
I felt them as mystical moments.

Looking back with retrospective insight, I know

These soul encounters with the sacred shaped my life.
Gave my life meaning, defines me now.

Section 1

Eye Surgery, World War II, Many Moves, Promises to God

Chapter 1

Above the Clouds – Depth Perception

My first vivid memory is of being on an airplane and pressing my nose against the window. I was in the sky above the clouds. Wonder and delight! I imagine that I excitedly turned to my mother to show her. We were on a DC-3, going across the continent in an overnight sleeper. Seats were transformed into curtained beds for us at night. My mother and I were flying across the country from Los Angeles to New York City to have my eyes operated on by doctors she trusted. It was my first up-up-and-away adventure. I was between three and four years old.

Cosmetically, the surgery was immediately successful. My eyes looked as if they were tracking together, and appeared to work together. I no longer was "cross-eyed." Ordinarily, each eye sees the same object from a slightly different angle, the brain merges the two, resulting in depth perception. Or, as I came to appreciate, depth is the result of having binocular vision, something that I might be able to achieve through eye exercises.

Depth perception is a theme and a metaphor that runs through my life. The eye problem I was born with and the efforts to correct it influenced me to "see" people in depth through seeing what acted upon them from outside and what shaped them from inside. It led me to develop the psychological theory of personality that I wrote about in *Goddesses in Everywoman* and *Gods in Everyman*, which I described as "binocular vision." It is seeing how every one of us is shaped by two powerful forces (stereotypes and archetypes) that act on us and in us—forces of which we usually are unconscious. Stereotypes are projected on us by family and culture. They are the roles we are supposed to inhabit: how girls and women, and boys and men, fit expectations and gain approval or not. Archetypes are patterns of being and behaving within us that influence how we react to what is meaningful, and are personality traits that are natural to us.

I could "see" with psychological "binocular vision" because of the time and place where I trained to be a psychiatrist. It was in the mid-'60s and '70s when feminism arose and became a movement. Consciousness raising brought awareness of the inferior status and oppression of women. I was in San Francisco at the University of California Medical Center where I became acquainted with the psychology of C. G. Jung who described patterns inherent in human beings cross-culturally, as archetypes of the collective unconscious.

I have one other memory of this trip. It's morning, and the sun is coming into the high windows. I look down from where I am and see the entrance to the hospital. Someone is with me, maybe a nurse. I am eagerly waiting for my mother. My stay in the hospital was short. I hadn't been afraid or in pain. The operation had been done on my inward-turned eye. The surgery was to correct the *strabismus*, the muscle imbalance that meant that my two eyes did not track together. Surgery now made this possible, and I was no longer "cross-eyed," but to have binocular vision, I would have to do eye exercises when we went home.

My Doctor Mother

While there probably were excellent eye surgeons in Los Angeles, my mother brought me across the country to Columbia University's eye specialists. She graduated from Barnard College, a Phi Beta Kappa, and then from Columbia University College of Physicians and Surgeons as an Alpha Omega Alpha. Then she had come west and interned at Los Angeles County Hospital, the first person of Japanese ancestry to do so. She met my father and after they married went into private practice in Los Angeles' Nihonmachi (Little Tokyo).

My mother, Megumi Yamaguchi Shinoda, MD was a pioneer. She was the first Japanese-American physician to practice in Los Angeles. Racial prejudice made it impossible her to open an office elsewhere. It didn't matter that she was born in the United States or that her credentials were outstanding. In Los Angeles, people who were not white worked and shopped in ghettos. Property deeds had covenants in them, ownership in desirable areas was legally "restricted" to only Caucasians.

My mother had to adapt to prejudice in California that she did not grow up with in New York. She was born in Cleveland, Ohio in 1908, while my grandfather Minosuke Yamaguchi, went to the Medical School that became Ohio Wesleyan University. He came as a married student and had two children before my mother was born. It was unusual for medical students to be married, much less married with children; most of his classmates were young men who called him "Pops."

After he graduated, he moved his family to New York City, into the hilly, wooded top end of Manhattan, an area I recall hearing referred to as Inwood Park. My mother was the middle child in a family of seven: two older sisters, a brother, then my mother, followed by two younger sisters, and the last-born brother. My grandfather expected all of his children to go to college, which they did. Four followed his example and went on to medical school. Two sons and two daughters became MDs.

Some stories that stick in my mind about my mother's childhood. She almost died shortly after she was born. It was a medical crisis, prognosis was very bad, and there were no miracle drugs. There was, however, the power of prayer and faith. My grandparents prayed over her, and she survived. I think that her health was frail in early childhood, and the miracle that she lived was part of what made her special. Each of the Yamaguchi girls was named after a Christian virtue. "Megumi" translates into "Grace." She almost died, but by prayer and grace, she lived.

In her large family, some affinity or responsibility paired each of the older three siblings with one of the younger three. As the middle child, my mother had no pair. All except her shared a bedroom with a sibling. Theirs was a hospitable household. Dinners were large, guests came often, and their big house was a center of many social events for the small community of Japanese in New York City. She dreaded having houseguests; because she had the only single room in the house, she had to give it up.

The Japanese who came to the house had come to New York City as students, as businessmen who represented their companies, or as members of the diplomatic community, and were most likely all members of the Samurai class. The Japanese in the early twentieth century were as class conscious as the English, with lineages and arranged marriages going back many centuries. I had seen a scroll with the Yamaguchi lineage that I was told went back to the fourteenth century. The visitors who came to the Yamaguchi house had not come to America as permanent immigrants. Even my grandfather, who had established himself here, spoke of taking his family back to Japan someday.

Family Theme of Christianity

The basis of the arranged marriage between my maternal grandparents was unusual. My grandmother's brothers chose my grandfather for her because he was a Christian.

Missionaries did not have much success converting the Japanese to Christianity, even as the schools they established were welcomed. In instilling social class values, my grandmother, Yukiko Sasaki Yamaguchi, spoke of her family being Samurai with the status of being close to the Emperor, the inference being that she married a gradation below her social class. Since she had been raised to be the equivalent of a Lady-in-Waiting marriage to my grandfather required major adaptations. In accompanying him to Cleveland while he went to medical school, she would have been a stranger in a strange land, a young mother, separated from the support of family and friends, and without amenities with which she had grown up. And, as my mother tells it, she was humiliated by how she helped my grandfather support them: it was her role to be dressed in a kimono, while he gave lectures about Japan.

Christianity was the motivating theme on my father's side of the family as well. Their conversion to Christianity was the reason my Shinoda grandparents (Kumaichiro and Masuno Shinoda) left Japan and came to California. They came to stay, though the Asian Exclusion acts would not allow them citizenship or property ownership. They came from a village in a farming community that did not approve of their conversion to Christianity. My impression is that they came as the early pilgrims did, in order to worship as they pleased. There were three boys and two girls already born when they settled in the San Francisco Bay Area.

My father Joseph Shinoda—no middle name, or Japanese first name—was the first of their children who would be born in America. He and his younger brothers were given biblical names: Paul, Peter, and Daniel. I think that he symbolized and carried his father's hopes and expectations. Though he had older brothers, the privileges and responsibilities of a first-born son may have been on his shoulders. He did very well in school, made friends and good grades, gained admission to Pomona College class of '32, as I did years later. There, he was the editor of the college newspaper, an English major, and a member of the college debate team.

In his Junior year, my father went to Japan and returned with stories of feeling "at home," which I would hear, years later. This is what I anticipated feeling when I went to Japan with my parents one summer while I was in medical school. I fully expected to get off the plane, be surrounded by people who looked like us, and feel as my father did—at home. Not so. I thought Japan was an interesting, very foreign country. We stayed at the Imperial Hotel and mostly in Tokyo, where night and day, it seemed that the streets were crowded with people. In Tokyo and then later in Hong Kong, this gave me a sense of what "masses of humanity" felt like. It was strange to see empty sidewalks when we returned to Los Angeles where almost everyone seems to get around by car.

We paid a visit to my Aunt Aiko Takaoka, who lived in Kamakura. She was my mother's second older sister, born in Japan and raised in the United States. She went to Barnard College, married a young Japanese diplomat, and had an interesting life going with him wherever he was posted. I later helped her publish her memoir (*Memories at Sunset*) and sent a copy to Barnard. In the nineteen thirties and up to the outbreak of World War II, they were in Los Angeles, Buenos Aires, Madrid during the Spanish Civil War, and Manchuria. As a consul-general's wife, she had to give speeches, and she would pretend to read them. Though fluent in Japanese, she could not read the language.

It was like going back in time to go from Tokyo to Kamakura. We took the train and then were brought by a taxi to the beginning of the footpath, which led through trees and bamboo to her home. She lived in a house that looked like it could have been in a woodblock print.

Christianity changed the course of both sides of my family and had to do with my grandparents coming to America, where my parents were born, married, and had me. It also contributed to me being out of step with most of my own generation of Japanese-Americans. Major community events such as the Cherry Blossom Festivals, the O-Bon parades, and even team sports were affiliated with the Buddhist temple in Little Tokyo. We did not speak Japanese at home, and once war was declared between Japan and America, there was no motivation for us to learn the language. (I was in kindergarten when Pearl Harbor was bombed).

The biggest difference, however, was the Evacuation. Almost all Japanese in California were taken to internment camps. Most children of my age spent their elementary school years behind barbed wire in these concentration camps. My family did not. We became "internally displaced refugees" by staying a step ahead of the forced evacuation which placed all Japanese, American-born citizens or not, under military control. Once we were out of California, we had the rights and freedoms of being American citizens.

I went to elementary schools and Sunday schools in churches where I was the only child who looked like me. I was different, but assimilated—accepted, treated well, included, but I was also an exception. Later when we returned to California, when I was around people who looked like me—accepted, treated well, included, I often felt different inside, especially after adolescence when I could see that I was freer to imagine and be active in the world than they were.

Positive Marginality

My experience of being different and yet accepted in two worlds, was simply my reality, not something I thought about. That is, not until I heard about the concept of *positive marginality*—and had the aha! of applying it to myself. Usually, people who don't fit in are "marginalized" or at the edge of a group, while those who belong take belonging for granted. "Marginalized" has a connotation of being barely acceptable, on the outside looking in, pushed aside by those who set the standards and have the social power to exclude others. I didn't feel like I was like everybody else who belonged. I was different, yet I was included, and was used to being acceptable. Back then, and still, I am both an outsider looking in and an insider looking out. In many aspects of my life, I experience this, which is another variation of "binocular vision."

I suppose that if the surgery had corrected the strabismus and at the same time had given me binocular vision, I might not have given the concept of depth perception a second thought. Nor would it have become a central metaphor for psychological insight.

Eye exercises with a stereoscope had me concentrate on putting an image presented separately to each eye into one picture with depth. It was a challenge I was presented with many times. At the beginning of each round of appointments, each eye looked at the same postcard-like scene and I saw two separate images Then by moving the controls, and with effort, I could merge the two and see one scene in depth. It got harder when merging two entirely different images: one eye looked at a birdcage and the other at a bird; success came when my eyes could work together to put the bird in the cage. Stereoscopic vision was a physical accomplishment that never "stuck" in spite of the effort and exercises. Instead, my brain almost instantaneously decided on the larger or clearer image, which is how my vision works.

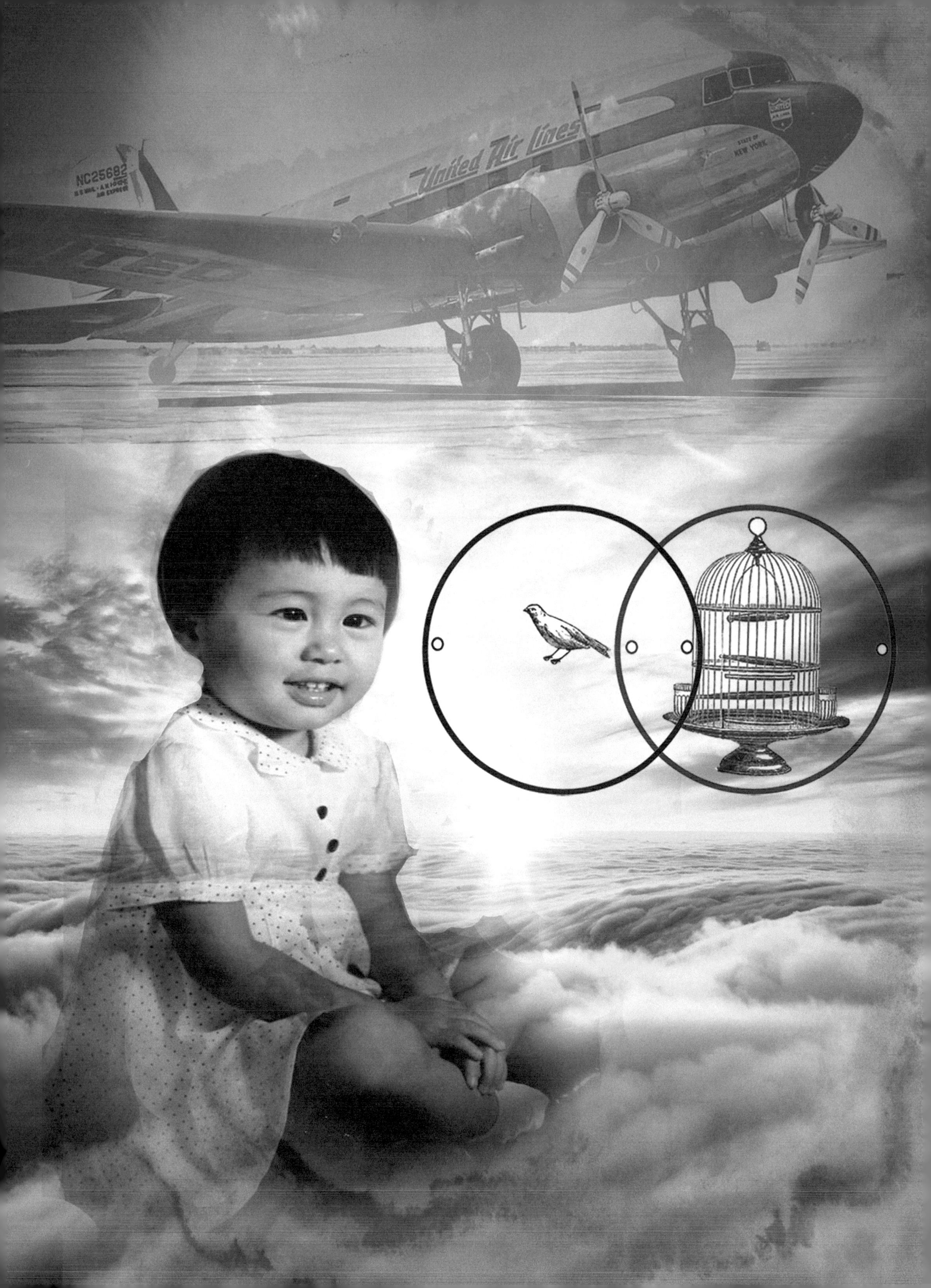
NC25682
United Air Lines
STATE OF
NEW YORK

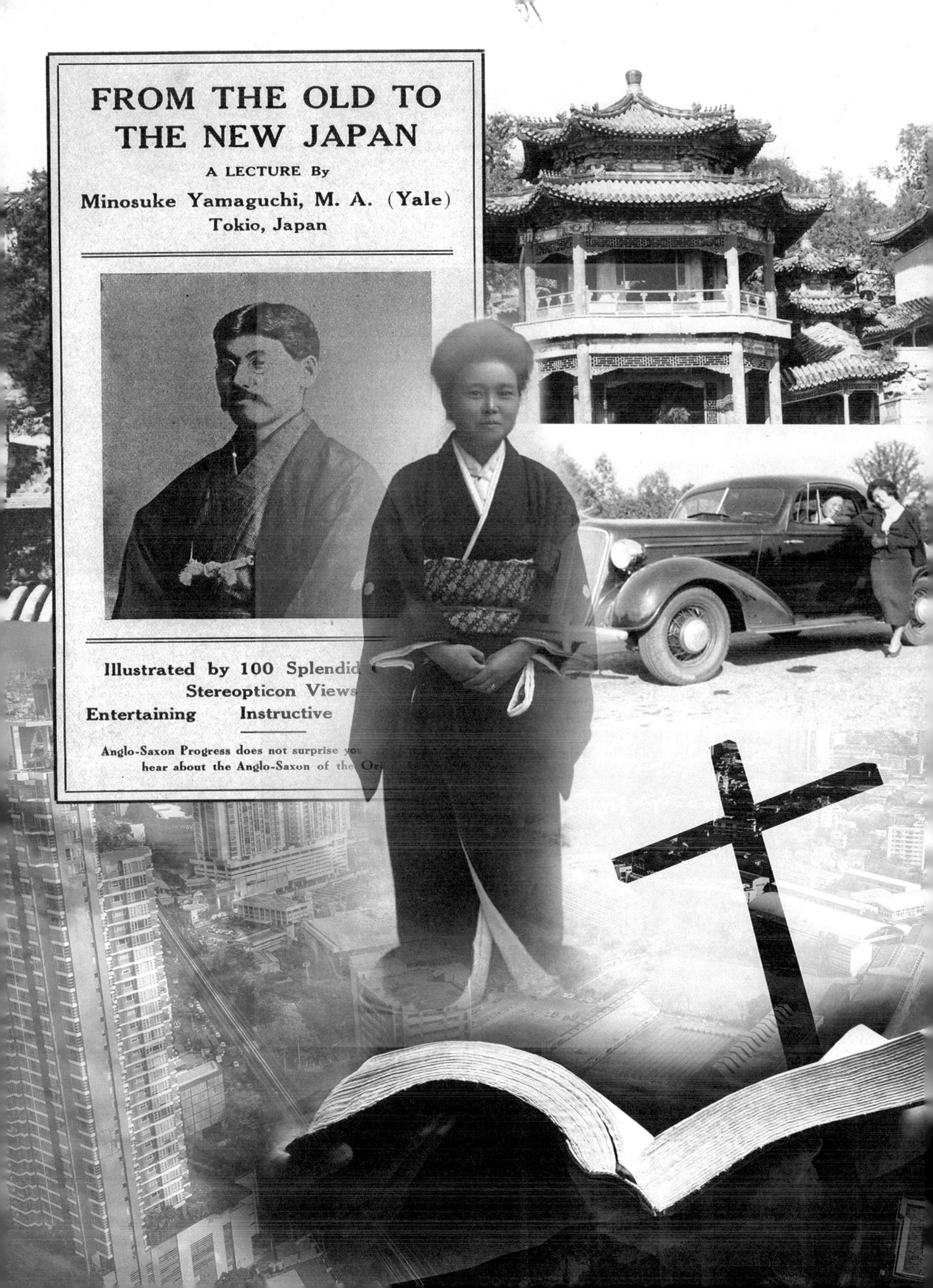
FROM THE OLD TO
THE NEW JAPAN
A LECTURE By
Minosuke Yamaguchi, M. A. (Yale)
Tokio, Japan
Illustrated by 100 Splendid
Stereopticon Views
Entertaining
Instructive
Anglo-Saxon Progress does not surprise
hear about the Anglo-Saxon of the

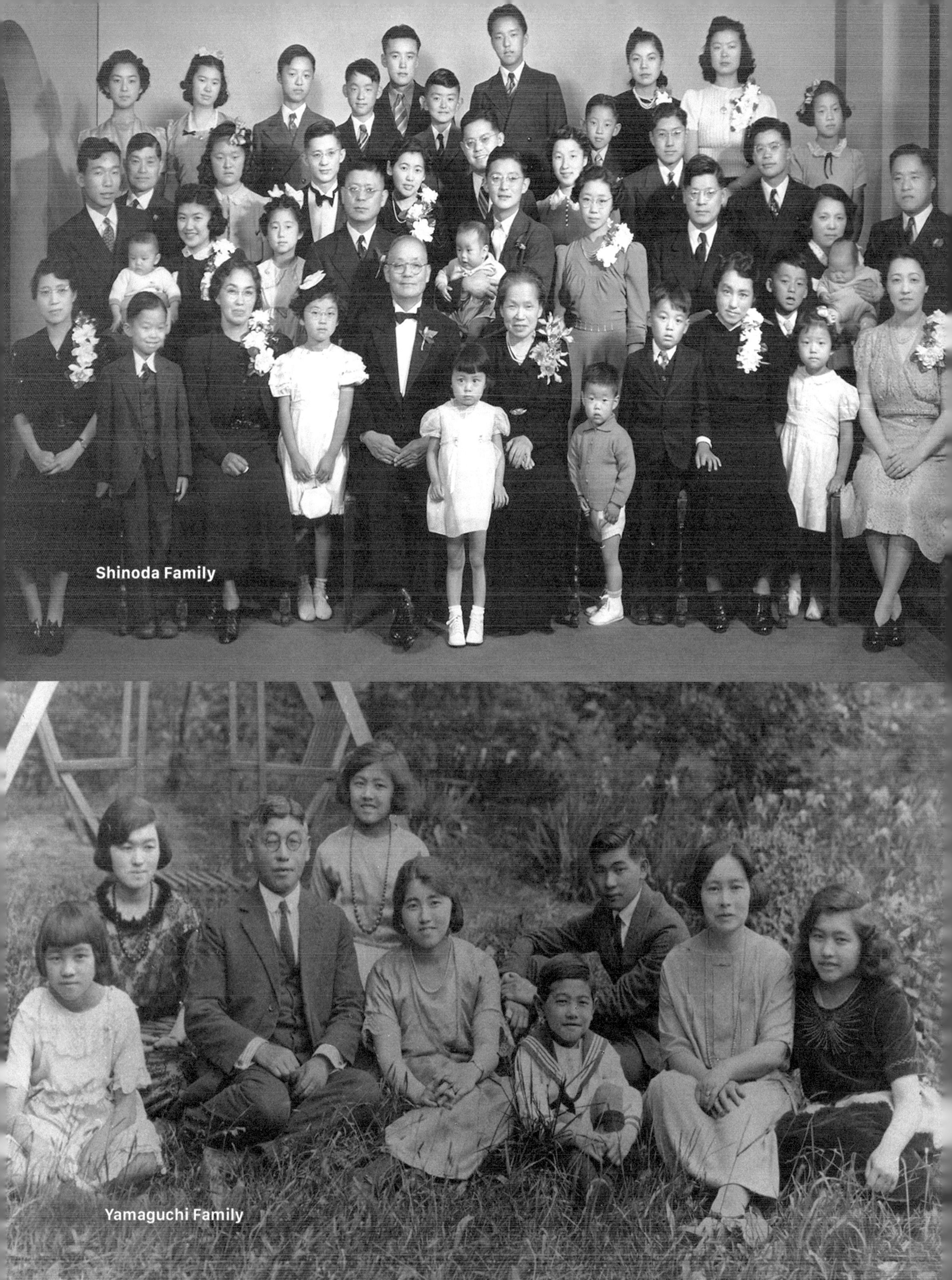
Shinoda Family
Yamaguchi Family

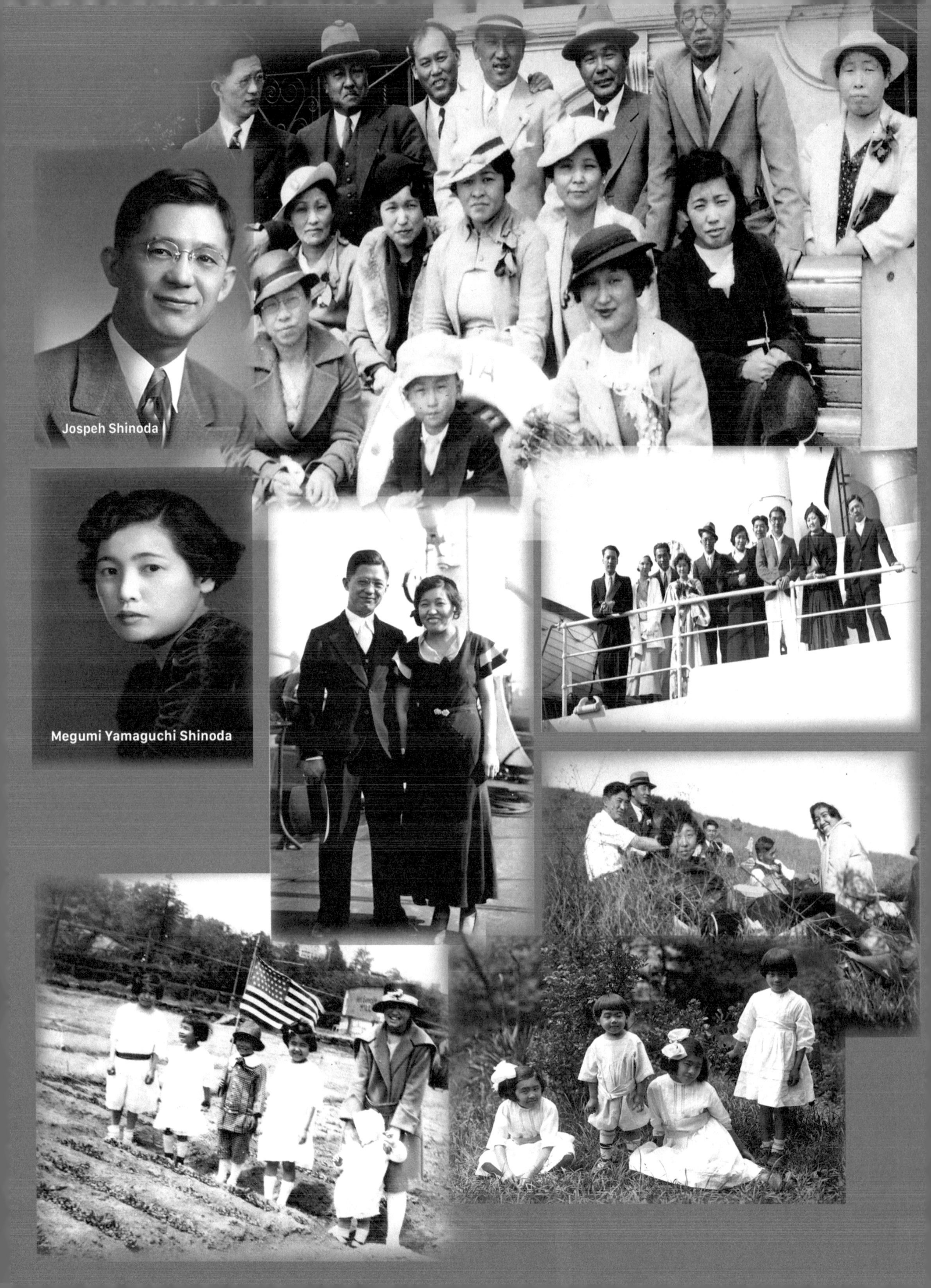

Jospeh Shinoda

Megumi Yamaguchi Shinoda

Chapter 2

My Parents - Pearl Harbor, the Evacuation

My parents married later than most people of their age did. They had met through Larry Tajiri, a journalist friend of my father and an acquaintance of my mother, as he had once dated her youngest sister. My father, Joseph Shinoda, had intended to go into law when he graduated college. Many of his editorials in the Pomona College newspaper addressed national issues, which were concerns of his. I wonder where his chosen course would have taken him had he not been summoned by his father to take over the family business, which was going bankrupt. The country was in the midst of the Great Depression. My grandfather had become an entrepreneur in seeking a means to be successful in America. For most immigrants, it's either hire out or start small businesses—which he did, several times before he began the San Lorenzo Nursery Company. Shortly after my father graduated from college, his brother Kiyoshi died. This was the older brother who had started the company with their father. I doubt that there was any question in either my grandfather's mind or my father's that if he was needed, this is what he had to do.

In the years that followed, my father put the company into Chapter 11, the bankruptcy code that allows time for a company to reorganize. While the growing end of the business was in San Lorenzo, a small community on the southeast edge of San Francisco Bay, the large wholesale market where flowers were sold to florists was in Los Angeles. There were two markets: the Japanese Market and the American Market. In each, growers rented space to sell the fresh flowers to retailers. My father established the San Lorenzo Nursery Company as a separate wholesale business and had flowers delivered to florists so they would not have to come down to the street at dawn when the flower markets opened. Joe Shinoda (everyone called my father Joe) took the company out of bankruptcy and made the business a success.

My mother had not expected to marry. Medical schools admitted very few women, and the expectation,, hers as well as theirs, was that a woman doctor or "hen medic" would devote herself to medicine. Otherwise, the education "would go to waste." My mother was not at all impressed by the eligible young Japanese men who came to their house to meet the five Yamaguchi daughters. She believed the stereotype of the Japanese male ego was true: that they had been raised to feel superior because they were male, and felt entitled to be waited on, more so depending on their family status.

Jung's psychological typology would probably peg my mother as introverted, sensate, thinking, while my father was extraverted, intuitive, feeling. Maybe theirs was an attraction of opposites. By typology, I took more after him, though I followed her footsteps into medicine. The quality they had in common was intelligence. The friend who introduced them must have challenged him to meet her, saying she was smarter than he was, which would hardly intrigue most men. However, not only did my father appreciate her brains, my father's father had once confided in him that he wished he had married someone smarter and advised my father to marry a smart woman.

I was born on June 29, 1936. My mother was 28. This was her first pregnancy. She would be considered an "elderly primip" (*primiparous*), the obstetrical term used to describe an older woman in labor for the first time. In my time as a medical student on obstetrics, it was written on the chart as an alert, because older first pregnancies often have more complications. Most women became pregnant for the first time in their late teens or early twenties, and 28 was considered old back then. The new fathers-to-be waited in the waiting room until the doctor came out to deliver the news. He would be able to see his wife for the first time after the delivery, after she had been cleaned and bathed, in a hospital gown and in a hospital bed; during visiting hours.

When my father came to visit my mother in her hospital bed, something was definitely wrong. She was not responding. He must have recognized that she was not asleep. He immediately called for help. She was hemorrhaging. Some part of the placenta must have been left in. If my father had not come to visit when he did, and not had the presence of mind to know something was wrong and take immediate action, she could have been one more woman to die in childbirth. My life would have been very different if she had died.

I was a small baby, but my parents were small people. My mother was barely five feet tall, and my father was five foot four. Other than size, I don't know why I was put into an incubator when I was born. My mother may have had a difficult delivery. I have no idea and can no longer ask her. I was born when middle class mothers bottle fed their babies. They had been sold the idea that only poor women breast-fed (and thus were like animal mothers). Babies drank formula from bottles sterilized in boiling water in the kitchen, and were put on a feeding schedule besides. A good mother followed the advice of male experts, who told them that good mothers did not feed babies on demand, and did not pick them up when they cried. They were to be the boss: teach discipline, and not be weak and give in. Wanting to be good mothers, women suppressed their maternal instincts and deprived both themselves and their children. Babies were to learn to comfort themselves, and I did. I sucked my thumb, as many babies growing up during this regime must have. There were many drug store remedies: bad tasting stuff that could be painted on the thumb, or mittens to cover the hands. Getting me to stop sucking my thumb was an ongoing struggle.

Doctor Spock (the famous pediatrician, not the pointy-eared Vulcan of *Star Wars*) wrote the book which was the bible for new mothers about breast feeding and feeding on demand, and revised it a decade after it could have done any good for me or my generation of babies. Mothers with the best of intentions deprived themselves and their babies of touch, instinctual responsiveness, bonding at a cellular level and perhaps even disempowered us: if we are hungry and cry and cry, but no one comes, we learn to be quiet. My generation of babies grew up to be the Silent Generation of the 1950s.

In the first years of my life, we moved from a small wood-frame house to a larger stucco house on a hilly street, both close to Sycamore Park, where I was taken to play. The Pasadena Freeway, which now is close to this little park, had not yet been built. My mother had resumed her medical practice in *Nihonmachi*, Japantown, once we were settled into the stucco house. An older Japanese woman became live-in help for me.

"Oba-sun" only spoke Japanese. I have no personal memories of her, though I do recall two stories I was told later. One was that I spoke Japanese to her, which gave me the hope that maybe it could come back to me, though it never happened. The other I remember because I recognize it as so me. My mother fed me before she left for her office. Regardless of how long it was until she came home, I wouldn't eat again until she returned. I may have been hungry, but I was more stubborn than hungry. From what I was told, vaguely feel, and from old photographs in which she held me, I know I was comfortable being left with Oba-san. But I knew who and what I wanted, and would wait. I think of this stubbornness as early signs of character and integrity that would lead to discernment and choice about what I would believe or take in, and who I would allow to be close to me (i.e., spiritually, emotionally or physically).

I was a happy child, a "Daddy's Little Girl," a princess (as the daughter of a favored son), and I had large round eyes. The girl next door, Elizabeth (who was older by a decade) was my friend when we lived at our first house, and Chrissy (the son of a fireman, who lived up the street) was my buddy friend. Whatever he thought was important, I echoed. He wanted an Erector set for Christmas so, of course, I wanted one, too. I got one. These are more than enough reasons from the first years of my life for me to have developed basic trust, to view the world and people as basically good, to make friends and to do what boys could do. I had lots of dolls to play with as well.

There was also a big dog in my life. He was a German shepherd named Rudy. I think he must have joined our household as a grown dog, not as a puppy, and I don't know what happened to him. He was in my life and then he was not. I was told that when I went down the street to play, the parents of my playmates had said: "Jeanie is welcome to be here, but don't bring Rudy!" I recall that he liked eating corn on the cob. Maybe it was Rudy who made me unafraid of dogs. I meet them as individuals, respecting them and their boundaries. It hurts my feelings when a dog doesn't like me. I think I speak Dog. As a child, I'd bark a friendly hello, to which dogs responded. Sometimes, when no one else is around, I still do.

I was either an oblivious child, or my parents kept me innocent of their worries on purpose. I know the latter to be so in regard to their biggest heartbreak, which was that something was wrong with my brother. Stephen Joseph Shinoda was born on November 4, 1940. His was a long and difficult delivery. With his head stuck in the birth passage, the doctor took forceps and forcibly pulled him out. There were large hematomas—swollen areas caused by the pressure of the forceps on either side of his head. His head seemed larger than normal then, and later as well, even after the swelling disappeared.

In the years that followed, questions arose. What was wrong with him? Did he have a brain injury from the forceps delivery? Was it psychological? Did it fit the newly created diagnosis of autism?

America's Entry into World War II

When Stephen came into the world in 1940, Hitler's armies had the upper hand in Europe; allied forces evacuated through Dunkirk; the bombing of London had begun; Germany, Italy and Japan were unified against the allied forces, and winning in Europe, North Africa and southeast Asia. Winston Churchill became prime minister of Great Britain. Roosevelt aided allies with equipment, but the United States was staying out of the war. Then Japan bombed Pearl Harbor on December 7, 1941.

The Evacuation

On February 19, 1942, ten weeks after Pearl Harbor, President Franklin D. Roosevelt signed Executive Order 9066, which authorized the military to define the need and removal all people of Japanese ancestry from sensitive areas, such as near military bases. The military defined the area as the entire west coast. By June 1943, 120,000 Japanese-Americans were relocated to internment camps. That the majority were American citizens did not matter. Hysteria against us, fear that we would aid Japan, newspaper stories that were, in fact, fake news (later proven by the FBI) all contributed to murderous acts against individuals just for being Japanese.

Much later, I learned that relatives of my father's secretary, farmers in the Imperial Valley of California, were murdered shortly after Pearl Harbor. These people had nothing to do with Pearl Harbor, except in the distorted minds of perpetrators. After the 9-11 Twin Towers attack, turban-wearing Sikhs were attacked in similar ways. Valarie Kaur told me about the murder of her uncle in the bombing of a Sikh Temple in Wisconsin, and how this led her to film and document many incidents that took place then, which led her to be an activist now.

My father had tried to rally the Japanese community to appeal to President Roosevelt after General DeWitt announced that under Executive Order 9066 every person of Japanese ancestry, whether citizens or not, would be evacuated from the entire west coast.. Meanwhile, Japanese were not evacuated from Hawaii, Honolulu, or Pearl Harbor, where the bombings occurred. As a result of speaking out, my father was called to testify before California's Un-American Activities Committee and questioned by the FBI. I was too young to know about such things. Later, I learned from him that leaders of the JACL (the Japanese-American Citizens League) at the time persuaded the community that we should demonstrate our loyalty by cooperating with the forced evacuation. My father was advised that if he continued to protest, he would go to jail.

Japanese-Americans were told to leave their homes and businesses, take one suitcase each, wear a label, and board trains and buses that would take them to assembling centers. The stables at Santa Anita Racetrack the center closest to us. From there they were transported to hastily built relocation camps to live in barrack-like tarpaper and wood buildings surrounded by barbed-wire fences, with armed guards. Quakers helped in ways they could. Possessions, property, and pets had to be given away or sold for next-to-nothing.

In 1944, the Supreme Court in a 6-3 decision upheld Executive Order 9066 in Korematsu v. United States. It has not been overturned. In response to the Japanese attack on Pearl Harbor, the United States required Japanese-Americans to move into relocations camps "as a matter of national security." Fred Koramatsu chose to stay home rather than obey the order, and was arrested and convicted of violating the order. He responded by arguing that the order violated the Fifth Amendment of the constitution. The majority of the court said the order "did not show racial prejudice," but was "martial necessity arising from the danger of espionage and sabotage."

In 1980, Congress established a commission to investigate the camps. The final report called the forced evacuation a "grave injustice," motivated by "racial prejudice, war hysteria and the failure of political leadership." Japanese-Americans then serving in Congress helped turn the report into legislative action to provide for tax-free compensation and a formal apology. In 1988, after a decade-long campaign led by the JACL, President Reagan signed the Civil Liberties Act which offered a formal apology and paid out $20,000 in compensation to each survivor. The redress effort was led by John Tateishi (married to my cousin Carol), who spoke of the evacuation as both humiliating and disorienting. In August, 2013, he told NPR, "We came out of those camps with a sense of shame and guilt, of having been considered betrayers of our country."

Once 9066 was signed, the army carried out the executive order. Designated areas to be evacuated would be announced, and the Japanese-Americans in that location would be under martial law and were not free to travel or have rights as citizens. Just before this applied to Los Angeles, we packed up and left for Central California, a step ahead of the forced evacuation. I was in kindergarten when Presidential Order 9066 was signed and then enforced. I was an oblivious, happy child who was suddenly living in a cheap hotel for itinerants in Del Rey, a two-story wooden building that faced a big, empty lot with weeds and paths that ran through it. Two families we knew had joined us. With the Japanese values of cleanliness, the women scrubbed and cleaned, while we children played tag on paths outside and in sight. There was no hot water in these rooms. Water was heated on the stove and I was bathed in a metal washtub.

It was only a matter of time before Japanese-Americans in Central California were next. I learned much later that my father went to Sacramento and got us papers from the Secretary of State's office that permitted our family to leave California for New York. He had also asked my uncle Mitsuya (Mits), the youngest Yamaguchi, then an intern at a New York hospital, to go to Mayor La Guardia's office to get another document that said we had a place to stay and would not need financial assistance from the city.

Leaving California

Armed with proper papers, we returned to Los Angeles in order to take the train from Grand Central Station across the continent to New York City. No one looked at us, and no one asked for the papers. We boarded the train, and once out of California we were again free American citizens. When I found all of this out much later, the family explanation was that everyone who saw us must have assumed we were Chinese. We got out — which meant that we missed the experience of being forced evacuees and then prisoners in a "relocation camp." We called them "concentration camps" which is what internment camps were called in my house.

During the cross-country train trip, though I didn't have a word for anxiety, that was the feeling in the air. My parents took turns doing whatever might help quiet my brother, who made sounds, was hyperactive, and didn't sleep easily. They didn't want to draw attention to us, they did not want us to be noticed. Though we had made it out of California, we were "Japs." My awareness of being an "other," of having a negative identity and that I could be the recipient of sudden hostility, began on this trip. I became aware and cautious around white strangers. I unconsciously and automatically learned to be disarming, especially when there was anger in the air. This would be something I had to "unlearn" to be a psychiatrist.

On arrival in New York City, we temporarily stayed in my mother's parents' apartment, until my father found us a place in Kew Gardens, a complex of apartment buildings in Queens on Long Island. They enrolled me in school, which I took to easily. It was good that I liked school, did well, and never approached a new school situation with fear and trepidation. Between the first and third grade, I would go to schools in Kew Gardens, New York, Blackfoot, Idaho, Grand Junction, Colorado, Denver, Colorado, and Monrovia, California. I was on my own a lot of the time. These were years when children went out to play and would come home in time for dinner. America was a safe place for a child. Around Kew Gardens, there was ongoing construction with concrete pipes tall enough for all the children in my neighborhood to stand in. In each new location, I played and explored, made friends, adapted.

While I was occupied with school and play, I was unaware that my mother was taking my brother to Columbia Physicians & Surgeons Medical Center, where there were no satisfactory answers about what was wrong or what might help. Meanwhile, my father was seeking ways to get his parents, siblings and their families out of internment camps. He was also running San Lorenzo Nursery Company from afar, which he was able to do all through the war years. This was possible because Mr. Swift was his general manager. While most employees were Japanese, Mr. Swift was Caucasian—a white person of European origin—a word I don't hear anymore. Mr. Swift's loyalty meant that there would be a business to return to and assets that remained.

Artemis and My Psychology

My father and mother were positive role models. Both influenced and shaped how I reacted to our changing circumstances. While they managed as they did, I now realize that without the vocabulary, without any idea that there are archetypal patterns that can resemble ancient goddesses, how children and adults behave and react has to do with what and who they came into the world to be. Babies have personalities—they aren't "blank screens" to be programmed. Artemis, the Greek goddess of the Hunt and Moon, is the archetype in a little girl who can play by herself outside, likes animals, and can compete with boys and feels equal to them. And she can, like Artemis, the archer with unerring aim, focus on targets or goals of her own choosing and shut out what would distract someone else.

Another child with a different archetype would naturally respond differently to the tensions and difficulties in the air around me. Artemis' domain was the wilderness, which can be a metaphor for any unknown terrain, and so my response was to explore with curiosity, common sense, and courage, as one would on entering a physical wilderness. Each new school, each new place to live, and each new situation was for me a new and unknown wilderness. I could be emotionally self-sufficient, adapt to change with curiosity, and make my way outside home on my own.

I didn't know what the matter was with my brother and only in retrospect do I know how important an influence he was on my life. My parents did not expect me to take care of him. He was the impaired child who got their attention because he needed it. I was healthy and smart, I would be a good girl, and I would not cause my parents any worry. In the way that young children unconsciously do, I became who they needed me to be, which I could because of the Artemis archetype.

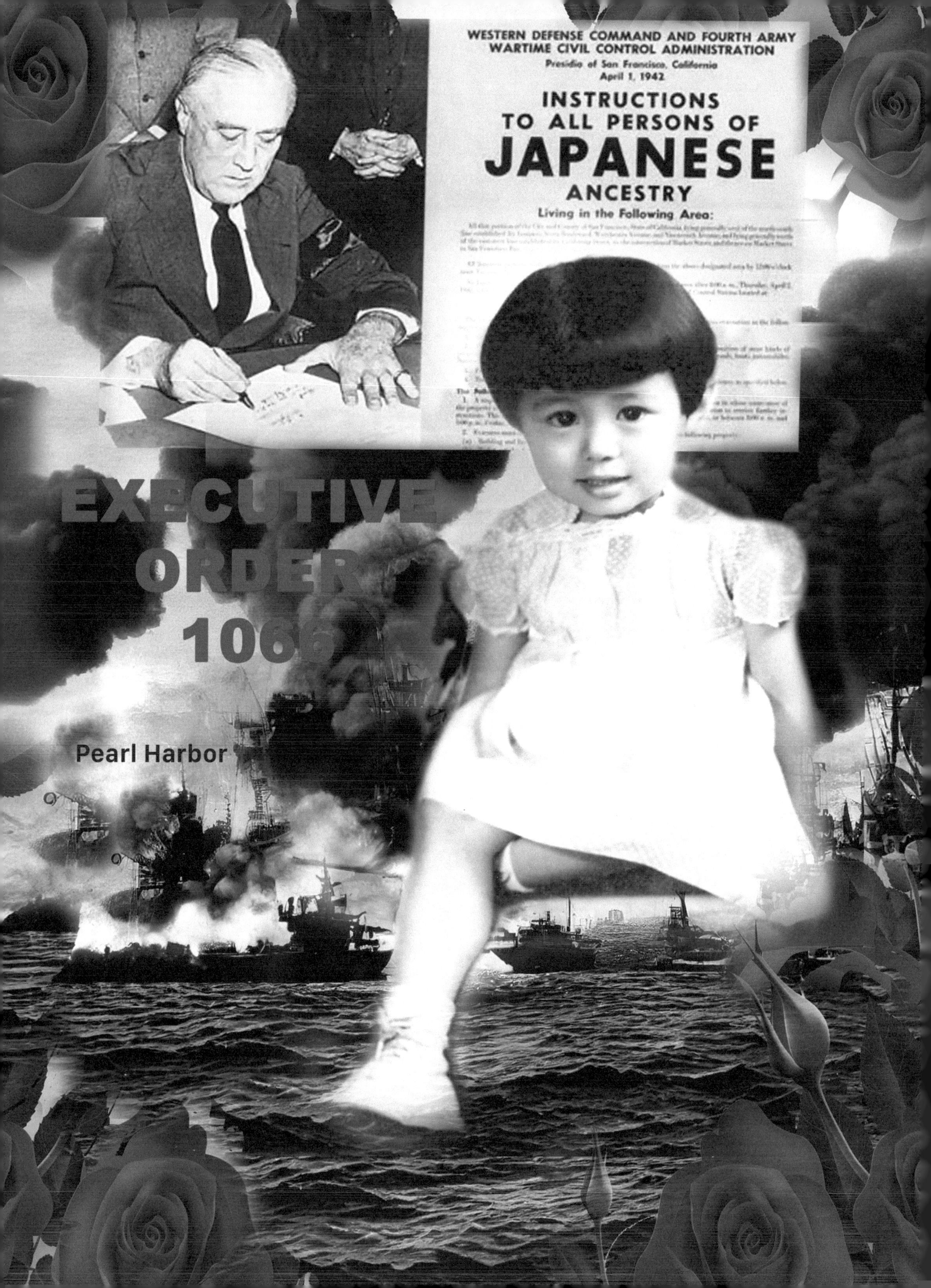
WESTERN DEFENSE COMMAND AND FOURTH ARMY
WARTIME CIVIL CONTROL ADMINISTRATION
Presidio of San Francisco, California
April 1, 1942
INSTRUCTIONS
TO ALL PERSONS OF
JAPANESE
ANCESTRY
Living in the Following Area:
EXECUTIVE
ORDER
1066
Pearl Harbor

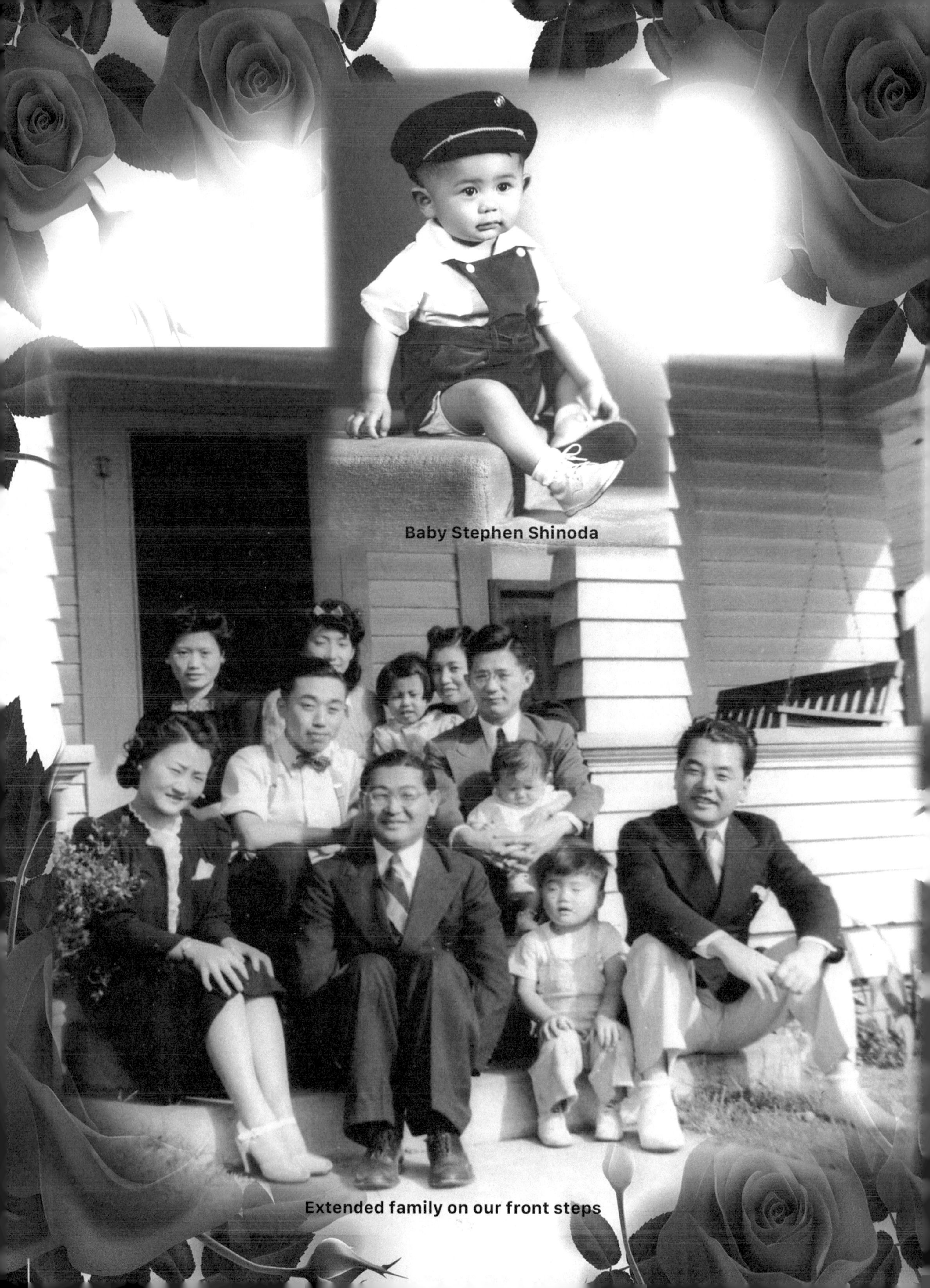

Baby Stephen Shinoda

Extended family on our front steps

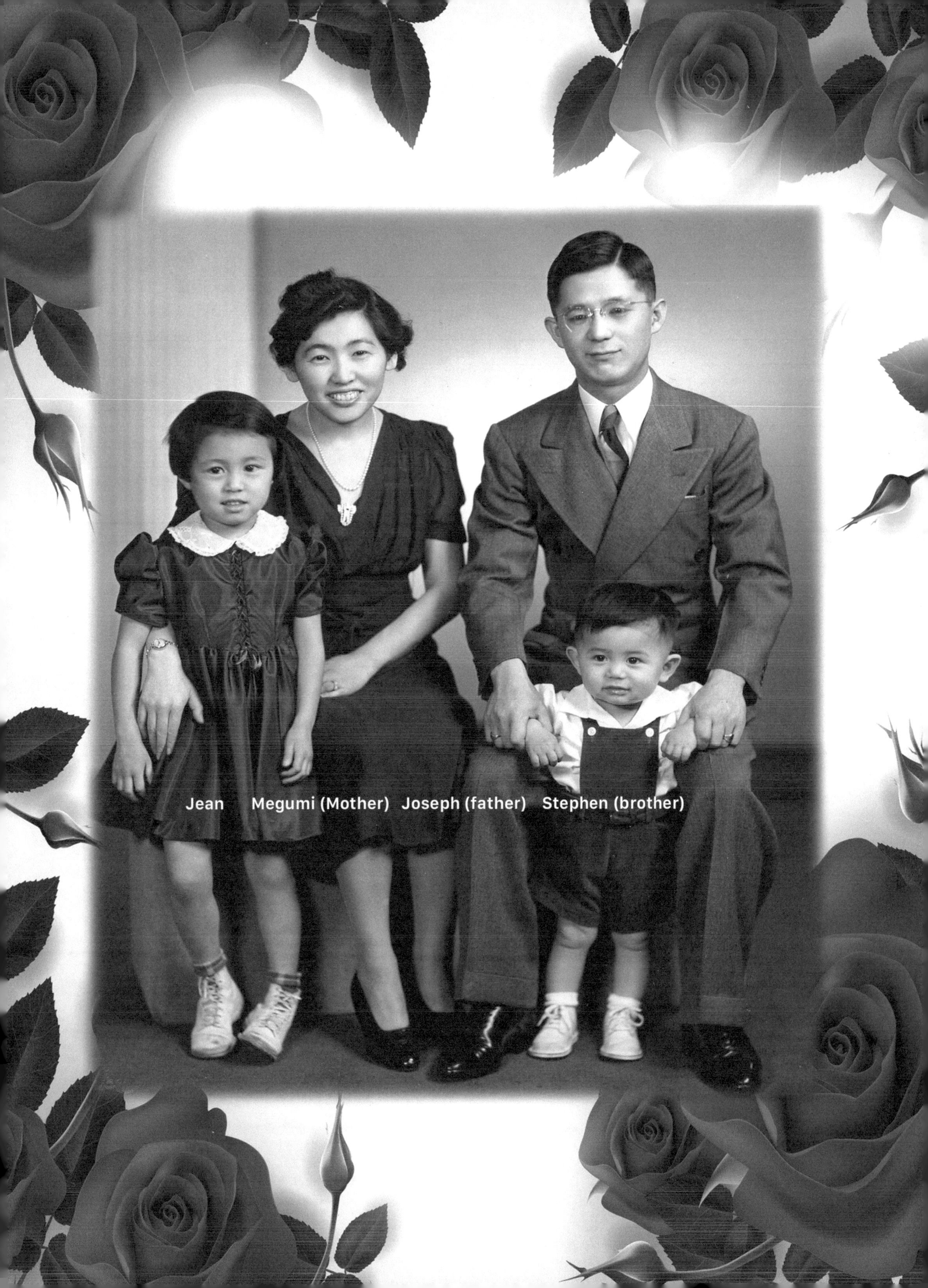
Jean
Megumi (Mother)
Joseph (father)
Stephen (brother)

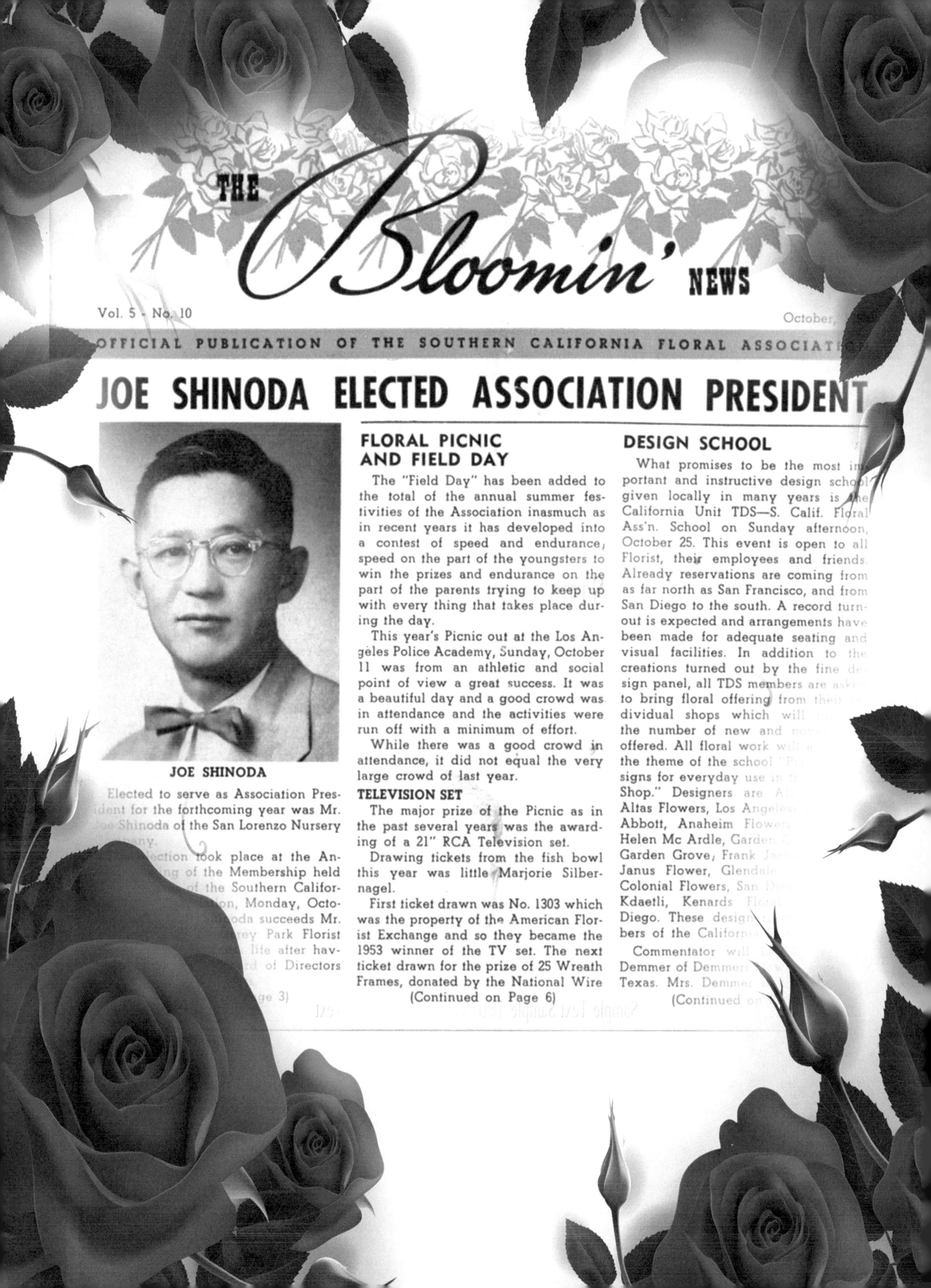

THE *Bloomin'* NEWS

Vol. 5 - No. 10 October,

OFFICIAL PUBLICATION OF THE SOUTHERN CALIFORNIA FLORAL ASSOCIAT

JOE SHINODA ELECTED ASSOCIATION PRESIDENT

JOE SHINODA

Elected to serve as Association President for the forthcoming year was Mr. Joe Shinoda of the San Lorenzo Nursery ...pany.

...lection took place at the An... ...ing of the Membership held ... of the Southern Califor... ...on, Monday, Octo... ...noda succeeds Mr. ...rey Park Florist ... life after hav... ...d of Directors

...ge 3)

FLORAL PICNIC AND FIELD DAY

The "Field Day" has been added to the total of the annual summer festivities of the Association inasmuch as in recent years it has developed into a contest of speed and endurance, speed on the part of the youngsters to win the prizes and endurance on the part of the parents trying to keep up with every thing that takes place during the day.

This year's Picnic out at the Los Angeles Police Academy, Sunday, October 11 was from an athletic and social point of view a great success. It was a beautiful day and a good crowd was in attendance and the activities were run off with a minimum of effort.

While there was a good crowd in attendance, it did not equal the very large crowd of last year.

TELEVISION SET

The major prize of the Picnic as in the past several years was the awarding of a 21" RCA Television set.

Drawing tickets from the fish bowl this year was little Marjorie Silbernagel.

First ticket drawn was No. 1303 which was the property of the American Florist Exchange and so they became the 1953 winner of the TV set. The next ticket drawn for the prize of 25 Wreath Frames, donated by the National Wire

(Continued on Page 6)

DESIGN SCHOOL

What promises to be the most important and instructive design school given locally in many years is the California Unit TDS—S. Calif. Floral Ass'n. School on Sunday afternoon, October 25. This event is open to all Florist, their employees and friends. Already reservations are coming from as far north as San Francisco, and from San Diego to the south. A record turnout is expected and arrangements have been made for adequate seating and visual facilities. In addition to the creations turned out by the fine design panel, all TDS members are aske... to bring floral offering from their in... dividual shops which will ... the number of new and nov... offered. All floral work will ... the theme of the school "P... signs for everyday use in ... Shop." Designers are ... Altas Flowers, Los Angele... Abbott, Anaheim Flowers, ... Helen Mc Ardle, Garden ... Garden Grove, Frank Ja... Janus Flower, Glendale, ... Colonial Flowers, San Di... Kdaetli, Kenards Floral ... Diego. These designers ... bers of the California ...

Commentator will ... Demmer of Demmers ... Texas. Mrs. Demmer ...

(Continued on ...

Chapter 3

Wartime – Living in Many Places

For a brief period, my family lived in a New York City apartment that typically belonged to relatives who took part in the exchanges between the US and Japan. Two of my mother's sisters and their children were to travel with their repatriated husbands on a ship, the *M.S. Gripsholm,* across the Atlantic, around Africa, and onward to Japan. My cousins were two little girls close to me in age. Keiko, a year older, puzzled me because she often clung to her mother, turning her face away as if she were scared or shy. Yohko, a year younger, became a playmate while the adults talked. Many years later when I visited Japan with my parents, I met Yohko again. She had just graduated from Keio University and would have liked to work, but this wasn't an option for her at the time. I invited her to live with me and two of my medical school classmates in San Francisco.

My cousins and their families were waiting to board the *Gripsholm*, a Swedish cruise ship chartered by the U.S. government to transport civilians and POWs during World War II. Between 1942 and 1946, the "Mercy Ship" participated in a dozen exchanges between the U.S. and its wartime enemies: Germany, Italy and Japan. There were just two exchanges of civilians with Japan in June 1942 and September 1943. Approximately 3,000 men, women and children of Japanese ancestry took part in those exchanges.

Yohko's family had to leave their dog behind, a small wire-haired terrier, which became mine. I thought his name was "Chummie," or "my little chum," which he became. Much later, I learned that his name was *Cha-mai,* a Japanese name.

Except for my mother, all of the Yamaguchi sisters married Japanese nationals. Her two older sisters were born a year apart in Japan and came to the United States as infants, and her two younger sisters were born in the U.S. Aunt Fumiko, my mother's oldest sister and the first of her siblings to go to medical school, married Kageyasu Amano; the two Doctor Amanos had a medical practice in Tokyo. My Aunt Aiko married the diplomat Teiichiro Takaoka, who had been teasingly referred to as "tapioca" by her sisters when he courted her. With the ascendency of the war party in political Japan, Takaoka had been relieved of further diplomatic postings. The two younger sisters were in New York when war between the two countries was declared. Aunt Etsuko had married Kosuki Konishi, a Mitsui Company man (Keiko's parents). Aunt Shizuko's husband, Yoichi Hiraoka, was a member of the New York Philharmonic orchestra.

My aunts, who were among those exchanged for Americans in Japan, were American-born citizens, as were my cousins. Once America entered the war, Japan soon would be on the losing end of it, and America was the enemy. Fortunately, Japanese was spoken in their respective homes, my cousins were very young, and my aunts' language and behavior did not give them away as Americans. Food was scarce, and all signs were of course, in Japanese, a language they could not read. My aunt Etsuko's husband was sent by the Mitsui Company to the Philippines, where the Japanese were hated, and as the war progressed and Japan was in retreat, he disappeared and was thought to have been murdered. Yoichi Hiraoka, my aunt Shizu's, husband became famous as a xylophone virtuoso in concerts after the war.

Blackfoot, Idaho

Shortly after my mother's sisters and their families left for Japan on the Gripsholm, we also left New York. We travelled across the country by train to Blackfoot, Idaho, a small town in the southeast corner of the state between Pocatello and Idaho Falls. I went to another new school. Many of my classmates were bussed from the reservation. For the short time that we lived there, I went to school with Blackfoot Indians. This was the first time that I came in contact with Native Americans. Much later, when I learned their history of displacement and removal to reservations, the parallels to the treatment of Japanese-Americans were obvious.

From the vantage point of my age now, as I write about this first contact, I see the journey through life as a spiral path. There will be many more turns to go. With each subsequent contact, as my appreciation for Indigenous wisdom and spirituality grew, so did my affinity with them. This was helped along by being mistaken for one of them when I travelled to Hopi and Navaho lands in the 1990s. There was after all, a land bridge that once connected North America to Asia, over which the ancestors and genes of all the Indigenous peoples in the Americas crossed. Japanese and Native Americans share a Mongol heritage. Heart-beat drumming, campfires, and Girl Scouts all fostered a sense of oneness in nature as I was growing up. Empathy for others came from stories, such as imagining walking a day in another's moccasins. Much later, I led retreats at the Feathered Pipe Ranch outside of Helena, Montana, with Brooke Medicine Eagle as a co-leader, and participated in the sweat lodge and sacred ceremony led by a pipe carrier.

We came to Blackfoot, Idaho due to my father's concern for his aged parents, and his effort to get them and other family members out of a nearby internment camp. During the war, farming was an essential industry. Japanese-Americans in the concentration camps could be released if they had jobs in an essential industry. My father made arrangements for these jobs, and thus was able to gain freedom for his parents, brothers, sisters and their families.

Blackfoot is in Jerome County, Idaho, as was the Minidoka War Relocation Center, which is now a National Historic Site. I assume that this was the camp since I no longer have living relatives to ask. One short description: "Nine thousand Japanese-Americans were imprisoned there. The environment was described as extremely harsh, with temperatures ranging from 30 degrees below zero to as high as 115 degrees. They also had to contend with blinding dust storms and ankle-deep mud when it rained."

We stayed in Blackfoot, Idaho, while my father somehow arranged their freedom. To do so, he must have also established that they had work in an essential industry. He must have travelled back and forth to Grand Junction, Colorado, moving relatives there after securing housing and farmland and taken responsibility for them. After this, we also moved there.

Grand Junction, Colorado

We lived in a one-story stucco house at the end of a gravel road. Furniture was sparse, and alfalfa fields bordered the front yard. I had a room of my own with a tree outside my window that I looked at before falling asleep. I walked to school. With gas rationing, nearly everyone did. School was on the other side of a highway. A shortcut took me across a field, a jump over a drainage ditch that was at the bottom of a culvert, into a neighboring field, past a mulberry tree, and onto another gravel road. The road intersected with the highway, which I carefully crossed, then took the path that brought me to the school. My schoolmates were the children of lumbermen, farmers, and railroad men. Railroad workers had a higher status, it seemed. My mother once told me that I had come home and said I wished Daddy worked for the railroad instead of being a farmer. Teachers liked me, I did well in school, and I had friends. Lunch was provided in the cafeteria, where we had to eat everything that we were served, and I was introduced to cottage cheese which I detested at the time.

My life had settled down. I was by now in the second grade. I remember being there in the spring and summer, when the mulberry tree bore fruit and I climbed the tree to eat them.. I also remember harvest times when large green tomatoes were carefully put in sectionalized boxes to be shipped, so they would become ripe and red by the time they reached grocery stores, and when the corn was picked and packed, and potatoes were dug up and bagged, and all was kept in the packing shed until they were trucked away. I remember seeing the fields after the harvest, plowed in furrows before anything grew in them. I can't recall seeing the fields covered in snow, but then this would be when they lay fallow.

The only wariness I recall about being Japanese was during a school drive to support the war effort. Children went from house to house and rang doorbells to collect coins in special cans. Near the highway there was a cluster of houses where somebody lived who was "prejudiced against Japs." When I rang doorbells there, I braced myself for an unknown unpleasantness, which didn't happen. My world was not without warnings that bad things (no details) could happen to little girls, and that some people were hostile to Japanese. I was told to run away if a man called me from a car or gestured to come closer to him. These were important exceptions to being polite and respecting adults, which was how I was raised. I did knock on strangers' doors to help with the war effort, but I was with schoolmates, and there may have been a supervising adult with us in the background.

Our house, our farmlands, and my school were in a broad flat valley between the town of Grand Junction and Grand Mesa, a flat-topped high mountain in a mountain range at the far end of the valley. A tributary of the Rio Grande River was a water source. There were big ditches that carried water to the fields. I liked being there. I liked that I could disappear after I came home from school, change out of a dress, and be gone until dinner time. I had cousins within walking distance, which meant going out the back door, up and over and down to a culvert, where I could jump over a narrowed place before it opened into a small marsh with cattails, skirt someone else's field that sloped uphill toward a sandstone ridge (a local landmark), jump another ditch, and get to the paved road which paralleled the ridge to my cousin Puzzie's house.

Puzzie (Paul Shinoda, Jr.) was a year younger than me and we were buddies. He had a younger brother, Davey, who always wanted to join us and who we, from time to time, were mean to and "ditched." Carol Ann was their baby sister. Puzzie and I spent time outside. There was a local cemetery near his house with many different gravestones and sculptured headstones. When it snowed, the wide swath of down-slope lawn which had gravestones areas on each side was perfect for sledding. We explored and played made-up games out-of-doors.

Puzzie and I once got in big trouble when we decided to run away from home. We didn't return to our respective houses for dinner and weren't home after dark. The adults went out looking for us. Obviously, they were worried. They found us hiding up toward the rafters in the packing shed on top of boxes of produce. Puzzie's dad was furious, and Puzzie got spanked. My mother and father took me home and talked to me instead. I probably heard about the worry that they had felt and how thoughtless I had been. My parents didn't spank me. Talking as discipline was their way, and I can recall saying out loud and definitely thinking when reprimanded, "Why don't you just spank me!" If they spanked me, I could be mad, instead of feeling that I done something bad or beneath their expectations. Their way was pretty effective. By telling me how they had felt when I hadn't come home, they were teaching me empathy and compassion, which are qualities that are needed to do the work I do in therapy and analysis. Over the years, it is a heart-connected way for me to know how another person feels, not just the individual in therapy, but their significant others as well.

When we lived in Grand Junction and I was going to or from my cousins' house on my own, I challenged myself to take risks when no one was watching. I jumped over ditches where I knew I could slip and fall into the water (and never did). There was one up toward Puzzie's house that might have resulted in a dangerous fall. There also were the trees that I climbed up into the high branches and, on coming down, couldn't find a foothold. So I would have to slide and drop to a branch below my feet, each time relieved when I did. Or those times when I instinctively telegraphed that I was harmless, and gave unfriendly guard dogs a wide berth if I failed to charm them. Or when I warily knocked on doors to raise money for the war effort. These were challenges or potential dangers that I didn't talk about at home. I came home when expected and had good marks for behavior and good grades. I gave my parents no cause to worry about me. They had their hands full.

My parents did not talk about their problems around me. I never heard them raise their voices in anger at each other or be in a heated argument. Maybe they did when I was out of the house. My brother was not developing normally. I didn't think about this or know how much of a concern he was to them. He played outside in water and dirt and ran around. He still didn't talk, but sometimes he would repeat a word that was said to him. At some point, he called himself "Tutu" and called me "Jin-jin." Sometimes I would be asked to watch him for a while, which I would do. But mostly, my parents made it clear that he was their problem, not mine to worry about.

The Grand Junction period in my life lasted through second and part of third grade. During the week, I went to school, which was fine. I had wished my mother would be more like other mothers and be active in the PTA—something I did tell her. Still, I clearly fit in and had school friends. Puzzie went to another elementary school close to his house, and I can't recall other Japanese-American kids who may have been there.

On weekends and school breaks, I spent most of my time with relatives who lived in a different part of the wide valley, in a semi-rural area nearer the town of Grand Junction. Here there were more houses built closer together, dairies, farmlands, barns, and fences. All of them lived close to the same two-way traffic country highway that ran by the Shinoda dairy. Four of my father's brothers, two sisters, and their families had settled within a couple of miles of each other. By then, he four surviving siblings who had been born in Japan, Uncle Tom, Uncle Masa, Aunt Kimiye, and Aunt Mary Shigeya, had teenaged and adult children. My father's younger brothers lived in two farmhouses at the dairy. My Uncle Peter and his family lived in one, and my father's youngest brother Uncle Dan, his wife Aunt Yuri, and my paternal grandparents (Kumaichiro and Masuno Shinoda), lived in the other.

The dairy farm was a wonderful place. In the summer, I gathered wild asparagus and explored. It had a pond that froze over in the winter to skate on, around which we made snow forts, and played goose-goose on paths in the shape of a wheel with spokes. The barns were warmed by the black and white cows in them. Everyone seemed to be a relative, a cousin, an uncle or an aunt. While I was one of the younger ones, I was the oldest cousin born to the oldest Shinoda brother born in the USA and I was an age and in a place where I could explore and learn new things.

Here I also got close to some Japanese traditions that I never would have known otherwise. There was a *Furo*—a Japanese bath in its own bathhouse at the dairy. It was a deep tub heated by a fire that was under it and could be tended from outside. Then there was *mochi,* which now is sold year around and in multiple flavors. Back then in my childhood, this was a very special New Year's treat. As New Year's approached, the men got together at the dairy to make *mochi*, which was made by pounding steamed sweet rice in a special container with a mallet. Everyone got a box of *mochi* to take home.

Life for me in the Grand Junction had a settled feeling. I liked living on a farm in the country. I was fine being a good girl and good student in school, and a tomboy after school. I liked being at the extended Shinoda Clan events at the dairy and having cousins and aunts and uncles around. I liked to listen to Sunday afternoon radio dramas with my cousin Helen ("who knows what evil lurks in the hearts of men… The Shadow Knows"). All this changed when we moved again.

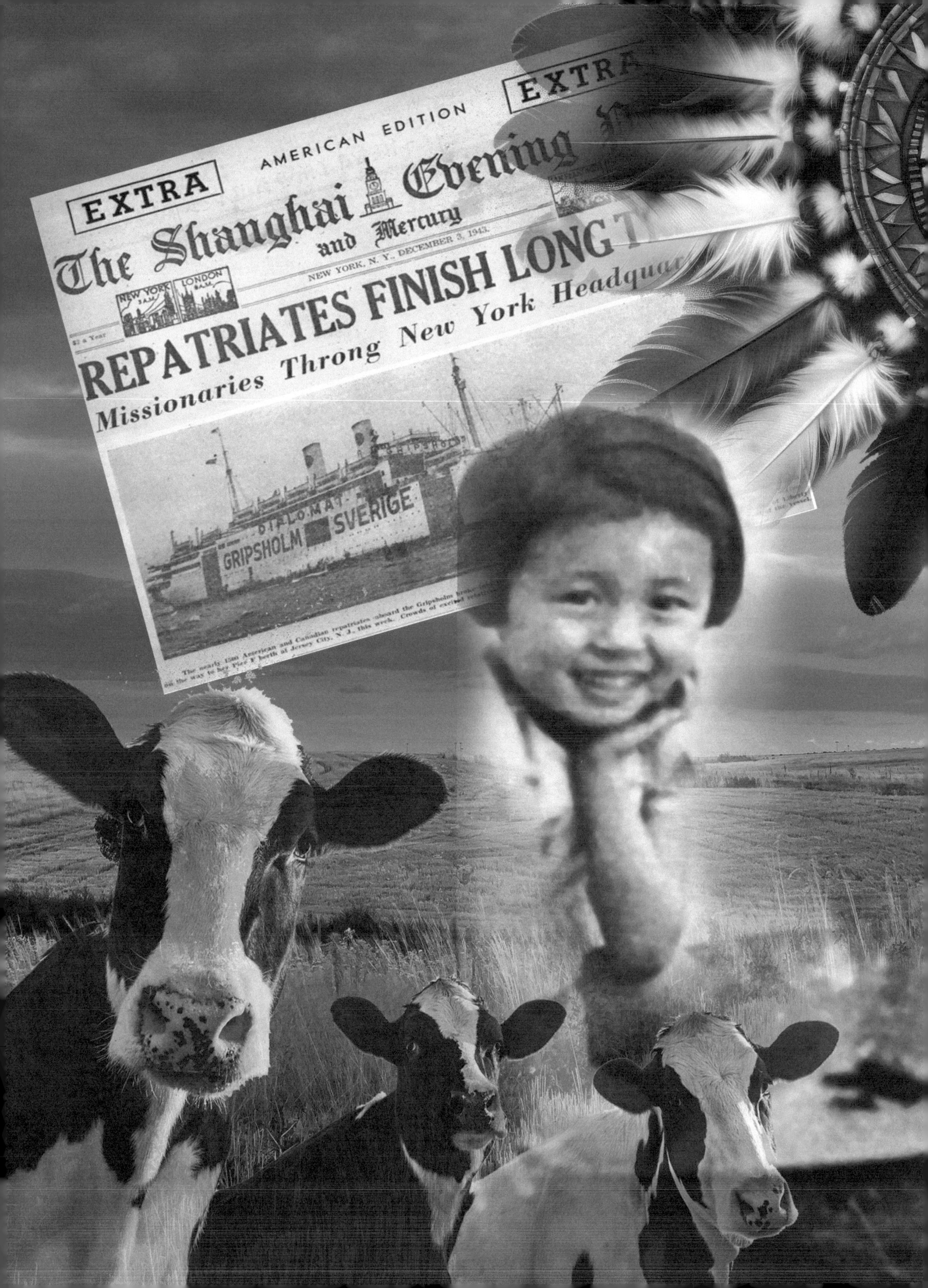
EXTRA
AMERICAN EDITION
EXTRA
The Shanghai Evening
and Mercury
NEW YORK, N. Y., DECEMBER 3, 1943.
NEW YORK
LONDON
REPATRIATES FINISH LONG
Missionaries Throng New York
GRIPSHOLM
SVERIGE
DIPLOMAT
The nearly 1500 American and Canadian repatriates aboard the Gripsholm
on the way to her Pier F berth at Jersey City, N. J., this week. Crowds of

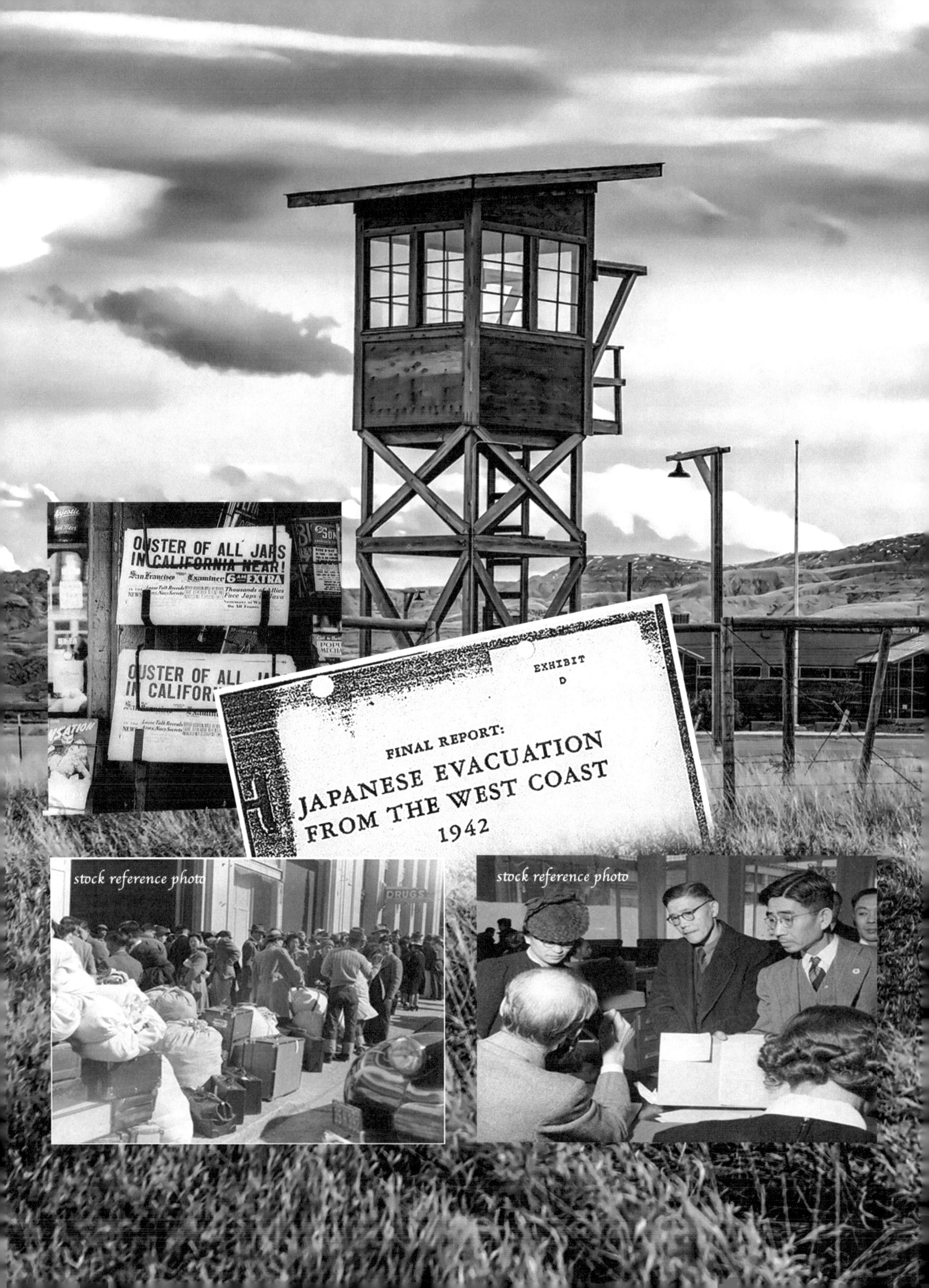
OUSTER OF ALL JAPS IN CALIFORNIA NEAR!
San Francisco Examiner
6 AM EXTRA
Loose Talk Reveals Army, Navy Secrets
Thousands of Allies Face Japs in Java
OUSTER OF ALL JA
IN CALIFOR
EXHIBIT
D
FINAL REPORT:
JAPANESE EVACUATION FROM THE WEST COAST
1942
stock reference photo
DRUGS
stock reference photo

During WW!! the Shinoda family moved near internment camps in Colorado and Idaho in order to help others, but avoided being intered themselves due to her parents planning and resourcefulness.

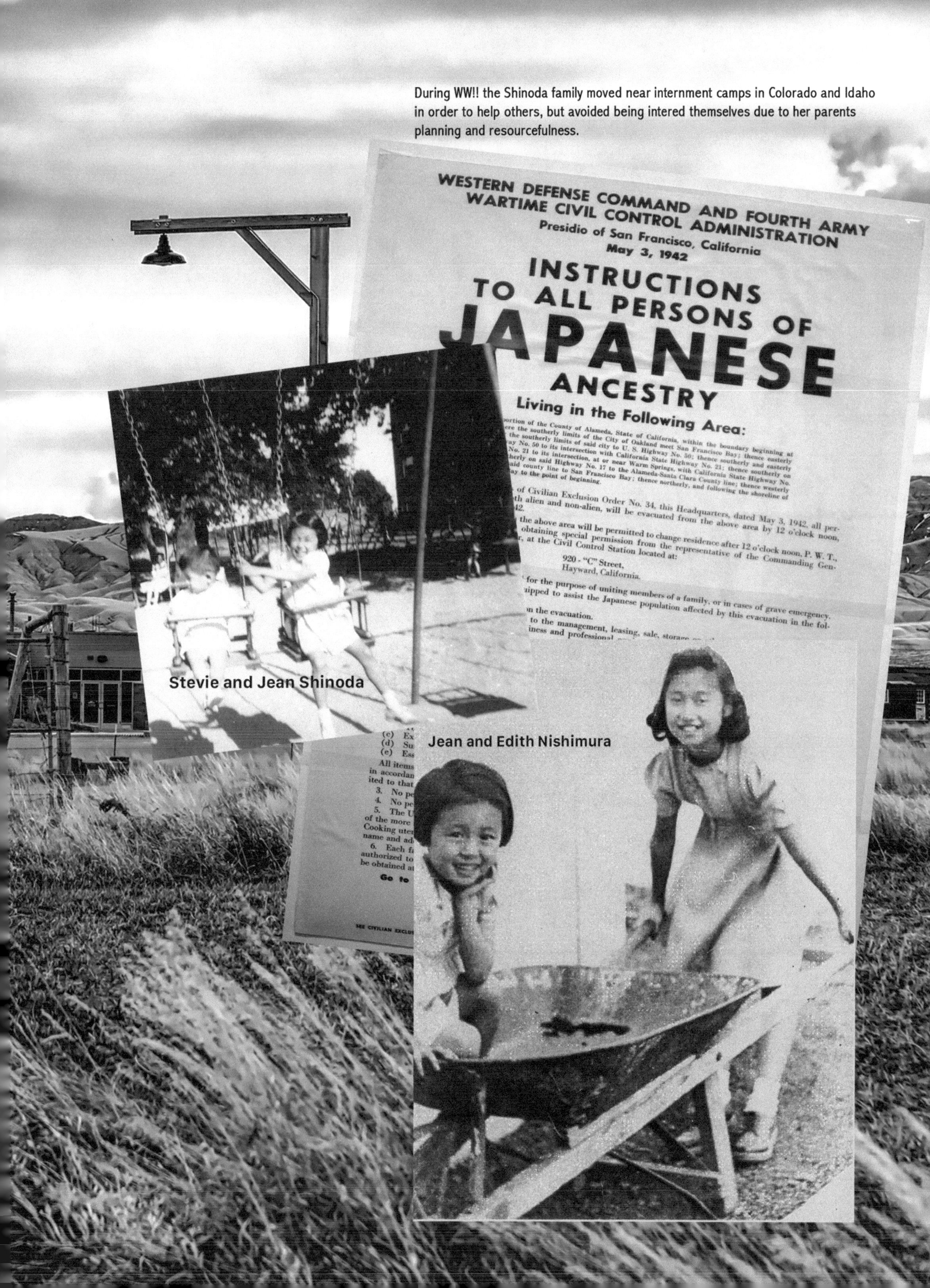

WESTERN DEFENSE COMMAND AND FOURTH ARMY
WARTIME CIVIL CONTROL ADMINISTRATION
Presidio of San Francisco, California
May 3, 1942

INSTRUCTIONS
TO ALL PERSONS OF
JAPANESE
ANCESTRY
Living in the Following Area:

portion of the County of Alameda, State of California, within the boundary beginning at
ere the southerly limits of the City of Oakland meet San Francisco Bay; thence easterly
the southerly limits of said city to U. S. Highway No. 50; thence southerly and easterly
ay No. 50 to its intersection with California State Highway No. 21; thence southerly on
No. 21 to its intersection, at or near Warm Springs, with California State Highway No.
herly on said Highway No. 17 to the Alameda-Santa Clara County line; thence westerly
aid county line to San Francisco Bay; thence northerly, and following the shoreline of
ay to the point of beginning.

of Civilian Exclusion Order No. 34, this Headquarters, dated May 3, 1942, all per-
th alien and non-alien, will be evacuated from the above area by 12 o'clock noon,
42.

the above area will be permitted to change residence after 12 o'clock noon, P. W. T.,
obtaining special permission from the representative of the Commanding Gen-
r, at the Civil Control Station located at:

920 - "C" Street,
Hayward, California.

for the purpose of uniting members of a family, or in cases of grave emergency.
ipped to assist the Japanese population affected by this evacuation in the fol-

n the evacuation.
to the management, leasing, sale, storage
iness and professional

Stevie and Jean Shinoda

Jean and Edith Nishimura

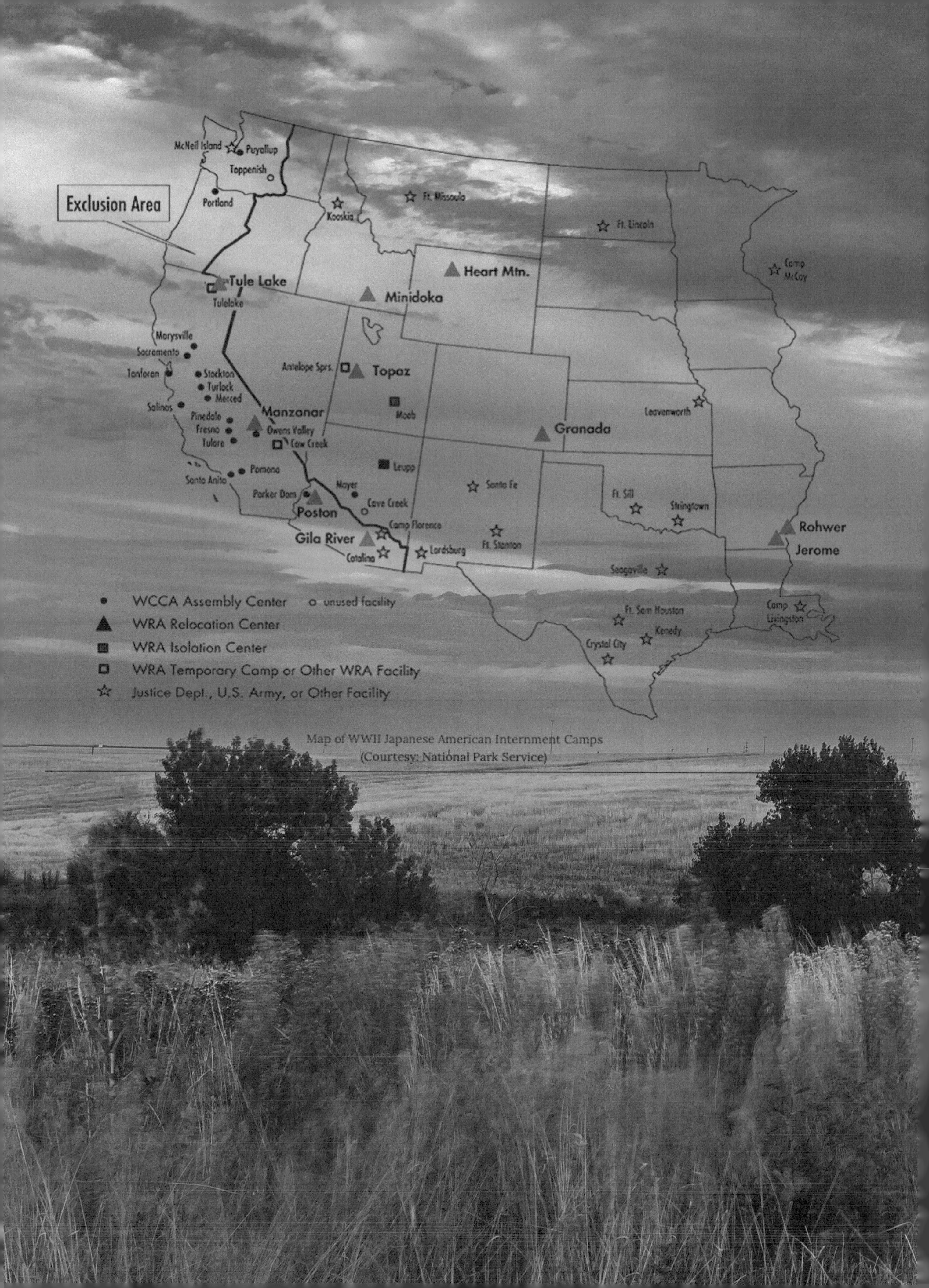

Map of WWII Japanese American Internment Camps
(Courtesy: National Park Service)

Chapter 4
From the Farm to the City

It turned out we would not be in Grand Junction "for the duration." I heard this phrase often. It meant this was temporary: until the war was over, until we could move back to California, until we could go home. My mother, brother, and I moved to Denver. My father stayed in Grand Junction during the week and came to Denver on weekends. We moved into a large two-story house in a neighborhood in the Capital Hill Area of the city. We lived downstairs, and another Japanese-American family lived upstairs with an agreement to take care of my brother.

I was not aware that my mother had been unhappy in Grand Junction. I can certainly see now that she was not cut out to be a housebound farmer's wife whose only outside conversations were with relatives—usually with the women, while the men had separate conversations. She was in all ways a city-person. She had been raised in New York City, and always walked like a New Yorker on sidewalks—fast paced, on her way somewhere. She was not a casual person; strolling was a foreign notion, as much as hiking would be.

Once she asked my father and me to pronounce "marry, merry, and Mary," which were distinctly different when she said them. My father pronounced all three the same, which is what most Californians do. I could say "marry" distinctly, but merry and the name Mary sounded alike. It seemed to mean something to my mother, and though I don't know why, it was a subtle sign that I had absorbed something of each parent and where they were from. Even now, after writing this and saying the three words to myself, it's still two out of three.

My mother's mind and preferences for city life resembled Athena. Athena was the Greek Goddess of Wisdom and Crafts. Her realm was the city. She was the patron goddess of Athens and of her chosen heroes. She was portrayed either as a warrior in armor, carrying a shield and a weapon, or unarmored with a spindle. Thinking strategically on the battlefield, being well-armored intellectually, or creating a tapestry on a loom all require having a practical mind that can utilize resources at hand, plan purposely and accomplish the goal. A housewife and farmer's wife was not who she was. She tried. I remember the day she spent canning tomatoes and trying to make ketchup. The project did not turn out well, but it was good for a laugh.

We moved to Denver after my mother had applied to and been accepted in a psychiatric residency there. Now she had something to do, and was studying what mattered to her. This was the era of Freudian dominance in psychiatric thought, when everything wrong with a child was blamed on the mother. I think that trying to learn what was wrong with Stephen and what might help him must have been part of her motivation for this residency.

The residency was at Colorado Psychopathic Hospital, which has had a name change and is now part of the University of Colorado Medical Center. This was before antipsychotic drugs were developed to help patients who hallucinated and were delusional and sometimes violent. Locked wards and locked isolation rooms were common. Sedation and ECT (electroconvulsive therapy) were about the only treatments available. After I became a psychiatrist, my mother told me about the harrowing time she had at Colorado Psychopathic, working in a locked ward of psychotic women. One patient had a son who was in the armed services in the Pacific. After the patient found out she was Japanese, whenever my mother came on the ward, this woman would shout "JAP!" and obscenities at her. This riled up the other women, who chimed in, all shouting "JAP!" My mother became the face of the enemy. It must have been an awful experience. I can imagine the scene because I have worked in locked wards with isolation rooms; those at San Francisco General Hospital immediately come to mind.

Every time we moved, I began attending a new school. I can't recall starting school at the beginning of a semester or beginning of a school year. I would enter my new classroom, the teacher would introduce me, probably suggesting that I be welcomed, show me to my desk, and proceed with the lesson. I was the new kid, and I was Japanese among non-Asians, which made me different. Between their friendliness and curiosity about me, and my friendliness and curiosity about them, I would soon sit with new friends at lunch, and have company at recess.

On Being a Minority of One: Exotic "Other"

I think of my experience of being accepted had to do with being an exception or an exotic in a positive way. I was an "other" who arrived and was introduced to kids with open minds, mostly because I may have been the first person they'd ever met who looked like me. After the novelty wore off, I became just me. I was welcomed as I later saw foreign students on exchange programs in secondary schools and colleges welcomed. It mattered that I stood out as an exception, rather than lumped into a group of people who were other than white, and either looked down upon or feared.

When I went to Pomona College in the mid-50s, we had an exchange program with Fisk University, a private historically Black university in Tennessee. Two Black Fisk students came to our campus, and two white students went to theirs. This was before the Civil Rights Movement, and before integration. They were welcomed and took classes with everyone else; they encountered friendly curiosity and acceptance —just as I had as in elementary schools.

Innocent comments (mostly from ignorant adults) that I found offensive were variations of "*My, you speak English well.*" Brought up to be polite, I would explain that I was born in America, as were my parents. The campaign to create fear of the Japanese was focused on the west coast to justify the forced evacuation. Most people in the rest of the United States were not even aware of the forced evacuation. If they wondered about me at all, most thought of me as an "Oriental."

Childhood and Family Life in Denver

In Grand Junction, I had had the freedom to roam and explore. I roamed in Denver, but instead of fields and nature, I now lived in a city that was laid out in orderly blocks with sidewalks. Our house was two blocks from my school. The bigger street with stores, streetcars, and the local movie theater was close by. I could take the streetcar into downtown to explore, which I did from time to time, or I would stop at the public library. There I browsed and chose the books I would take home to read. It was easy for me to became absorbed in what I was reading because the settings and characters became real in my imagination. I identified with the main character in the stories I read, who may have been boys (*Tom Sawyer*) or girls (Jo in *Little Women*) or animals (a horse in *Black Beauty*).

The empathy with which I listen to people in psychotherapy or analysis began in my childhood as a reader. It's second nature for me to be as attentive during sessions with people in my office as I was in my imagination when I read. Reading grabbed my attention, so much so that my parents knew that if I had my nose in a book, that they might have to speak to me more than once or even twice. I learned to respond to hearing them loudly say "Knock-knock," which went with the knock-knock gesture.

Outside of the house, I was trusted to take care of myself. I was what might be called a latch key child. I came home from school at lunch time to heat soup on the stove if I hadn't made a sandwich that morning and brought my lunch. I later once told my mother that this was "benign neglect." The family who took care of my brother lived upstairs, so it wasn't exactly an empty house. I think that then I was much the same as I am now. I have a need for "alone time" to refuel. Too much relating to others, especially at the chit-chat level of small talk, is tiring and takes effort and energy. I liked coming home by myself at lunchtime.

It was a different time then compared to now—most children were safe on their own back then. Benign neglect was much better for me than the "mother-hovering" I hear about. "Helicopter mothers" are usually stay-at-home middle-upper class mothers whose children's successful academic and social accomplishments can become the source of their self-esteem and a measure of how well they are doing as mothers. Children are driven to and from school, have a multitude of arranged afterschool activities, including play dates, lessons and tutoring. I wonder how a naturally introverted, dreamy child manages.

I remember talking with my daughter's kindergarten and first grade teachers about how introverted children differ from extraverted ones, which was about differences in processing new experiences, not whether a child is friendly or has social graces. I drew an example from Frances G. Wickes' *The Inner World of Childhood* which I paraphrase now, as I did then. A teacher enthuses, "Who wants to learn this new game?" Hands go up—extraverted kids respond. They learn the game as they participate, as they also find that they either like it or not. An introverted child prefers to watch, figure out what the rules are or how it is played, and then will decide whether they want to play it.

Meanwhile, an adult may be saying, "Don't be shy!" or "What's the matter, don't you want to play?" To be able to say "no" and have the "no" respected, early, makes it easier later, to not go along with the crowd, to not go against your own grain (your truth), and to not be intimidated by "don't be shy or don't be a scaredy-cat." In the larger world which comes with adolescence, learning about relationships and people by observing, rather than first-hand, often turns out to be a wise strategy.

Family tensions register on children subliminally even in the absence of fighting, crying or angry words. I can only imagine and infer retrospectively that my father was caught between his own father's expectations to look after the needs of the extended Shinoda family, my mother's unhappiness with farm life, and my brother's needs. My father ran the San Lorenzo Nursery Company from this distance, and from time to time, he would go to Salt Lake City to meet with his general manager, Mr. Swift. My grandfather was ailing. When we went to the dairy, we stopped first to say hello to Grandpa. I would go into his room where he lay in a tall bed that must have been a hospital bed. I'd come in to say my hello, and then I was excused to go play. My grandfather had had a series of strokes and died in Grand Junction before the war ended.

Our house in Denver was a two-story house in a shade of yellow-orange with a roof over the entry porch. It was on a corner. On the one side was the street, and on the other side was another two-story house. The steep eaves of both roofs hung over a narrow space between the two houses. I remember this because of the icicles that hung down from them in the winter. I slept in a partitioned-off part of the dining room. There was a fence in backyard, where nothing much grew, and a dimly lit kitchen. I read books. School wasn't difficult. My parents put up a Christmas tree, probably for me. It was minimally decorated with hardy ornaments, because my brother might put them in his mouth, or break them, or knock the tree down. Around this time, grown-ups might ask me questions, one of which was usually, "Do you have any brothers and sisters?" I would say, " I have a brother." If another question about him followed, I'd say, "He had a birth injury," which ended questioning.

In Grand Junction, my playmates were either only at-school friends or cousins. Now with my elementary school only blocks away, I was aware that life at my house was different, and I didn't invite anyone over to play. When summer came, my mother enrolled me in a summer art school, which was several blocks beyond my elementary school, but I could easily walk to classes. With good weather outdoors and something that I loved to do, I was a happy child outside of my house and, I think, a stressed child at home. Perhaps this this was me being unhappy, or perhaps I was picking up on my mother's tension when she came back from the hospital, or perhaps I was tuning into stress and worry between my parents when my father was there. I couldn't say, especially in retrospect and from this distance of time.

I certainly knew not to cause my parents any trouble. They had expectations of me which included doing well in school. One time I came home with my straight A's on my report card, and told them I had classmates whose parents gave them a dime for each good grade, so didn't I deserve that, too? The answer was something to the effect of "This is what we expect of you." Much later, when I became a psychiatrist, I read a study about how working for a tangible reward diminishes caring about or feeling positive about succeeding at the task itself.

Looking back, I did find a way to get attention, especially my mother's attention. I had asthma and patches of eczema on my elbows. I understood this as taking after my father, who had bad eczema on both legs, which trousers kept out of sight. I had no idea then that this was stress-connected. My mother, the doctor, knew it was part of an inheritable triad of atopic dermatitis, hay fever, and asthma. When I was in microbiology as a first-year medical student, this was supported by the presence of eosinophils, a type of white blood cells in my sample, which allergic people have and otherwise may not appear. Like so many physical conditions, the psychological situation has a lot to do with whether such conditions flared up or remained quiet. When I was in my psychiatric residency, I read an article that theorized that a child's asthmatic wheezing was the result of being angry and dependent. I could accept this theory for myself as a compromise and a solution—if I was suppressing unconscious anger at feeling neglected, the symptom came out as a wheeze and got my mother's attention, which is what I must have wanted.

The expression "letting something get under your skin" makes sense as leading to itching, scratching, and rashes. Now we have steroids that are an effective treatment, which is good. What is not good about finding an ointment, pill or an injection that works on this physical symptom, is that the psychological, spiritual, or relationship pain that underlies the symptom is skipped over. This can be the reason the eczema or rash keeps returning or spreading.

When physical-biological-genetic predisposition exists and can stay dormant or flare depending on psychological triggers, both need to be attended to. This is another version of the binocular vision metaphor: looking at something from two angles. Physical symptoms often do occur in a psychological or relationship field and need to be seen in order to help or heal.

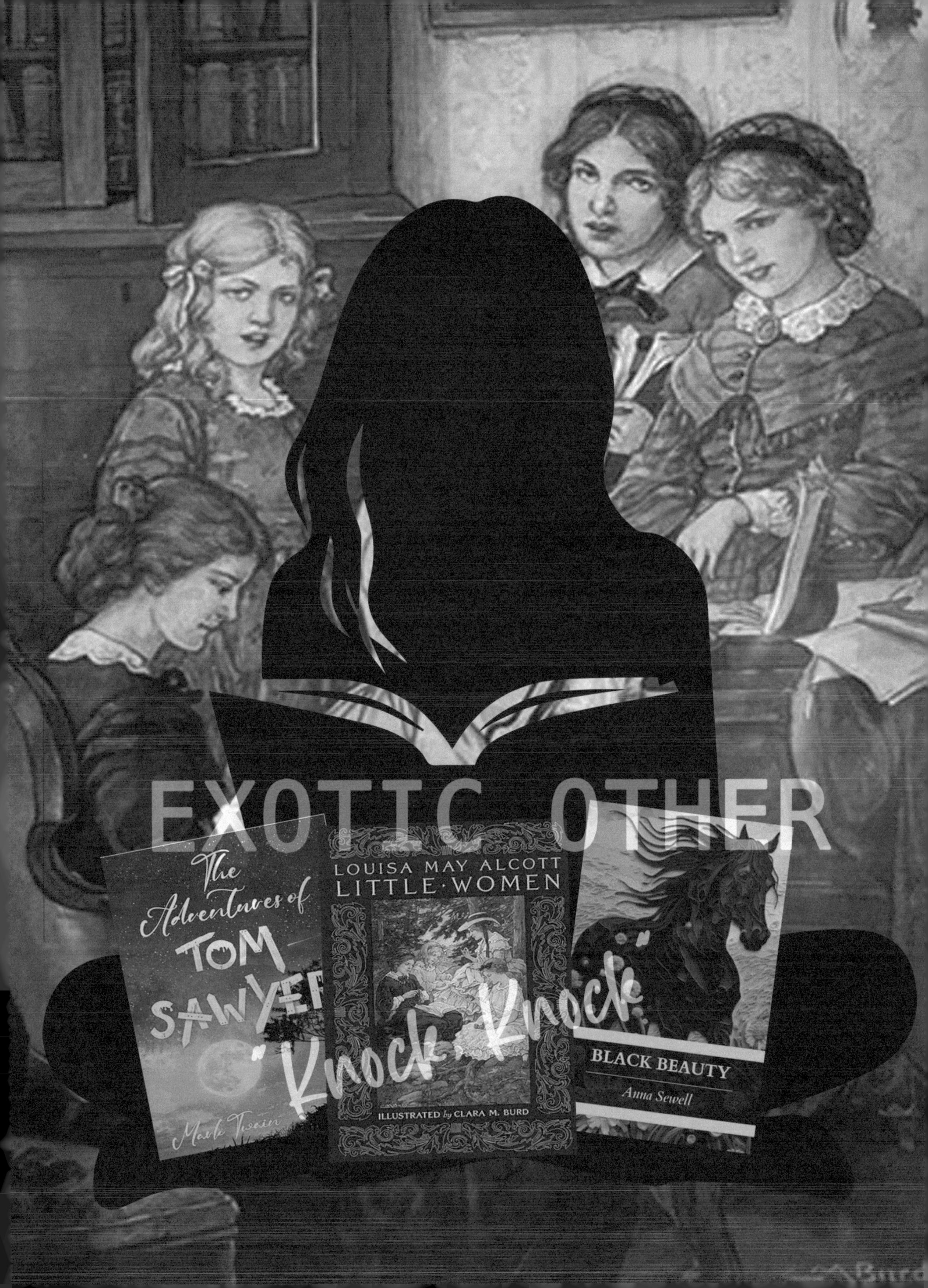

EXOTIC OTHER

The Adventures of
TOM
SAWYER
Mark Twain

LOUISA MAY ALCOTT
LITTLE·WOMEN
ILLUSTRATED by CLARA M. BURD

BLACK BEAUTY
Anna Sewell

Knock Knock

Burd

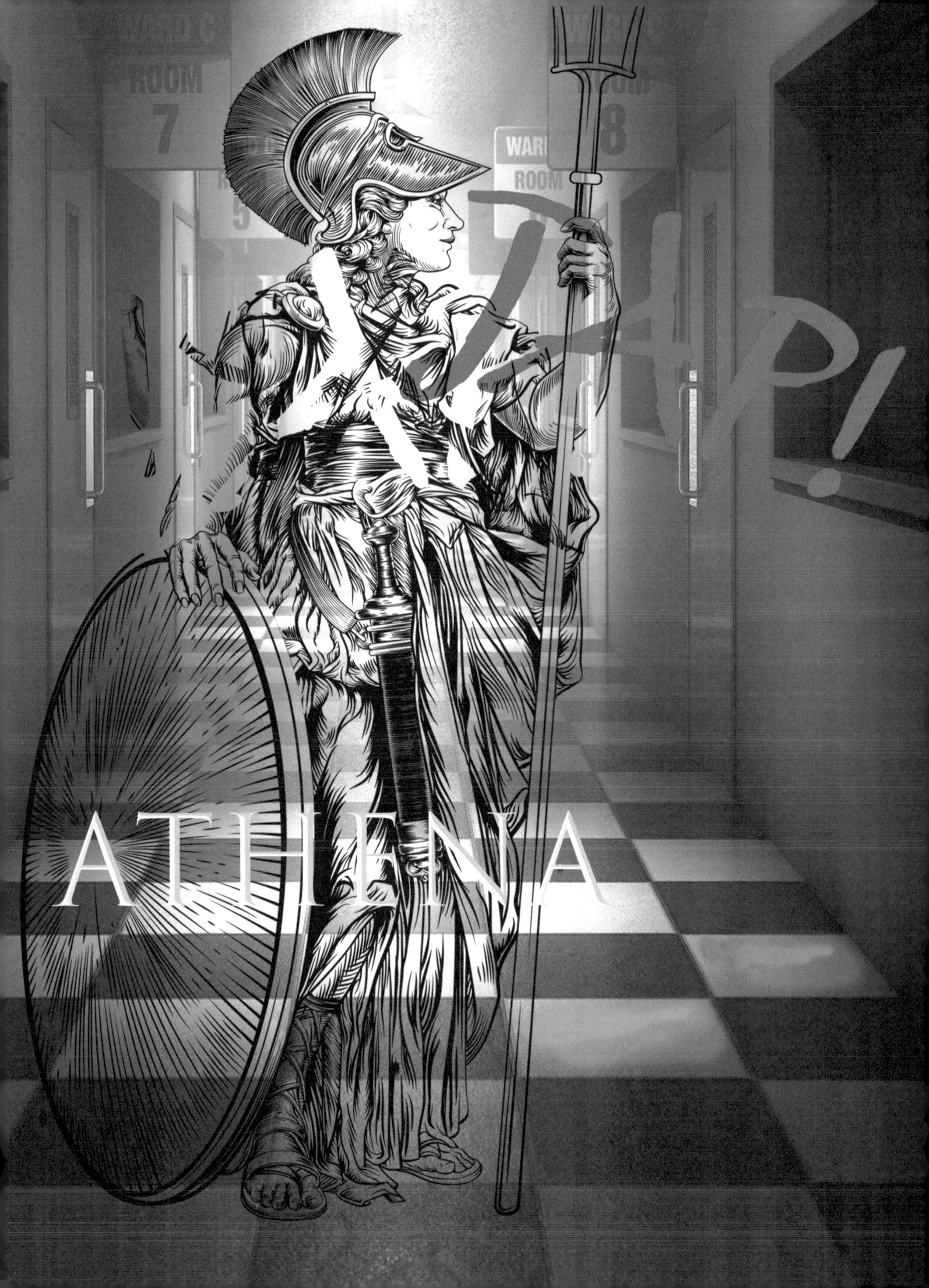
ROOM
7
ATHENA

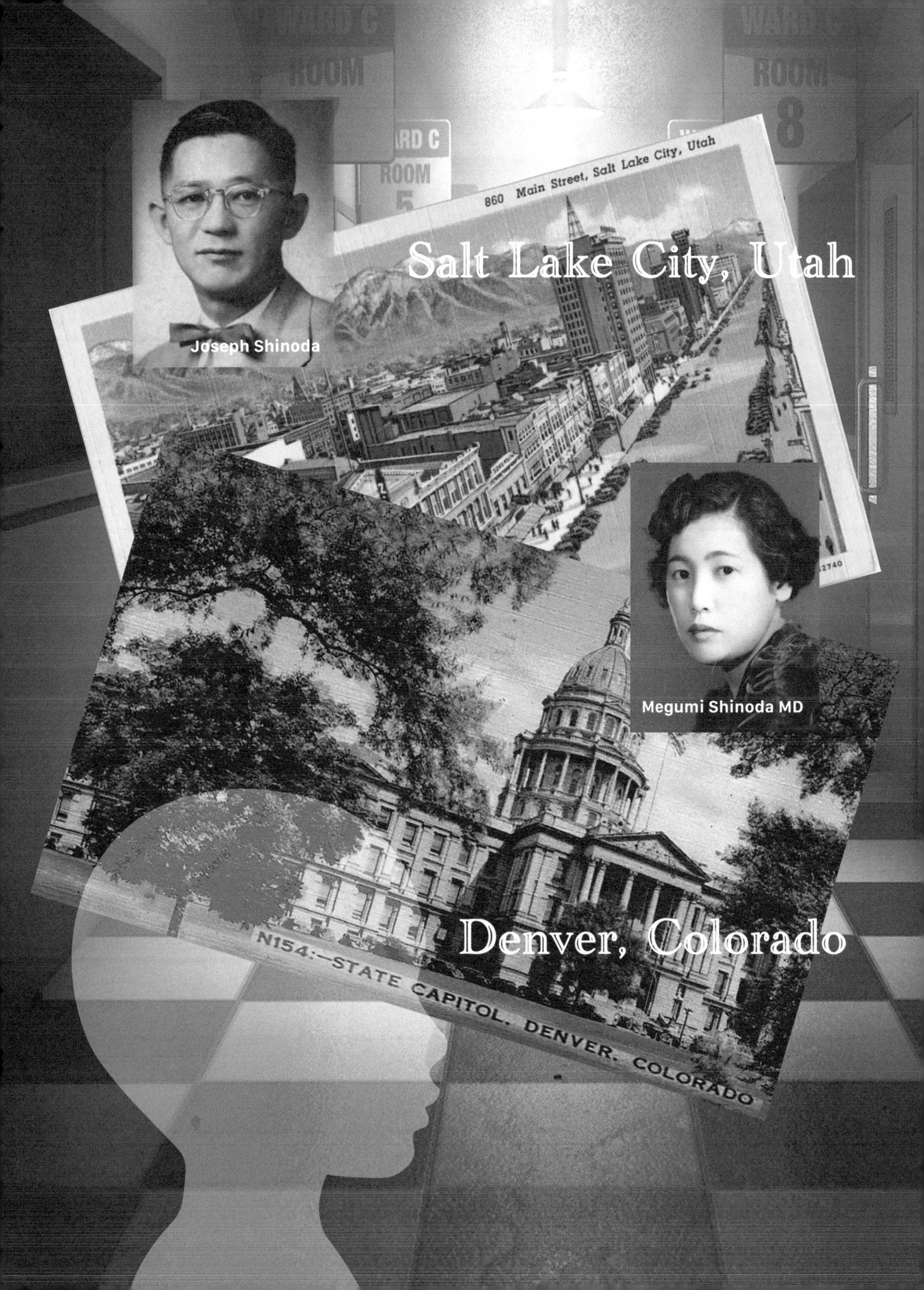

WARD C
ROOM
5
WARD
ROOM
8
860 Main Street, Salt Lake City, Utah
Salt Lake City, Utah
Joseph Shinoda
Megumi Shinoda MD
N154:—STATE CAPITOL, DENVER, COLORADO
Denver, Colorado

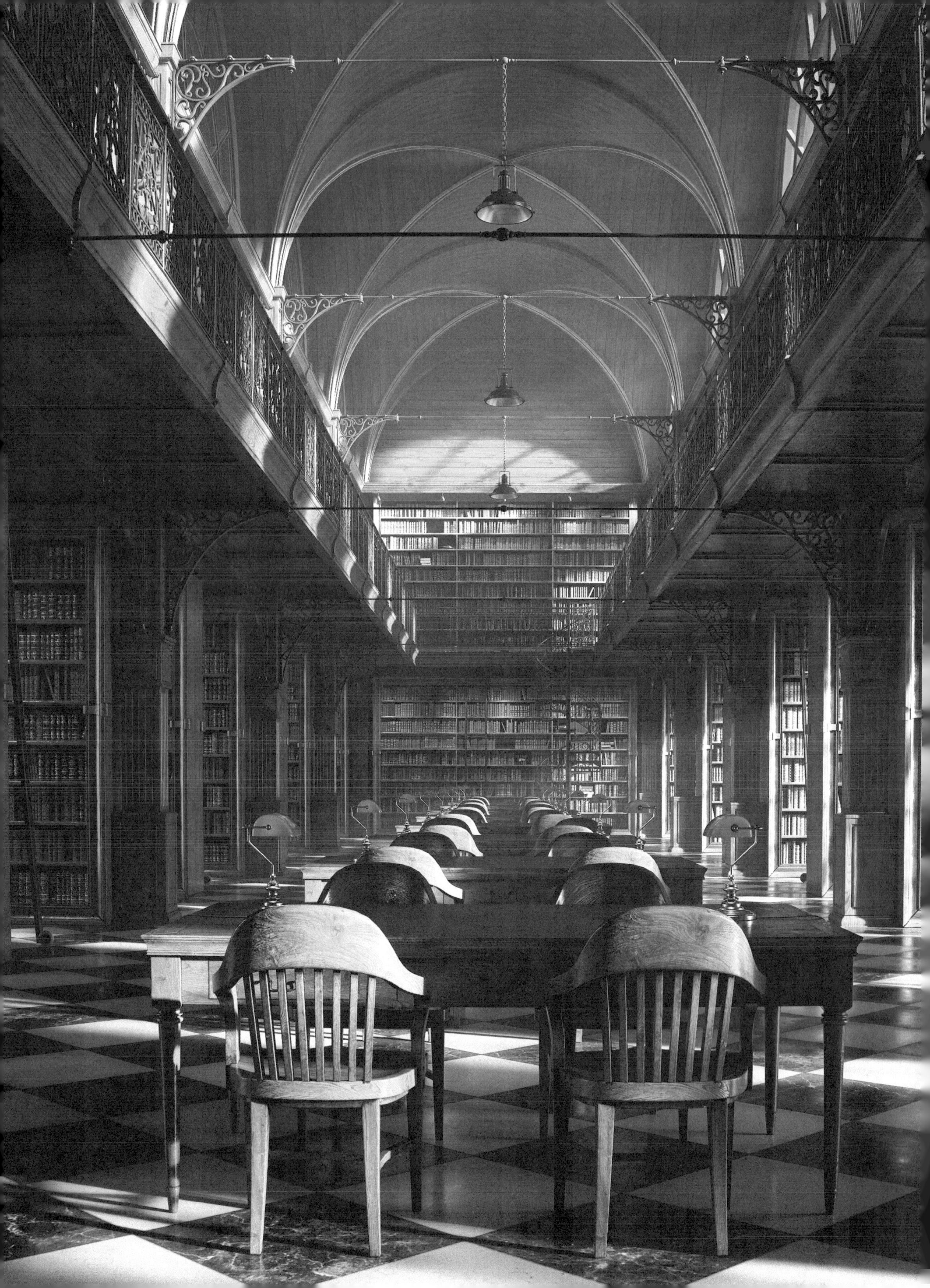

Chapter 5

End of World War II – Sky Mother

The newsreels I saw at the neighborhood theater in Denver were my source of news about the war. The local movie theater was usually packed with kids who would be entertained for most of the afternoon. A second-run movie along with the featured film made it a double feature, with one or two cartoons, and then a grainy black and white newsreel with theme music and a somber male voice describing what we were seeing. It cost nine cents for a child under twelve. The first-run movie house in downtown Denver charged twenty-five cents. It must have been a babysitting godsend for working mothers, since many women worked jobs during World War II and, in addition, would also have housework to do. Life was made more difficult with shortages of everything and rationing, which meant standing in long lines when something became available.

The "News of the World" onscreen at the movies didn't seem real. While America's entry into the war had disrupted my young life, my father's exemption status meant that our family was intact. This kept the war from being close to home, which it had to be for others whose husbands, fathers, sons or brothers were on active duty. As the war went on, the casualties and deaths affected more and more families. Before it ended, The number of families affected was huge, as World War II was the deadliest military conflict in history in absolute terms of total casualties.

In June 1944, British and American forces launched the D-Day Invasion and landed on the Normandy beaches of German-occupied France. Germany surrendered in May 1945. V-E Day, May 8, 1945, was the day on which Allied forces declared victory in Europe. The war against Japan continued with heavy fighting in the Pacific, liberating islands held by Japan. By late spring 1945, Allied forces began heavily bombing major Japanese cities. In early August 1945, the United States dropped atomic bombs on Hiroshima and Nagasaki. Japan surrendered a few days later. V-J Day, August 15, 1945, was the day on which the Allies declared victory over Japan.

On September 4, 1945, the Western Defense Command issued Public Proclamation Number 24, revoking all individual exclusion orders and all further military restrictions against persons of Japanese descent. This meant my family could return to California and, shortly after, we did. It was another interim move. We settled in Monrovia, California, to live on property owned by San Lorenzo Nursery Company in a canyon in the foothills of Southern California. Here plants and flowers could be grown year around, sheltered under lath which were thin strips of wood that offered some shade protection from Southern California's sun, dry heat, and wind. For me, this was another move, another house, another school.

This time, I was enrolled in the fourth grade at Mayflower Elementary School in Monrovia until we could make a permanent move to Los Angeles. Sometimes I would get a ride to or from school, but more often, I would walk by myself. Our neighbors in the canyon were relatives, the walk was not very long and spending time on my own seemed to suit me then. It still does. Once, on a drive with my parents, they pointed out the Santa Anita Racetrack. It was in Arcadia, the next and closest town to Monrovia, which we passed going into Los Angeles. After they had been taken from their homes and held under military guard, Japanese-Americans were temporarily housed at the stables at Santa Anita. When I learned this, the racetrack stood out like a historical monument, marking a place where something bad happened.

Sky Mother

When I thought about the many schools I had attended due to becoming internally displaced refugees, I became aware how smoothly my entries to each new school had been. What I did not see at the time was that every time I went to a new school, my mother had gone first to arrange my enrollment. There weren't test scores that placed children in classes back then. Every time I went to a new school, I believe she paved the way and, as a result, I was placed in classes with the smarter kids.

She also ensured that I got music lessons. I had a small violin and took violin lessons once a week, which had to be arranged for me, just as arrangements were made for me to go to art school in the summer and on many Saturdays. My mother probably knew this was something I would take to, which I did. In the summer I spent Saturdays in art classes which, as a child, I took for granted. She saw to what I might need to occupy myself and had expectations of me that I could meet, and she was right.

My mother looked after me and made arrangements that I did not see, just as I couldn't see the connection between the newsreels and what happened to my family and me. There was a direct connection between the bombing of Pearl Harbor, America's entry into the war, and why we packed up and left Los Angeles, lived many places. As written in the 1983 report of the Commission of Wartime Relocation and Internment of Civilians: "There were decisions made that were based on race prejudice, war hysteria, and a failure of political leadership."

My mother was what I now call a "Sky Mother." "Earth Mother" is a common expression, and as a type of mother, she is usually obvious. An Earth Mother is very present, near and visible, and physically expressive: she provides a lap and hugs, is a nurturer and provider of food and comfort. A Sky Mother's care for her children includes an overview of qualities that need to be developed or discouraged. She finds out what is available that would help her child grow, and identifies good influences.

Over the years of listening to people talk about their mothers, I came to the conclusion that the Sky Mother's maternal style is exemplified by Samurai mothers and New England white Anglo-Saxon Protestants mothers. Both are undemonstrative, and their love is usually understated. A Sky Mother is usually objective about her child's qualities. She assumes responsibility to shape character as well as behavior that reflects well on the family. She gets help as needed. She can delegate caretaking, which would be a deprivation for an Earth Mother. Sky Mothers encourage children to be independent, which can feel like benign neglect. Earth Mothers do the opposite, and can sometimes do too much for a child, which can foster dependency or feel like smothering. She may not see her child clearly and feel loss when her child needs her less.

In the independent-dependent continuum, it's hard for moms to get it just right. "Good enough" will do, which my mother was. The phrase "good enough mother" was first coined in 1953 by Donald Winnicott, a British pediatrician and psychoanalyst. Winnicott observed thousands of babies and their mothers, and over time he came to realize that babies and children benefit when their mothers fail them in manageable ways, which help them cope with the outer world.

Since I am now defining my mother as a Sky Mother, it's fitting that my first vivid memory was of flying across the continent with her for eye surgery to correct my vision. I was both cross-eyed and vision-compromised. Despite my challenges with my vision, in drawing class, I had no trouble getting the perspective right. I could create the illusion of three dimensions (depth) on a two-dimensional (flat) piece of paper. Others had some difficulty with this, presumably they had ordinary eyesight and stereoscopic vision. Maybe this is another variation of positive marginality. I don't have what they have (I am not the same as they are) but I can see how to illustrate and appreciate what it is that they take for granted.

When my eyes were tested after we returned to California, the vision in my two eyes differed: I was nearsighted in one, and farsighted in the other. I saw well because my brain selected the best or clearest image between the two, which means I alternated eyes, using my nearsighted eye to read or look closely at something, and the farsighted one for distance. If I had had a dominant eye and favored it, the other eye would be mostly unused; the right and left occipital lobes of my brain would not be in continual use, and I wouldn't have an internal switch that chose which eye and image I would see. My visual back and forth is similar to how I am writing about my childhood experiences: there are the close ups—what I remember or was told—and a view of the larger forces of history that had personal consequences to me.

A Permanent Home

Our next and final move was to a house in the Silver Lake area of Los Angeles that became our family's permanent home. I lived here from most of the fourth grade through my first semester of college, after which I mostly was away. My father spent the rest of his life in this house, and it was where he took his last breath. My mother did, as well—but that would be over forty years later.

It was a large, solid, square wood-sided house with a front porch. Our street had been cut into the side of a steep hill, and the house had been built on the hillside, above the street, on the part of the property that was relatively flat. The street began its descent gently in front of the house before it then resembled a sled run straight down to the bottom of the hill. The winning elements of this house were the size of the property, its natural privacy, and with the addition of an unobtrusive chain link fence, my brother's safety. At that time, I was nine and he was a hyperactive five. He liked to run, both in the house and outside. The basement was converted into a living space for live-in help for my brother when my parents were at work.

The yard was huge and overgrown. I sometimes called it "the jungle." There were many fruit-bearing trees: apricots, guavas, pomegranates, grapefruit, avocado, and also large pines and a huge pepper tree that I climbed and would sit in with my imagination to keep me company. In spring, weeds grew and went from green to dry yellow, and the Fire Department would send out a fire-hazard notice. I went to Micheltorena Street School, on a street which ended at Sunset Boulevard at the bottom of the even steeper street above ours.

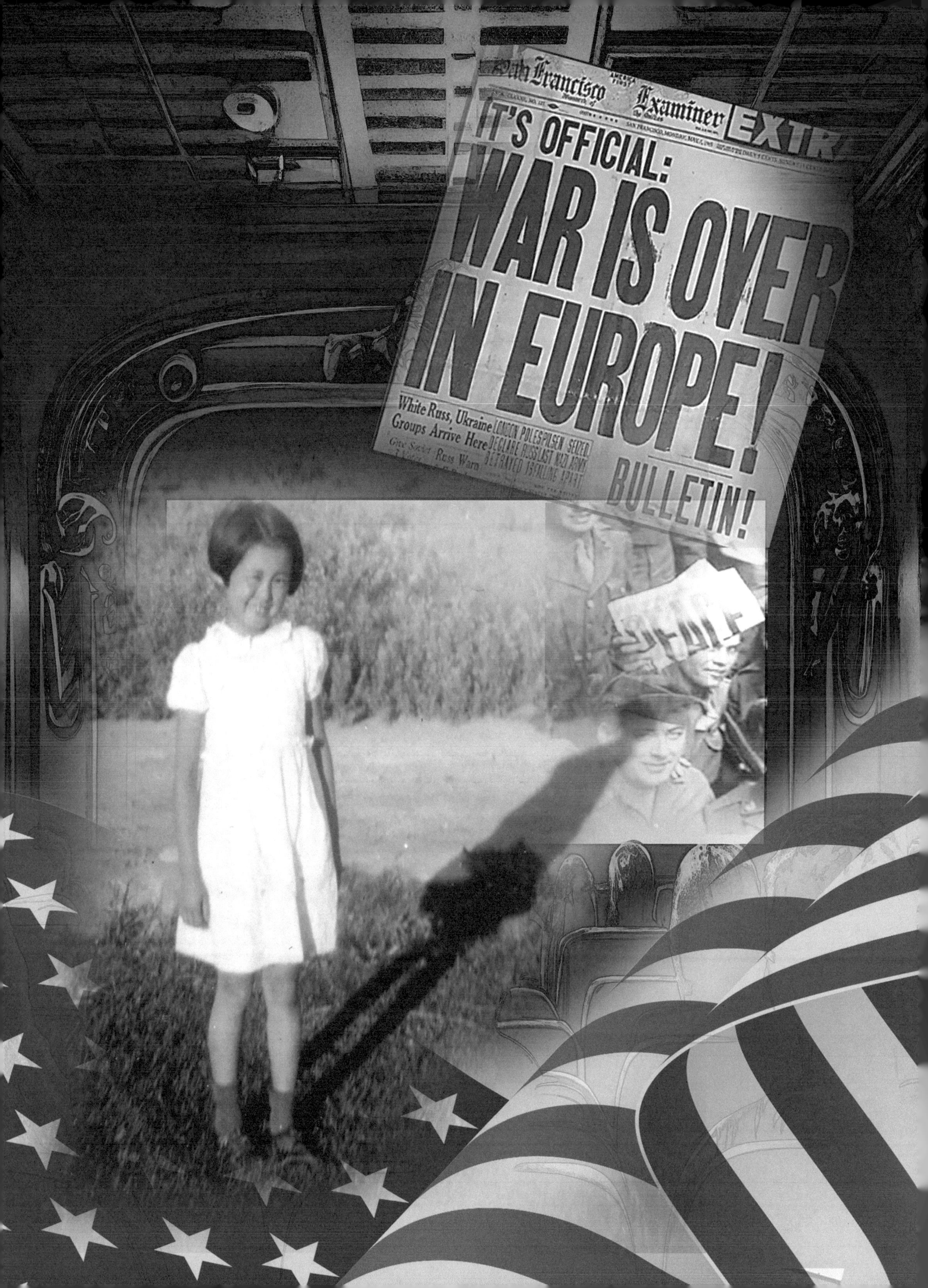
Examiner
WAR IS OVER
IN EUROPE!
BULLETIN!
White Russ, Ukraine
Groups Arrive Here
LONDON POLES
DECLARE RUSS
BETRAYED

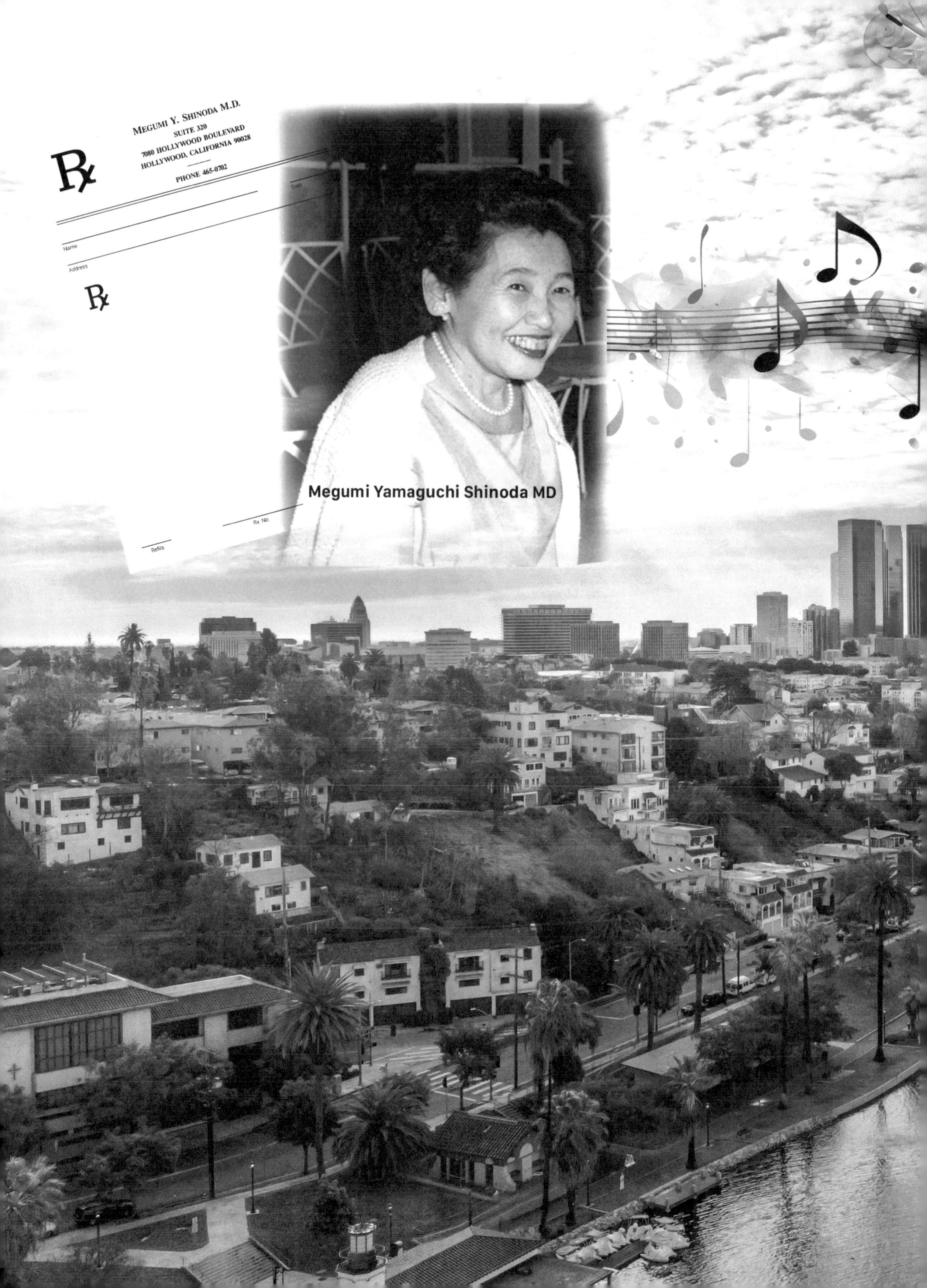

Megumi Yamaguchi Shinoda MD

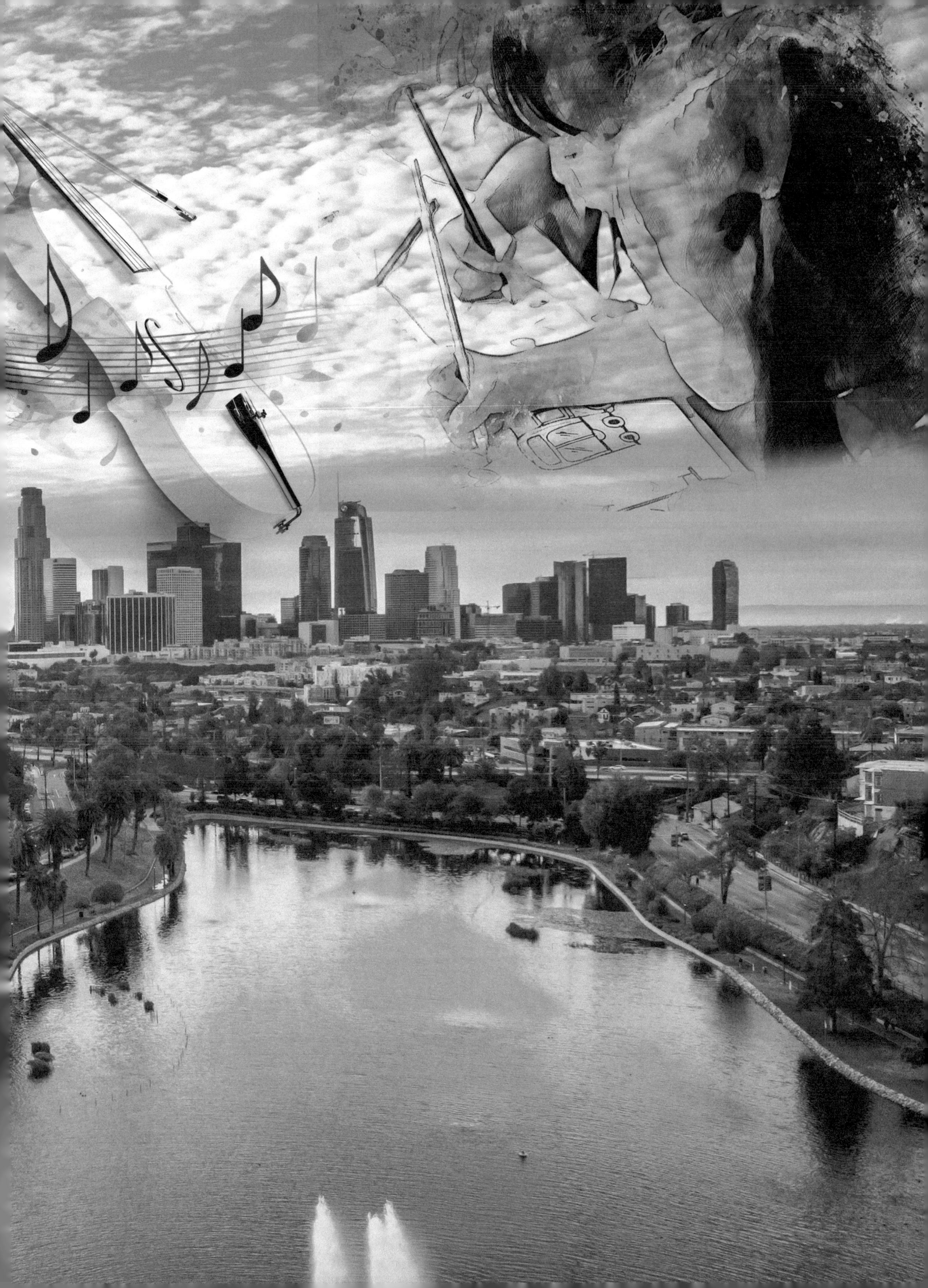

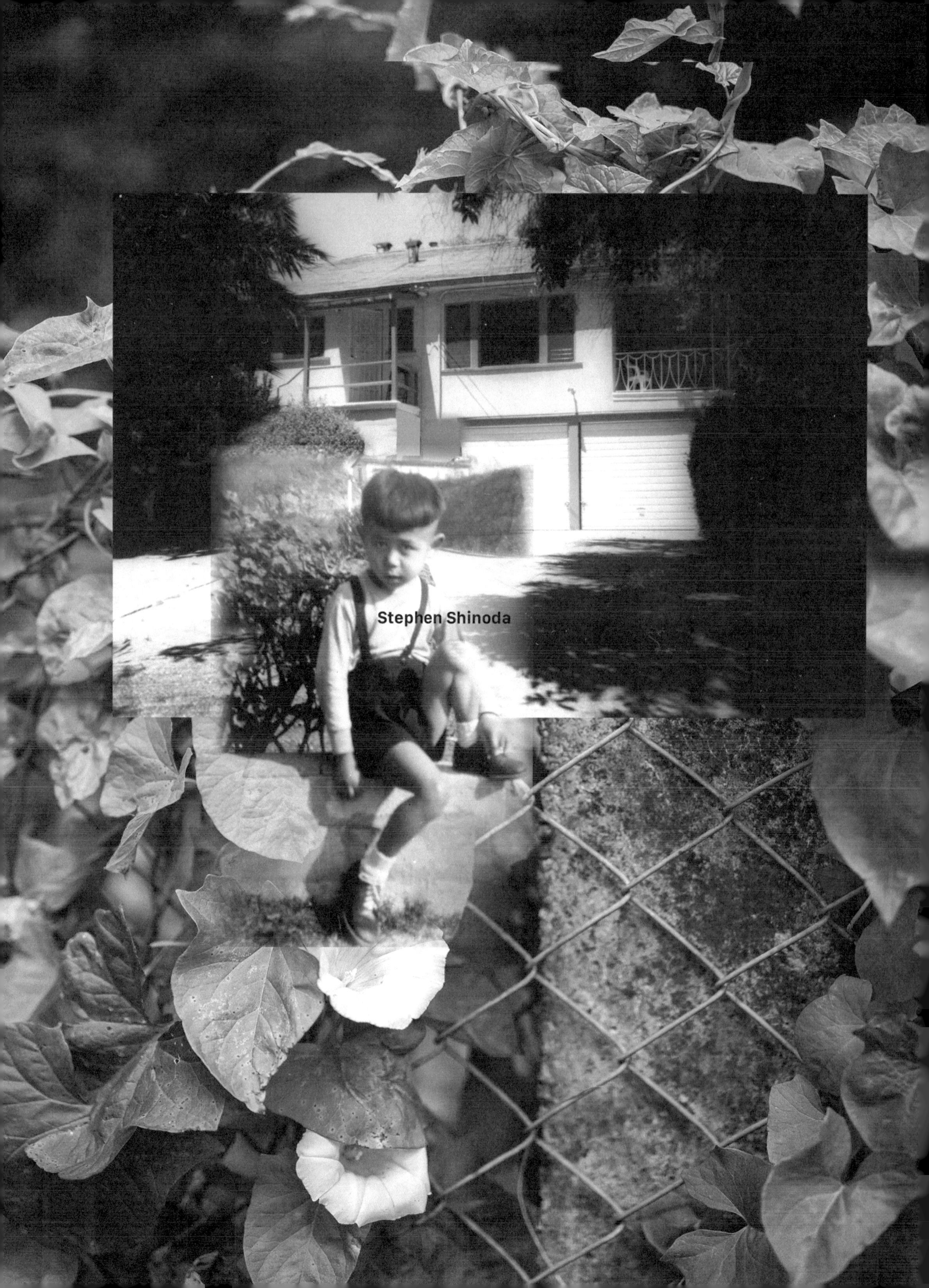

Stephen Shinoda

Chapter 6
Initiations

In addition to the usual elementary school curriculum, at the end of the fourth grade, girls, with signed permission from parents, watched a film about menstruation and the physical changes we could anticipate happening to us. This was helpful information and meant we knew what was happening when we bled for the first time. When it happened to me, I remember having a vague sense of its significance, beyond and besides physiology. It was an initiation, just as first intercourse and first pregnancy can be, when "something" stirs in the deeper layers of the psyche in response to an experience. This was a glimmering, the personal ground of knowing—the "something" that responded decades later when I heard about a Native American ritual-celebration from a colleague, a child psychiatrist who spoke about her daughter's first menstruation and of the ritual that was held in the backyard of their home.

These stirrings were inklings into an awareness that there is more than one way of knowing. There is intellectual, scientific knowledge, what we know for a fact, and can rationally back up. This is what the ancient Greeks called *logos*. They had another word for knowledge of a different kind, that which we subjectively know to be true for us, called *gnosis,* that is deeply felt and/or intuitive knowledge. It is what we know "in our bones," or in our heart or soul. This part of us can know something that is impossible to have known rationally. I had only a vague inkling when I had my first indication that menses was beginning. I may have known that something more could be happening beyond this physical sign. It is a significant change. It is *menarche*, the first of the blood mysteries. A girl is becoming a woman when she bleeds for the first time. After this, *menstruation* will soon become monthly, she and other menstruating women will bleed every month—at the same time, if they are exposed to moonlight. Menarche, menstruation, and menopause are all derived from *meno*, or "moon" in Latin.

When menses begins its often a secret between daughter and mother. I told my mother, who had previously given me a book about menstruation, and who now introduced me to Kotex pads and the need to use cold water to wash blood out of my underpants. Anything else (a celebration, a ritual, an announcement at the dinner table) would have really felt weird. There was no conscious cultural context to mark this as a deeply meaningful event in the first half of the twentieth century, not in a Christian-American context, anyway. The colloquial expressions were negative. Menstruation was "the curse" or "being on the rag."

Rituals call upon the invisible to bless, or deepen, or signify the importance of a rite of passage. Or, as can often be the case, the ritual is itself the rite of passage. Around the same time of this physical initiation that was the beginning of a monthly inconvenience, I took part in two formal initiation. One was religious and Presbyterian, the other was a Girl Scout Investiture. Each marked a formal beginning of a lifetime exploration into sources of personal meaning that began when I was in the fourth to sixth grade at Micheltorena school. They had nothing at all to do with what I was taught there, and everything to do with what I was doing outside of school.

Girl Scouts

The Girl Scout Investiture was a solemn evening occasion held in Mrs. Titus's living room. We had signed up to join Troop 788 and had met after school to learn about becoming a Girl Scout. There was a handbook, rules (or laws) to learn, and an oath to make. For this ritual, we were in full green uniforms, stood in a circle, and held a candle. I think we each in turn recited one of the laws and lit our candle. I draw from memory the oath (while holding up three fingers of the right hand) that must have become etched in my mind: "On my honor, I promise to do my duty to God and my country, to help other people at all times, and to obey the Girl Scout law." I also took to heart the words to a song that I can still sing: "When ere you make a promise, remember well its importance, and when made, engrave it upon your heart."

At regular afterschool Girl Scout meetings we giggled, made things, earned badges, and occasionally went places as a troop. Nothing felt particularly significant about our meetings, and yet from the pledge of allegiance to the Girl Scout code, values were put into words.

I knew Girl Scout Camp was significant, and I began attending the summer after the fourth grade. "Camp Osito," the Los Angeles Area Girl Scout Camp, was close to Big Bear Lake in the San Bernadino Mountains. It was a rustic camp, with girls of the same age in small units named after Native American tribes or native plants, and each unit had a couple of camp counselors. We slept out of doors, in sleeping bags on metal army surplus beds with a thin mattress. We kept our clothes in the one tent, which held our possessions, and where we could change clothes, and could go to if it rained, but it never did. We wore "greenies": short-sleeved shirts and shorts. Around us were towering Jeffrey pines with bark that smelled like vanilla, red-branched Manzanita bushes, and not much else. We had a bathhouse with latrines and cold showers. We had duties to help clean our own unit, and various chores in the kitchen, bathhouse, and outdoor eating areas. We sang around the campfire every night, we sang when we hiked together on a road, and often sang at mealtimes. We were often challenged to learn new skills, from tying knots, to setting up a campfire, to chopping wood. There were plants in the meadow to identify and star constellations to learn. Girls came from all over Los Angeles. Those who came back, as I did, loved being there. As a result, we had camp-friends and school friends.

Cosmos Initiation

Most nights, we went to sleep with the Milky Way above us. It was awesome to see the stars, so close, and so many, and so beautiful! I'd never gone to sleep out of doors before, and though a few stars and the moon were visible from Los Angeles, there is too much light from the city for the stars to be seen. It may have been the second or third summer that I had my first liminal, spiritual experience. I had been paying attention to the star-filled sky, looking for a shooting star. Every so often, we might see a streak of light, sometimes slightly colored, which was probably a meteor. If you saw one, you could make a wish. That night, the sky had my full attention. I was awake and alert. The stars were up there and they were beautiful. I was looking at them, and something shifted in me. I was no longer an observer—a girl looking up at the stars. In a shift of consciousness, I suddenly knew (*gnosis*) that I was part of this beautiful awesome universe. That it and I were one. This wordless revelation stayed with me as a deep in my soul. I couldn't express it until I had the vocabulary, much later.

Other authors have written about moments in which they had a profound shift in perception while alone and out of doors. In *Zen of Seeing*, Fredrick Franck wrote of such a moment, when he was around the same age I was. He was walking between fields of curly kale, it had just begun raining, when he suddenly knew that everything he was seeing was inside of him. Barbara Ehrenreich described mystical visions she had had as a teenager and never spoke of them until she wrote *Living with a Wild God.* She talked with Terry Gross about it on NPR's Fresh Air: "I was just staring the woods when something happened. It's like a layer peeled off the world . . . it wasn't scary. . . I couldn't tell anybody. I had enough sense to think that this would be seen as crazy." The second vision she had, "the only words I can put to it after all these years is . . . that the world flamed into life. Everything was alive…"

For me, as it seems in others, what we looked at became much more than a visual experience. Vision was suddenly imbued with meaning, and ordinary reality shifted into something subjectively much more. I received *gnosis* information for the first time. It was a spiritual experience, not a religious one. I associated religion with church.

Religious Ritual: Presbyterian Communion

During the forced evacuation and our many moves, I occasionally had been to a church, but it was not until we had returned to Los Angeles and settled into our permanent home that I began going to Sunday School at the neighborhood Presbyterian Church regularly. This was about the same time that I became a Girl Scout. One of my parents would drop me off and pick me up to take me home after church. Sunday school was in the basement of the church. When I was ten or eleven, I was baptized and confirmed at the same service with others in my Sunday school class.

After I was baptized and confirmed as a member of my local Presbyterian church, I participated in the communion Service. Welch's grape juice was served in individual thimble sized glasses, and white bread was cut into cubes to represent the bread and wine served at the Last Supper, the final meal that Jesus shared with his disciples on the night before his arrest and crucifixion. On the back of each of the wooden pews were holders for the Hymnal and Bible used during every service, and a thin shelf with round holes to put the small empty glasses after we had taken communion. Communion was about remembrance for Presbyterians, who did not have mystical-magical beliefs that the bread and grape juice was transformed into the actual blood and body of Christ. In Sunday school we learned bible stories from the Old and New Testaments. In the Sunday Church Service, the sermon was usually preceded by a reading from verses in the King James Bible on which the sermon was based. Some verses became familiar sources of solace.

Junior High School

After we moved to Los Angeles, I went to same elementary school and progressed with my classmates from fourth grade through sixth grade. We went on from there to Thomas Starr King Junior High School (seventh, eighth, ninth grades). These three years were smack-dab in the middle of the twentieth century (1949-1951). Girls were required to take home economic courses (sewing and cooking classes), and most of us also took typing. Boys had to take one of the shop courses (woodshop, print shop, or metal shop). Conformity to gender roles, getting-along, not making trouble—those were our priorities. I was part of a circle of friends from several homerooms. It was literally a circle, since we usually sat on the lawn in a circle while we ate our lunches. It was a friendship-based group, and most of us were active in school government and did well in academics. Many of these friendships continued into high school, several into college, and three of us of Marriam (Myrna Cramer) Ring, Katherine (Kay Hessen) Hensley and I stayed in touch into our eighties.

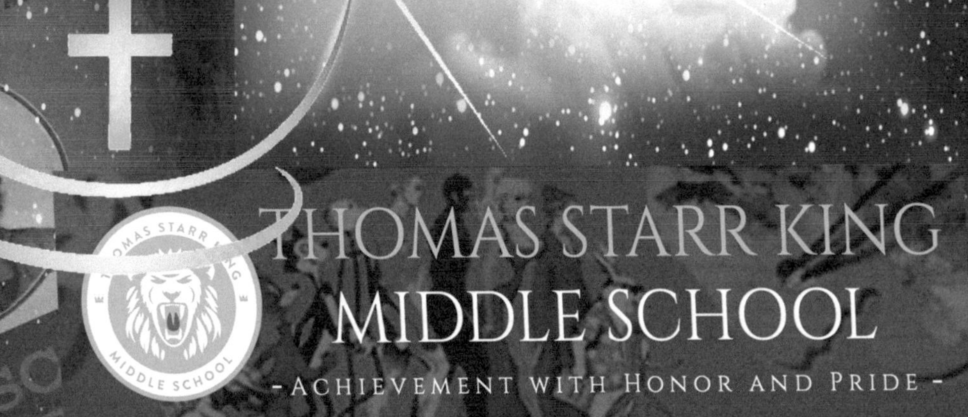
THOMAS STARR KING
MIDDLE SCHOOL
- ACHIEVEMENT WITH HONOR AND PRIDE -

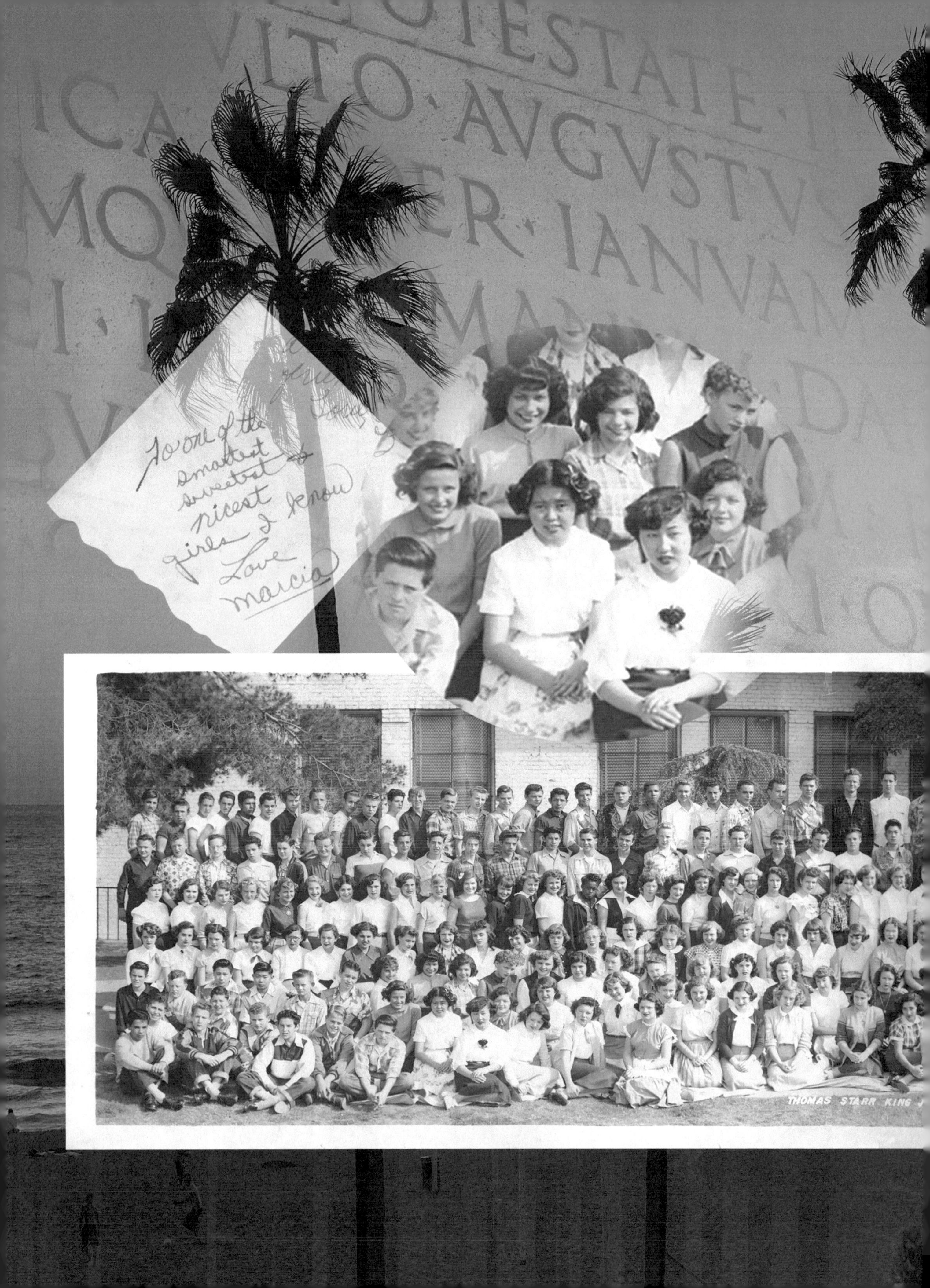

To one of the
smartest
sweetest &
nicest
girls I know
Love
Marcia
THOMAS STARR KING J

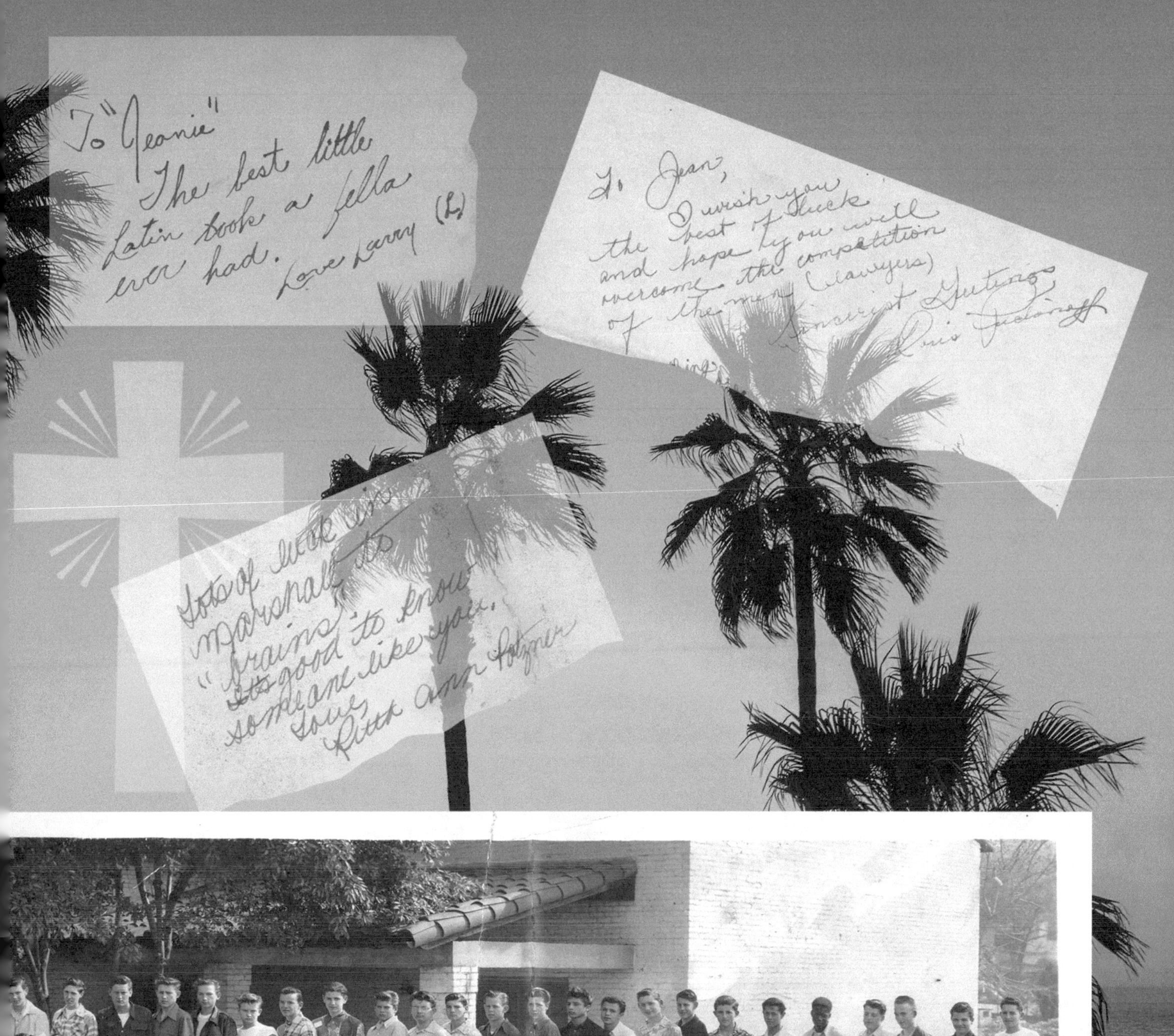
To "Jeanie"
The best little
Latin book a fella
ever had.
Love Larry (L)
To Jean,
I wish you
the best of luck
and hope you will
overcome the competition
of the men (lawyers)
Sincerest Greetings
Lots of luck in
Marshall its
"brains"
It's good to know
someone like you.
Love,

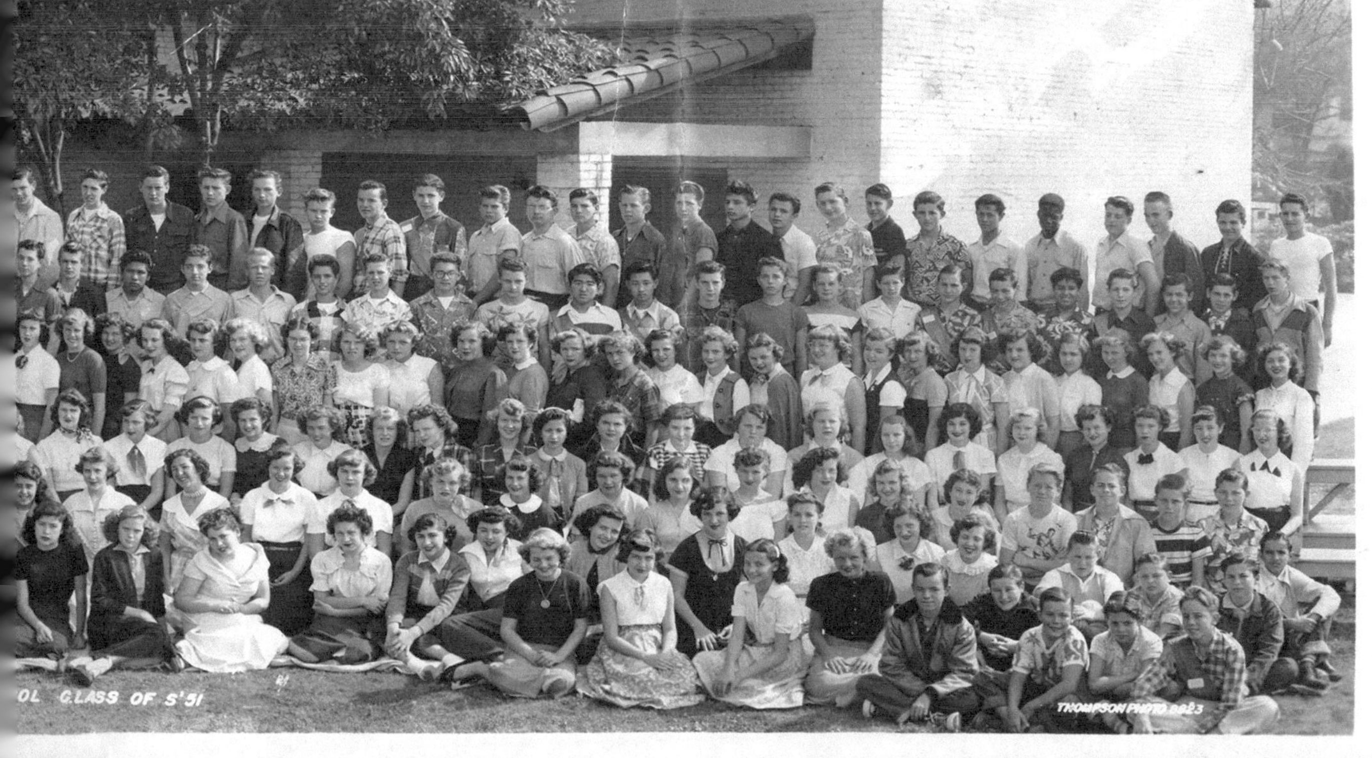
OL CLASS OF S'51
THOMPSON PHOTO 8823

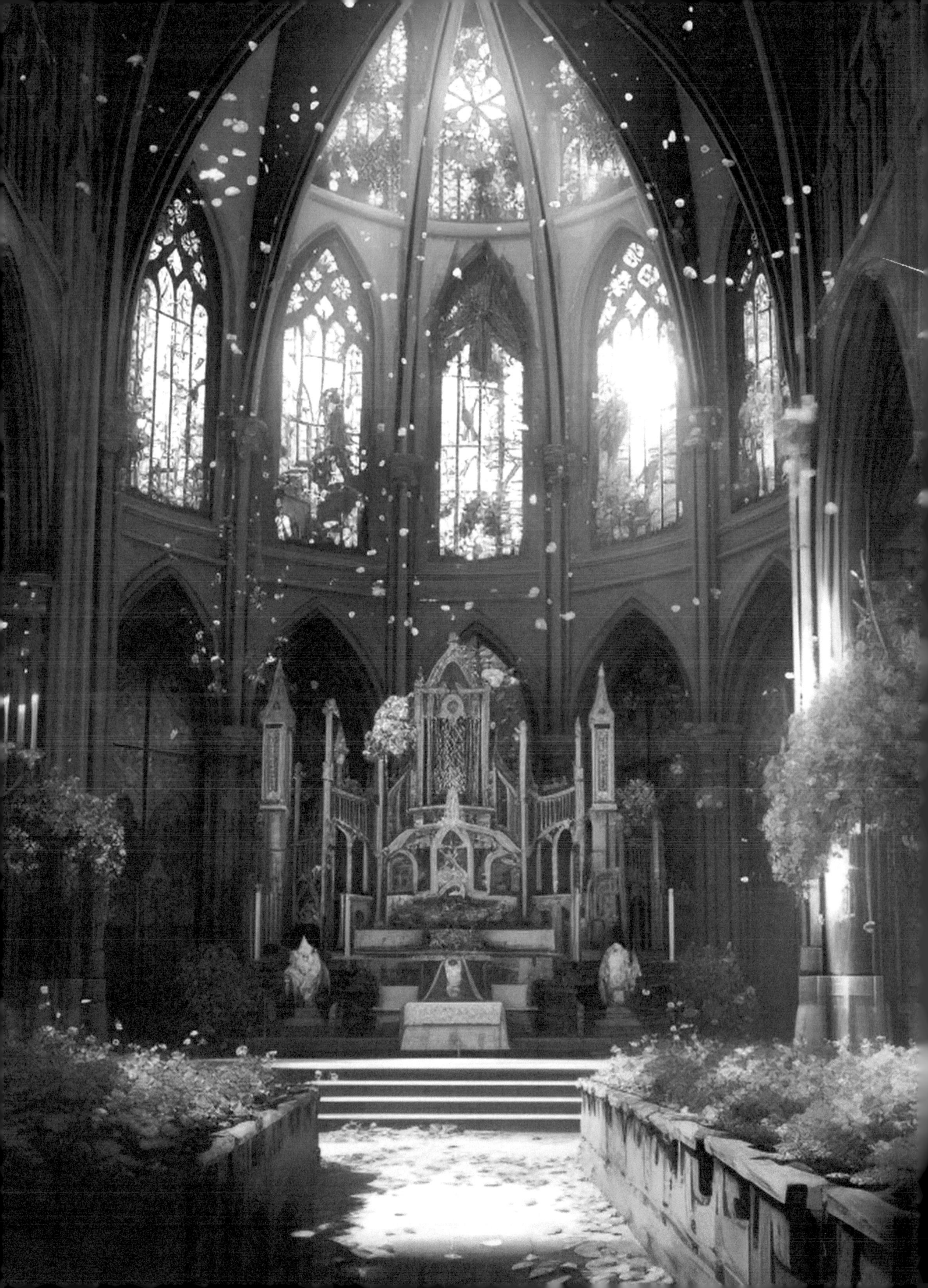

Chapter 7

My Brother – My Parents' Grief

Once we were back in Los Angeles, my school years became regular and predictable. While my life was going smoothly, my parents were in anguish about what could be done for my brother. My mother had noticed that when he was a baby, he never cooed and smiled like babies do. As he grew older, from time to time, he would do something that seemed hopeful, though it's unclear to me now what seemed encouraging. He was my strange little brother, who seemed to be in his own world and yet, he was sweet. My parents tried to find doctors who could help, but no treatment was offered, nor even a clear diagnosis. Doctors suggested it might be brain damage. As he grew older, they wondered if it might be a developmental disability caused by birth injury, then called "mental retardation." Doctors suggested or recommended that he be put away in an institution for the "mentally retarded," which my parents would not do.

This was a nothing-can-be-done sad state of affairs for my parents, as it was for parents of any infant or child who did not develop normally at the time. Then, parents who put their child in such institutions were not supposed to visit them; they were told that visits would disturb both the child and the parents. In the mid-forties, a psychiatrist described a new condition that raised the hope that deterioration was not inevitable, and a new surgical procedure was touted.

In 1943, autism was discovered and described as an exceedingly rare condition by Leo Kanner in his book *Autistic Disturbances of Affective Contact.* He described a distinct syndrome, instead of previous depictions of such children as "feeble-minded," "retarded," "moronic," "idiotic," or "schizoid," and cited eleven cases. Kanner's patients seemed to have autism from birth. He had borrowed the term "autism" from Eugene Bleuler, who had coined it to describe a symptom: an inward focus and self-absorption in some adult schizophrenics. Schizophrenia was also a condition that usually progressed, and when people with schizophrenia were hospitalized, they deteriorated in these institutions.

A month after World War II ended, the forced evacuation of people of Japanese ancestry from the entire west coast of the United States was officially over, and we could return to California safely. When we left Denver, which would have been as soon as we could, my mother had not completed a full residency in psychiatry at Colorado Psychopathic hospital. I don't know if she had learned of Kanner's paper while she was there. Quite likely, she did, and I am sure she would have shared this new diagnosis with my father.

After autism became more widely known, parents were blamed for the condition. The labels "refrigerator parents" and "refrigerator mothers" were coined around 1950 to describe parents of children with autism or schizophrenia. This led to the Refrigerator Mother theory: lack of maternal warmth as the cause of autism. The theory was promoted to the public by Bruno Bettleheim and supported by psychoanalysts. It became the accepted theory for the next two decades. Bettleheim became the director of the Orthogenic School for Troubled Children at the University of Chicago in 1943.

What mothers themselves had to say about their babies (that didn't make any difference to psychiatrists and psychoanalysts) is that children had a lot to do with how mothers respond to them, as well as vice versa. But this was a time when Freudian theory dominated psychiatric thinking, and so a time when children were seen as blank slates upon which mothers wrote and evoked the kind of children they became. This was also an era when men prided themselves "as never changing a diaper" and left raising children to women.

Besides being a mother herself, my mother was in general medical practice and saw lots of babies. My brother Stephen was different; there was no babbling and cooing, nor reaching up for hugs. He didn't want to be cuddled, and didn't make eye contact. As he got older, she tried to engage him in many ways, but nothing worked. In parent-child observations, mother and child are watched through two-way mirrors, and interactions between an autistic child and his mother couldn't be described as warm and close. "Aloof" or "cold" were the standard descriptions of mothers of autistic children.

I do not doubt that I was unconditionally loved by the same parents that Stephen had. It could be deduced from the emotional security I went into the world with as a child, and how they responded to needs I expressed in my teens and adulthood. I also see how much they devoted to taking care of him. Our parents were home on weekends, and with their separate work hours, one of them was usually home to be with and watch Stephen play with water, run back and forth, or run in circles, eat, or go for rides, which he seemed to like. Or, when he still was small enough, my father carried him on his shoulders, and then when bigger, on his back. Stephen liked movement. When I was home, I would occasionally be asked to watch him. Since he didn't interact or play, "watching" him was what I did.

My mother and father persisted in seeking help for Stephen. I don't know who they had consulted after discovering an autism diagnosis might apply to him. The experts also began to say that autism had a psychogenic cause. I don't know how much blame was put on or taken by my mother since the "refrigerator mother" was said to be the cause. I learned later that someone they had consulted suggested that Stephen's asocial withdrawal and lack of communication could have resulted from severe anxiety due to the forced evacuation and the many moves we made as a result.

In the mid-forties, a psychosurgical procedure to cut neural connections in the frontal part of the brain came into vogue and was used to treat psychiatric patients. The rationale was put forth by Walter K. Freedman, a neuropsychiatrist. He acknowledged that while no diseased brain tissue had been found to account for mental illness, obsessions, delusions, and other signs of mental morbidity could be caused by dysfunctions in the internal wiring of the brain. Cutting some of these connections, the white matter of the brain, had been pioneered in Europe and was called a leucotomy. Freeman needed a neurosurgeon to do a modified version to prove this theory, which became known as the Freedman-Watts prefrontal lobotomy procedure, first done by in 1937. It required drilling holes in the scalp that could only be done in an operating room by a neurosurgeon. James W. Watts was the neurosurgeon who was persuaded by Walter Freeman to undertake this and with Freeman was the co-author of *Psychosurgery, Intelligence, Emotion and Social Behavior Following Prefrontal Lobotomy for Medical Disorders* (1942).

Freeman believed that this surgery would be unavailable to those he saw as most needing it—the patients in state mental hospitals, which didn't have operating rooms, surgeons, or anesthesia, and were on limited budgets. Freeman was the medical director of St. Elizabeth's Hospital in Washington, DC. He invented another procedure that could be done through the eye sockets with an ice pick from his own kitchen. This new trans-orbital lobotomy involved lifting the upper eyelid and placing the point of the ice pick under the eyelid and against the top of the bony eye socket. A mallet was used to drive the instrument two inches into the brain, and then moved from side to side, and up and down, cutting the white fiber connections to the prefrontal cortex. A special tool to do this was later created.

Freeman performed the first trans-orbital lobotomy in 1946, and was exceedingly successful at promoting it. Between 1940 and 1944, there were 684 lobotomies performed in the United States. With development of the trans-orbital procedure, the numbers increased. In 1949, the peak year, 5,074 lobotomies were performed. It wasn't until a decade later, after antipsychotic, anti-anxiety, and anti-depressant drugs were introduced, that lobotomies went out of favor. By then 50,000 of them had been performed on people.

My brother was one of them. Stephen had a lobotomy at Cedars of Lebanon Hospital (now Cedars-Sinai) in Los Angeles. I was in junior high school and remember being picked up after school and taken to visit Stephen at the hospital several times. He was in a hospital bed, with a big bandage wrapped around his head that also went under his chin. In my mind's eye, it was in the shape of a football helmet kept in place by an under the chin-strap. He looked small. He was awake and as usual showed no signs that he was aware I had come. I would later learn it was my father who had high hopes for this procedure. When he talked to me about why Stephen was in the hospital, I saw tears in his eyes for the first time ever, which probably was after the surgery. I can recall hearing how good this neurosurgeon was, and that he also was a fine sculptor, which was his hobby. He had been carefully chosen, and the surgery had been carefully done, and not with an ice pick.

Freeman had promoted lobotomies as a procedure he could do in ten minutes. There had been glowing testimonials in the news from patients themselves as well as families after lobotomies. For some with overwhelming anxiety, it had been miraculous. I imagine that this positive news was what had raised hopes in my father, and in Joseph Kennedy, Sr., the father of Rosemary and patriarch of the famous Kennedys of Massachusetts. Joe Kennedy was used to making decisions, and at this point in his life, he had suffered no real tragedies, success had come relatively easily, and he relied on faith and prayer to see him through difficulties. Freeman himself performed the lobotomy on Rosemary. In her book about Rosemary, *The Missing Kennedy,* Elizabeth Koehler-Pentacoff described the procedure as such:

> In 1941, unbeknownst to his wife and family, Joe Kennedy took Rosemary to be examined by Dr. Walter Freeman, a neurologist and psychiatrist who was also a professor at George Washington University. Joe had read about the doctor's successes in *Life, Time*, and *Newsweek* magazines.
> "Dr. Freeman's diagnosis of Rosemary was "agitated depression." He claimed a lobotomy would not only relieve her of the rages she suffered but also render her happy and content. The prestigious doctor, an imposing six feet tall, bore a professorial-looking mustache and beard. He assured Joe that a lobotomy was the best option available for Rosemary. Joe said he wanted the doctor to go ahead.

Rosemary had been diagnosed as "mentally retarded" and did not have any signs of autism. She may have been brain damaged by efforts to keep the normal delivery from happening until the doctor arrived, during which time, her brain may have been deprived of oxygen. Another speculation was that she had been infected in the uterus by the influenza virus. In her family photographs, she is an attractive Kennedy, a young woman, not a child. Koehler-Pentacoff 's work is a poignant and sympathetic telling, including the possibility that Freeman (who often showed photographs of his patients when telling of his successes) had shown Kennedy before and after photographs of Emma Ager, a woman with the same diagnosis of "agitated depression." Ager looked miserable before the lobotomy and relaxed and content after.

After the procedure, Rosemary was like a two-year old who needed to learn basic skills such as how to walk, how to follow simple directions, how to talk, and even how to go to the toilet. Kennedy's decision to have Freeman perform the prefrontal lobotomy was done without his wife Rose's knowledge. She and the rest of the family did not learn of Rosemary's lobotomy for twenty years. Kennedy told Rose and his children that her behavior had worsened, and that doctors had advised that she be institutionalized for her own good and should have no visitors because they could disrupt and confuse her. It was not until 1961, after Joseph Kennedy had been incapacitated by a stroke and administrators could no longer talk with him, that Rose was contacted and reunited with her daughter.

Parents of developmentally disabled girls are especially concerned about sexual predators and the vulnerability of their daughters. Kennedy had the additional fear of kidnapping for ransom after the kidnapping of the Lindbergh infant. Rosemary had begun wandering, leaving the house on her own, and had become angry and difficult, which also made her more vulnerable. Freeman was a salesman and a doctor whose claims had been widely reported, and not by investigative reporters.

Lobotomies were far from miraculous. They had caused deaths, put some in vegetative states, made many others apathetic and passive. When I was a resident in psychiatry and read about the effects of lobotomies, besides the adverse physical and mental toll it could take, one example stuck in my mind: a wife described her husband whose surgery was successful. He was now free of his disabling anxiety, but he was not the same person anymore. It was as if he had lost his soul.

There were no positive results from Stephen's lobotomy. Whether there had been a loss of soul, no one could know. The lobotomy seemed to have little effect on him, and the surgical scars were the only visible sign that the procedure had been done. Soon after the s

urgery, however, he had a convulsion for the first time—a grand mal seizure. Now he had epilepsy as well as what he already had, but at least there were anti-convulsion meds. The convulsions had no effect on his personality, which was an inadvertent test of another psychiatric treatment for disabling anxiety, depression and some other psychiatric conditions. In electroconvulsive therapy (ECT), which was widely in use, convulsions were induced by sending electricity through the brain or via intravenous insulin, which caused the blood glucose to drop until the brain convulsed. I learned about this much later.

When Stephen came home, there was a sadness in the atmosphere. We all went about our business, and mine was to go to junior high school. Our house had undergone some remodeling after we moved in and the overgrown yard, aka "the Jungle," had gradually undergone change in part because watering plants or pulling weeds was what my parents could do outside while watching over my brother and his solitary activities.

There were no afterschool Girl Scout meetings in junior high. For a time, I was a member of a fan club for an actor and sex symbol; I was just the right age for this. I learned how to ride a horse and joined the California Rangers. We wore uniforms, assembled at the stables by Griffith Park, and after doing some drills together, rode on the horse paths in the park and in the Hollywood Christmas Parade. In the summers, I went to Camp Rancho Osito, which was part of another dual reality: school and camp were two different worlds for me, both of which took me away from home, where Stephen was the family painful secret, and the reason that I had never invited a friend to my house, though I had been to the homes of friends for birthday parties and even a slumber party. I now had a cocker spaniel that I named "Chummie" after the small dog I once had in New York.

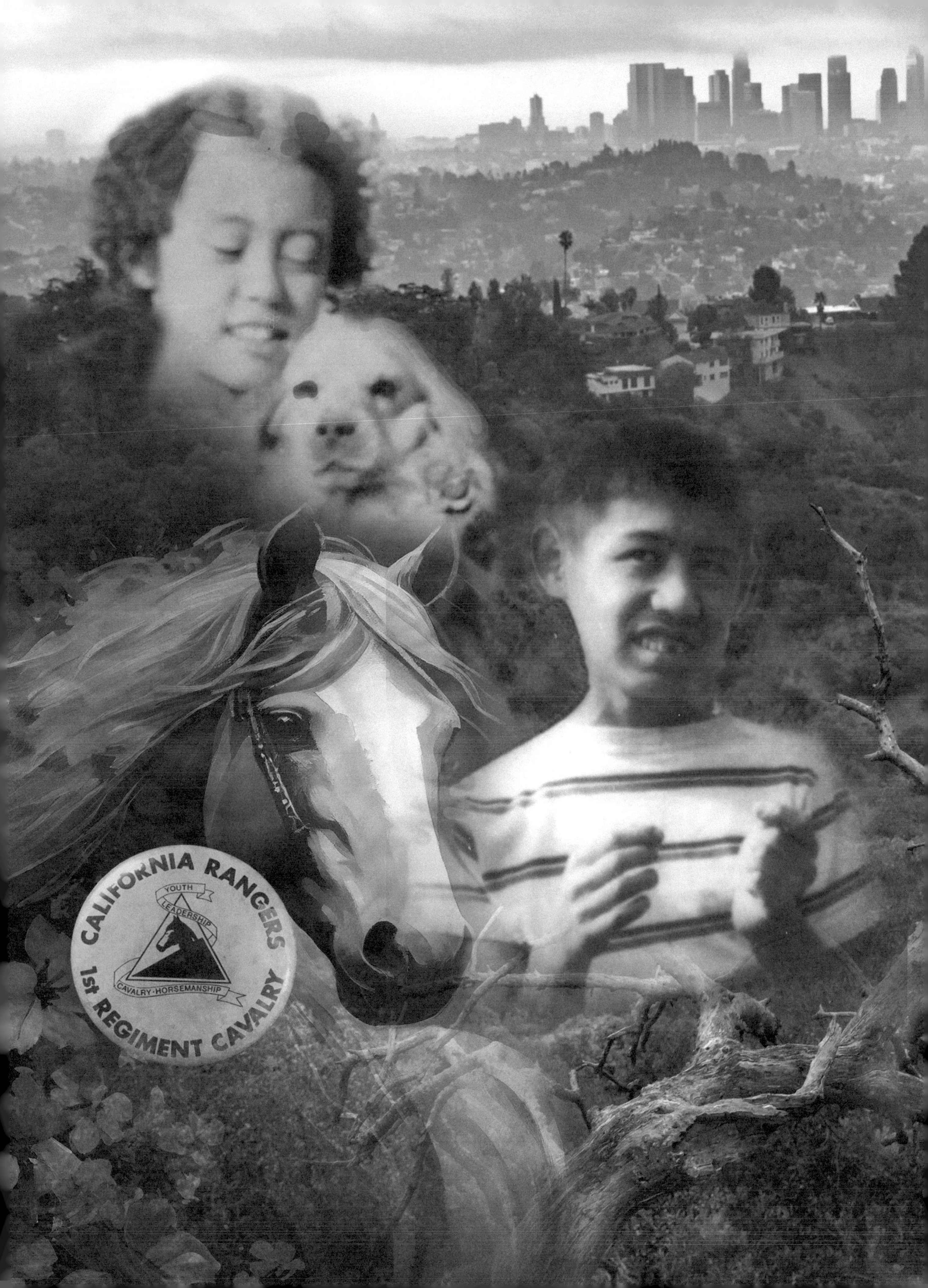
CALIFORNIA RANGERS
YOUTH
LEADERSHIP
CAVALRY·HORSEMANSHIP
1st REGIMENT CAVALRY

PSYCHOSURGERY, INTELLIGENCE, EMOTION AND SOCIAL BEHAVIOR FOLLOWING PREFRONTAL LOBOTOMY FOR MEDICAL DISORDERS

Walter K Friedman, 1942

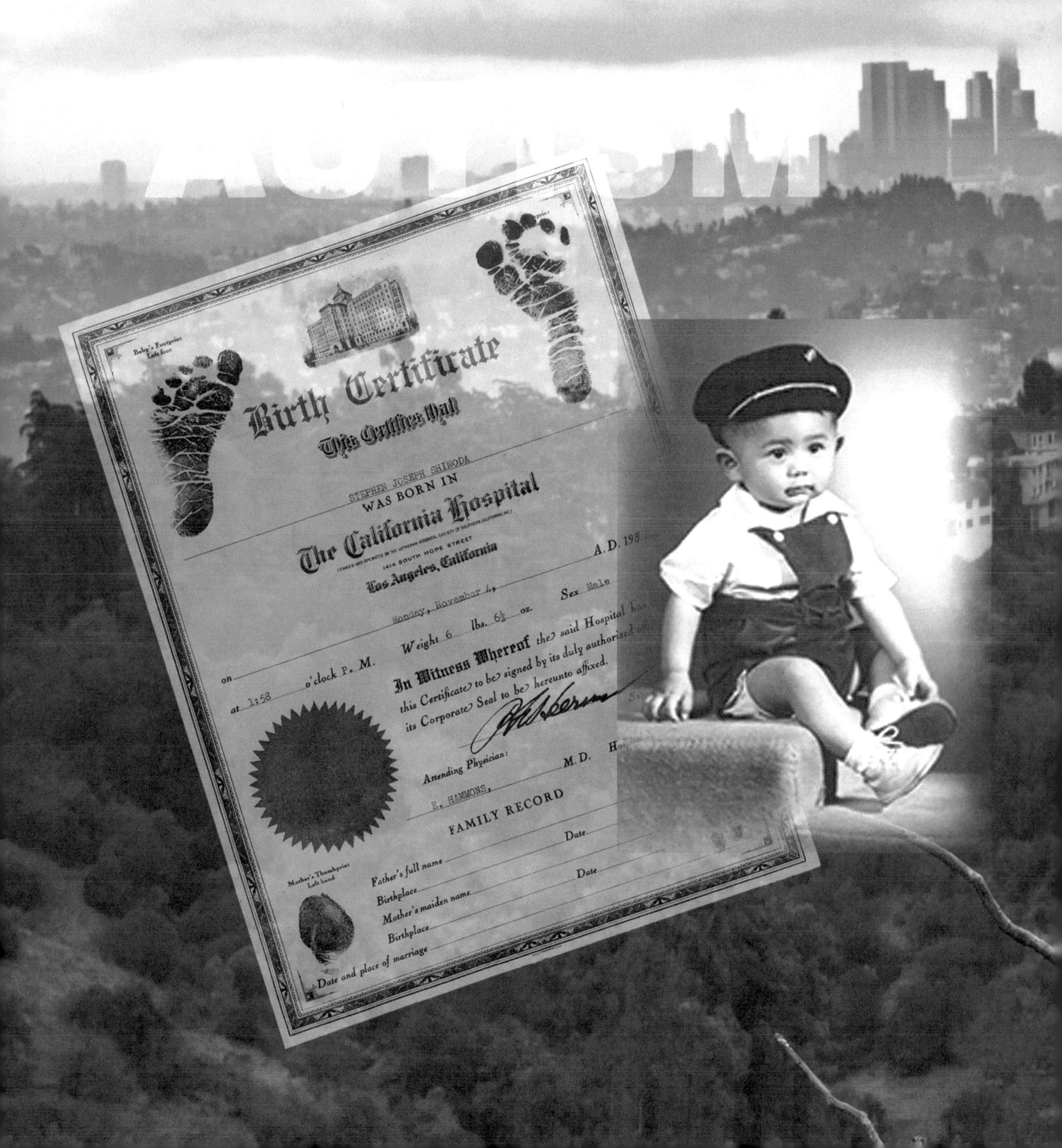

AUTISTIC DISTURBANCES OF AFFECTIVE CONTACT

Leo Kanner, 1943

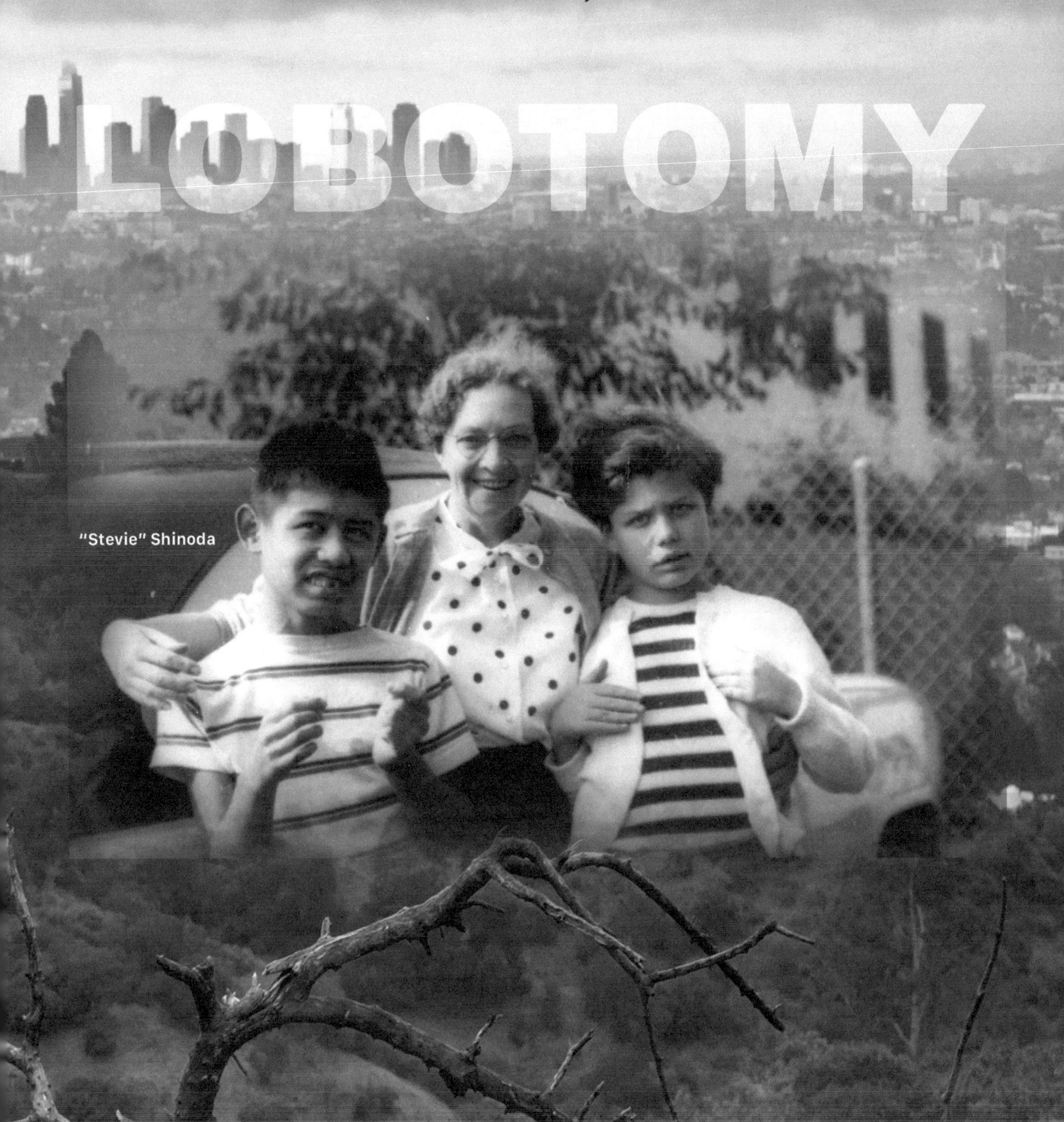

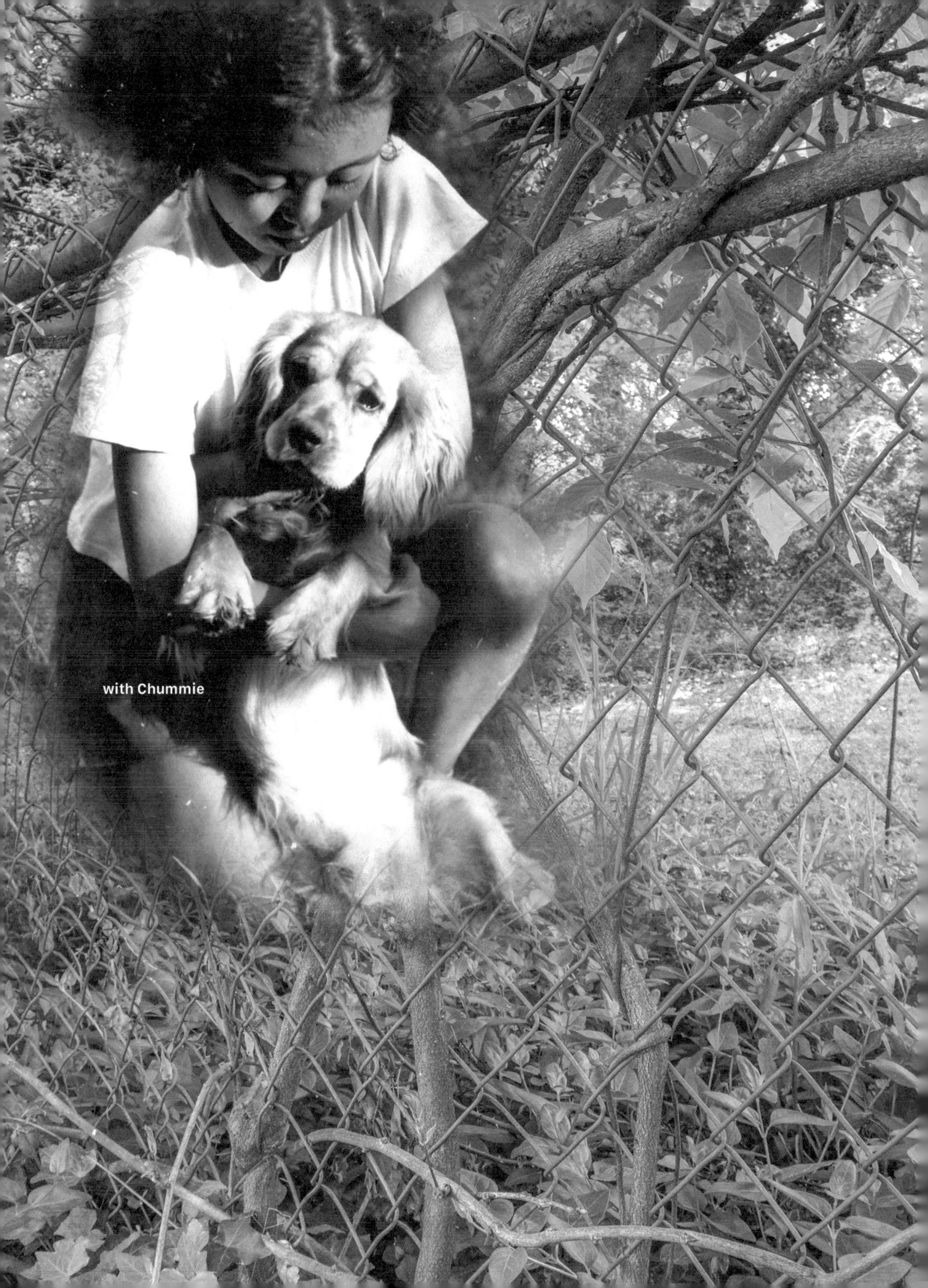

with Chummie

Chapter 8

High School Protester

I graduated from junior high school and in the fall went on to John Marshall High School as a member of the Class of '54. High schools in Los Angeles at the time were for three years (grades ten, eleven, and twelve). John Marshall was located close to Griffith Park, between the Los Feliz and Silverlake communities, which was not far from Hollywood.

These three years were personally significant. I made the decision to go into medicine rather than law, which came about unexpectedly and went against my natural talents and achievements. I changed churches after denouncing hypocrisy and anti-Semitism. I spoke truth to power on entering high school and paid a price for it three years later. High school extracurricular activities involved travel—across the country twice, and intrastate often. Travel is a theme in my life that began with flying across the continent for eye surgery, followed by the travels and moves my family made to avoid the forced evacuation and internment camp. Travel continues to be a theme in my life. I travel to teach, attend conferences and international events, to go on pilgrimages, and to lead groups.

John Marshall High School was named after the first Chief Justice of the United States. Our football team was "the Barristers," and the school mascot was a cartoon image of a boyish figure wearing a blue cap and gown. Our colors were light blue and dark blue, and our service organizations were named after groups involved in the American Revolution, the Continental Congress, and the founding of the United States. Coming into Marshall High School as a tenth grader, I could join the "Volunteers" and did. Miss Anderson was the teacher in charge of the Volunteers. At this point, I can't remember exactly what the circumstances were that made me speak up, be heard, and get in trouble. I recall it had to do with unfair discrimination. Those she favored came from the junior high school that was affluent and white, while others were more economically disadvantaged, and one was predominantly Mexican. There was a range of diversity in high school, social, racial, and class distinctions.

I was sent to the Girls' Vice Principal's office, to Miss Anderson, for speaking up with such passion about the unfairness or discrimination. I sat in her office and then outside of it for a long time after she spoke to me about my unacceptable behavior. I would not take back what I said. I would and could apologize for how I said it, since I had spoken in a judgmental and accusatory way, but I would not take back what I had said. That was why I was still sitting there when the bell rang announcing that school was over and she let me go.

The Girls' Vice Principal was in charge of the Student Government, which I participated in throughout high school. I brought honors back to the school when I was elected Lt. Governor of Girls' State as a Junior. In the twelfth grade, I was Student Body Vice President. Student Government met during a class period that I was in through my three years. I felt I had redeemed myself after my initial encounter with her.

There was a similar incident in church. I no longer was attending the neighborhood Presbyterian Church where I had been baptized and confirmed. I had continued there for a couple of years as a member of the youth group and quit when the leader of it persisted in making negative comments about "the Jews." I called him a hypocrite and quit after saying so in front of others. I changed churches, though I stayed a Presbyterian. I switched to Hollywood Presbyterian Church, which had an active high school and college program, was evangelical, and was affiliated with Forest Home Summer Camp.

In high school, I took the required courses for college admissions such as algebra, geometry, physics, chemistry, American history, and lots of English, which included public speaking and journalism. I also took Latin all three years. Three of my teachers, Mr. Hanks, Mr. Edwards, Mrs. Aguliar taught, mentored, and involved me in their respective extracurricular related activities. *Goddesses in Everywoman*, and *Gods in Everyman* were based upon the Greek and Roman gods and goddesses. After I wrote *Goddesses in Everywoman,* I sent a copy of it with a thank you to Mrs. Aguliar, my Latin teacher. She brought Dido and Aeneas, his journeys and encounters with Olympian divinities, and other mythic stories to life. We had fun wearing togas once a year, laughed and learned. As a result, Latin was not a dead language for me. It connected me with images and patterns that I later would learn fit C. G. Jung's description of archetypes in the collective unconscious.

Mr. Hanks taught public speaking and debate and was the coach of the Marshall High School National Forensic League teams. It was because of him that Marshall's debate teams were formidable in Southern California, either top ranked or one of the top three high schools, and were ranked nationally. At the beginning of an academic year, a national debate question would be announced, and those of us who debated would need to be prepared to debate either for or against in rounds with other schools. The tournaments also had competitions in oratory and extemporaneous speaking. At the beginning of the tenth grade, those of us who were interested met with Mr. Hanks, formed teams of two, and debated other newly formed teams. If we did well, we were chosen to represent Marshall and compete with others, as new at this as we were. Ena Dubnoff and I teamed up and did very well at this.

That year, Marshall High School qualified to go to the Nationals, and I was unexpectedly chosen to be on the debate team, even though I was only a sophomore. In my junior year, I chaired the Model United Nations in the council chambers of the Los Angeles City Hall. In my senior year, I won statewide titles in debate and in extemporaneous speaking and went to the Nationals again. In debate, the affirmative opening is prepared, and the three others who speak in turn, adapt. The point is to win by countering what the other side has just said, and supporting your side's position. It was no wonder that so many of the debaters intended to go into law. In doing the final rebuttal and summing up at the end of each debate, we felt like participants in a Perry Mason episode, another early, popular TV show.

Speaking in competition was excellent preparation for the lectures and workshops I do now, especially extemporaneous speaking. An hour before each of us was due to speak, we'd draw the subject, which would be from current events, and prepare an eight to ten-minute talk upon which we were judged. My strength was storytelling. I'd use a metaphor, a narrative, or even a myth to make the subject that I was supposed to talk knowledgeably about more interesting or understandable. It is still what I do.

My other mentor was Mr. Edwards, the journalism teacher who oversaw the school newspaper. I learned about the five Ws and H: who, what, when, where, why and how. It's what a journalist needs to know to report a story. Mr. Edwards had been my father's young journalism teacher at Franklin High School in Los Angeles, where he had been the editor of the paper—Mr. Edwards was by now on in age but he remembered my father. I was following in my father's footsteps.

Being part of the debate team was fun. Boys outnumbered girls and were in different classes, and as we travelled in cars and on trains depending on where the tournament was held, we got to know one another. During school, except for couples that were "going together," girls walked together between classes, spent the lunch hour in groups, and went to events with each other. Most of my friends were those from the big circle on the lawn in junior high school. There was one major area of exclusion for me, however. Marshall High School had sororities and fraternities; they didn't have Greek letter names, but this is what they were. There was no interracial dating in my world of school or family when I entered high school. Girls from my junior high crowd were "rushed," by the top sorority. Status was conferred when a senior boy let a girl, especially a sophomore, wear his fraternity jacket. It was a world I was not privy to and didn't think about. It was like knowing my friend Myrna Cramer went to a synagogue, while I went to church.

Many years later, I read Alix Kates Shulman's *Diary of an Ex-Prom Queen,* a novel that filled me in on what I had not missed. My ineligibility was a blessing, freeing me from anxiety about my social persona. Other girls struggled with what to wear, and who to be seen with, and the anxiety of being chosen or not, first by the sorority, and then at each important mixer. High school is a difficult obstacle course. There are hormones and major physical changes, learner's permits at sixteen, and then a driver's license and car, early drinking, and early sex. This was prior to feminism, so concepts and words such as date rape, sexual harassment, sexual predators, and pedophiles were not part of our language. I remember when Patsy, a high school cheerleader, became pregnant and left school, as pregnancy was a cause for expulsion. I was troubled when Joanie, a friendly and pretty girl in junior high school, whose body language now I can read retrospectively, became scared, inhibited, and withdrawn.

While I was in high school, the Korean War (1950-1953) was going on, with very little impact on my world. I was a member of a small generation of those born during the depression and before World War II, with male classmates too young to be drafted. This war began when North Korea invaded South Korea, supported by China and the Soviet Union. The United Nations, with the United States as the principle force, came to the aid of South Korea. An armistice ended the war after a bloody stalemate, with the front line close to the 38th parallel, where the war began. Some five million soldiers and civilians lost their lives during this war, and 38,000 were American soldiers.

On the national scene, I was in high school during the McCarthy Era. It was an era that originated with President Truman's Executive Order 9835 (1947) that began screening all federal civil service employees for "loyalty." During the mid-1950s, Republican Senator Joseph R. McCarthy held hearings, instigated investigations, removed book from the library program of the State Department, and gave demagogic speeches. Television on small black and white screens came into American homes during these same years, and went from children's programs (Howdy-Doody), variety (The Ed Sullivan Show), news of the day, to live televising of congressional hearings. We saw people denounced as communist sympathizers because of the organizations they had joined in college two decades before, or for signing petitions in the past. The takeaway message was "be apolitical and stay out of trouble." I remember hearing that one of my classmate's fathers was a Hollywood screenwriter who was denounced as a communist sympathizer and fired. ("McCarthyism" is now defined as "the practice of making accusations of subversion or treason without proper regard for evidence.") This must have had an effect on us, because as college students, we were labelled "The Silent Generation."

After my generation applied to college, the baby boomers flooded in. I and everyone who knew I had applied to Stanford assumed that I would get in. It was totally unexpected, a shock, to get the thin envelope that said I was not accepted. I had been so sure that I would get in that I had not applied anywhere else. It was a jarring lesson in pride going before a fall.

My father had my back. He flew to Stanford after making an appointment with the director of admissions, and learned that I had been "dinged" by the letter of recommendation that Mrs. Anderson, the student government sponsor, had sent on my behalf. More important to me was that my father would do this for me. When he found out why I had been turned down and wouldn't be going to Stanford, I could let go of it. I had no urge to apply again. I saw that in asking her to write a recommendation, there was an implicit suggestion of "I'll make you take back what you thought of me." It was arrogant of me, as well as naive. I did let Mrs. Anderson know what my father learned and that I knew what she had done. I also told others what had happened. Those who had rooted for me and had been shocked that I hadn't been accepted.

This rejection was the outcome of having some real agency for the first time in my life. My parents valued education, I had the green light from them to apply to any college or university I wanted to attend. Before this, every school I went to depended on where we lived, much of which had been a consequence of the forced evacuation. In contrast, where I applied and what I would study in college was up to me. Had I not wanted to have my abilities and achievements acknowledged by the one teacher in the school that I wanted to eat her earlier words, I would have very likely attended Stanford. It made me also realize how there are ripple effects on others, too. My high school best friend Myrna applied to Stanford because I urged her to do so. She was unsure that she would be accepted, but she was, while my hubris had set me on a different course.

I look back at the incident in which I confronted the unfairness and prejudice I perceived and spoke "truth to power," which was not a phrase or concept back then. It didn't cross my mind to take back what I was protesting and what I said then, or regret saying it when it turned out to be the reason I was not accepted into the college of my choice. It also did not silence the protestor-activist in me.

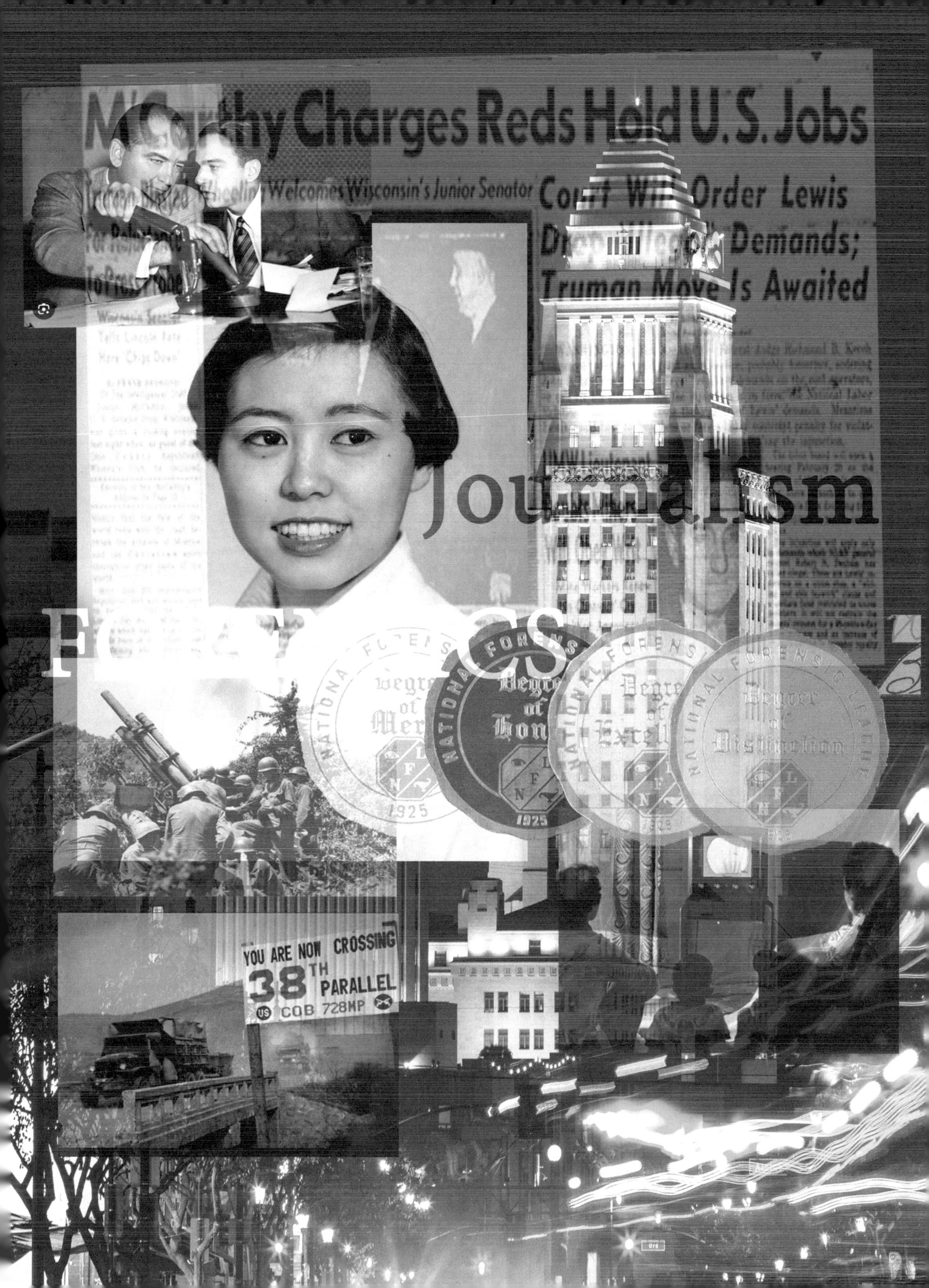

Charges Reds Hold U.S. Jobs
Welcomes Wisconsin's Junior Senator
Order Lewis
Demands;
Truman Move Is Awaited
NATIONAL FORENSIC LEAGUE
Degree of Distinction
1925
YOU ARE NOW CROSSING
38TH PARALLEL
COB 728MP

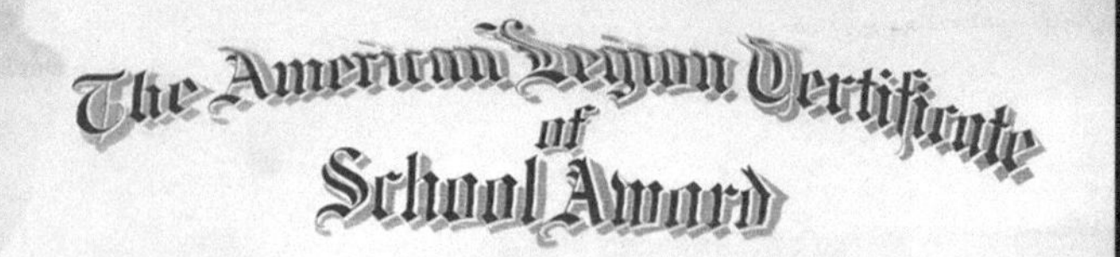

This Certificate of Distinguished Achievement
is awarded Jean Miye Shinoda
of John Marshall High School
in recognition of attainment acquired as winner of
The American Legion School Award
In Further Recognition
high qualities of Honor, Courage, Scholarship, Leadership,
Service, Companionship and Character
to the preservation and protection
tutions of our government and the advancement
This Award is made by
Post No. 353 The Department
The American Legion

The Ephebian Society

CERTIFICATE OF MEMBERSHIP

This is to certify that

JEAN MIYE SHINODA

by virtue of demonstrated qualities of scholarship, leadership, and character has been honored by election to membership in the Ephebian Society, and was administered the Ephebian Oath of Allegiance on this 11th day of June, in the year 1954.

President

Executive Secretary

Certificate of Appreciation

May it be Known that

Was the Guest Speaker at the

Griffith Park Lions Club

on February 16th 1954

As an Expression of Appreciation for Courtesies extended to this Club, we hereby present this Certificate.

Secretary President

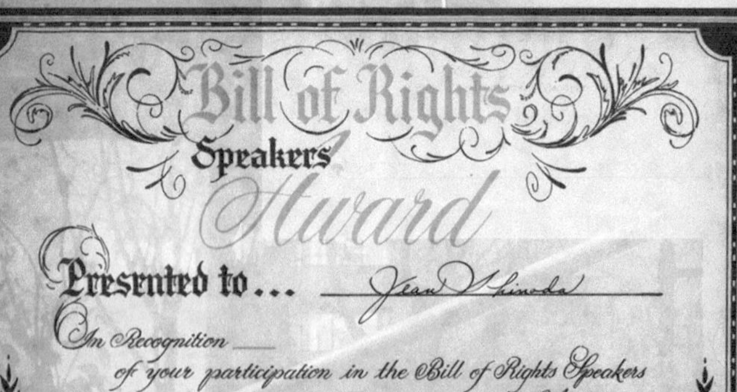

Award

for Community Service

To JEAN SHINODA

1953 Red Feather Student Speakers' Program

In recognition of services which have been helpful in the educational program of the Community Chest of Los Angeles Area, and to the 164 health and welfare services united in one annual campaign, this Award for Community Service is gratefully conferred.

Community Chest of Los Angeles Area

Maynard J. Toll, 1953-54 Campaign Chairman · Meldrim F. Burrill, Chairman, Schools Division · Robert Rivera, Chairman, Student Speakers' Bureau

YWCA · YMCA · USO

In recognition of first place award in a Zone Elimination Contest, held in connection with our 1953-54 Annual Student Speakers Program, WE, the members of the California-Nevada Association of Lions International,

Do Hereby Commend

An achievement on this level denotes previous first place award in a Community Contest.

Believing that the future well-being of America is dependent upon the adequate adjustment of each succeeding generation to problems of world-wide import, it is our feeling that this student's efforts relative to the subject:

"What the Constitution of the United States Means to Me"

constitutes a definite contribution to our annual Student Speakers Program.

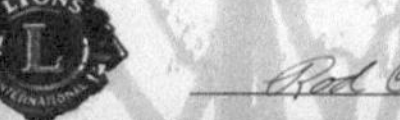

Zone Chairman District Governor

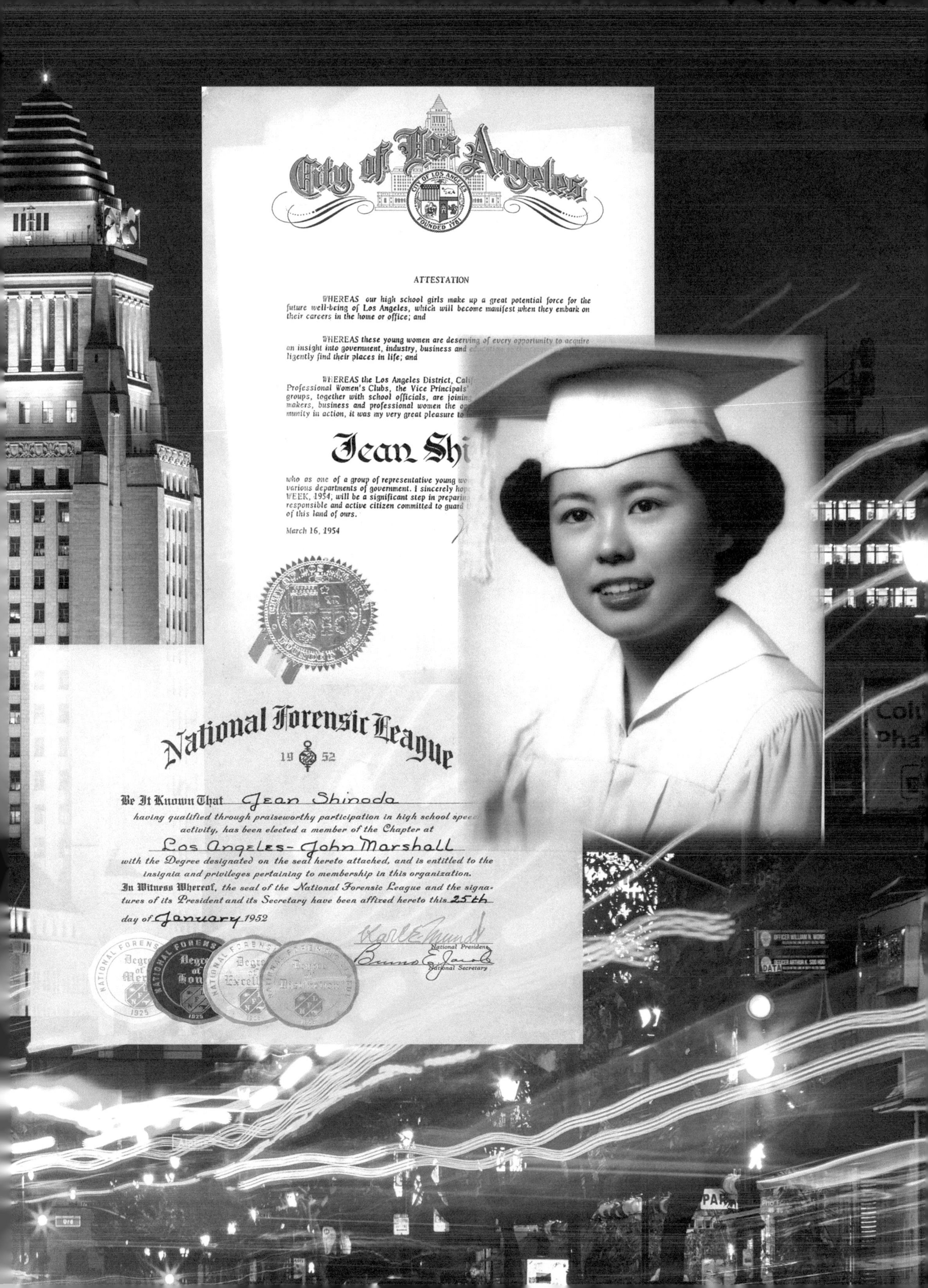
City of Los Angeles

FOUNDED 1781

ATTESTATION

WHEREAS our high school girls make up a great potential force for the future well-being of Los Angeles, which will become manifest when they embark on their careers in the home or office; and

WHEREAS these young women are deserving of every opportunity to acquire an insight into government, industry, business and
ligently find their places in life; and

WHEREAS the Los Angeles District, Cali
Professional Women's Clubs, the Vice Principals'
groups, together with school officials, are joinin
makers, business and professional women the o
munity in action, it was my very great pleasure to

Jean Shi

who as one of a group of representative young wo
various departments of government. I sincerely hop
WEEK, 1954, will be a significant step in preparin
responsible and active citizen committed to guard
of this land of ours.

March 16, 1954

National Forensic League

19 52

Be It Known That *Jean Shinoda*
having qualified through praiseworthy participation in high school spee
activity, has been elected a member of the Chapter at
Los Angeles- John Marshall
with the Degree designated on the seal hereto attached, and is entitled to the insignia and privileges pertaining to membership in this organization.
In Witness Whereof, the seal of the National Forensic League and the signatures of its President and its Secretary have been affixed hereto this *25th* day of *January* 1952

Karl E. Mundt
National President

Bruno E. Jacob
National Secretary

Degree of Merit
Degree of Honor
Degree of Excellence
Degree of Distinction

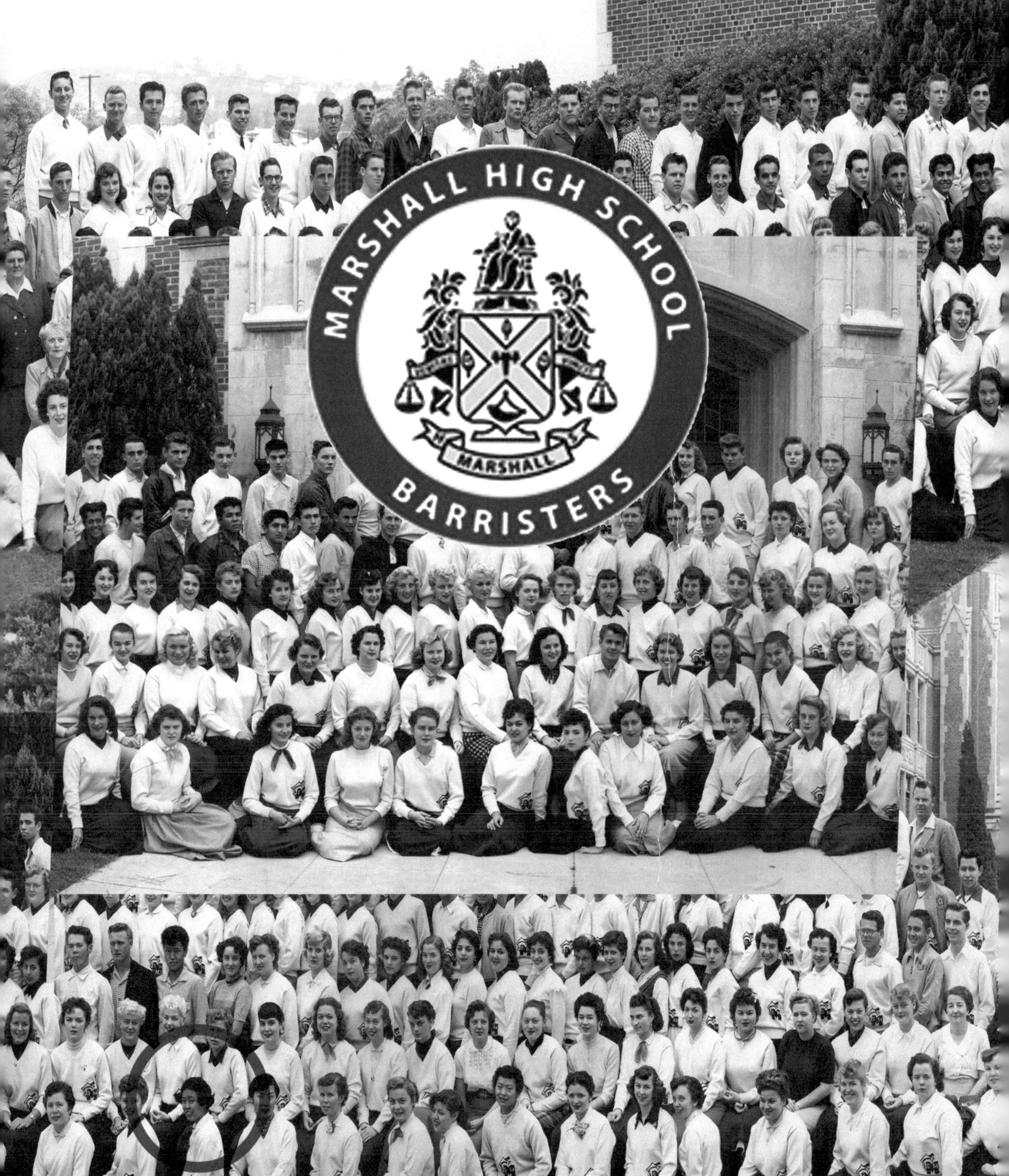

CLASS OF S'54

Chapter 9

Gratitude - Promises to God

The high school years were decisive in setting me on course of what I would do with my life and why. Most of this happened outside of school, in the mountains, and inside of me. It had to do with my relationship with God, Christianity—Protestant versus Catholic—and what the Bible said, all of which really mattered to me at the time.

I began to question my religion on the train that was taking the Marshall debate team and others from other Los Angeles high schools across the country to the national debate tournament in Washington DC. On the train, several of us got late night conversations with Kevin Robb, a debater from Loyola High School, who had decided to become a Jesuit priest. Bible study went along with going to Presbyterian churches, so words in the Bible were familiar to me. We were all earnest, the subject very personal, and all of us were debaters. Kevin, who was at a Jesuit school and had decided on this religious vocation, was much more knowledgeable than the rest of us on such matters, which made me want to learn more.

I had already had some questions of my own, especially about the Presbyterian belief of predestination. It had seemed to me that there was something inherently unfair that those who would be saved were predestined before birth to be so. I tried to wrap my mind around questions of predestination versus free will. I kept a mental tension between the two, since it didn't seem to be either/or. I could see this even then. I'd also thought for myself that there was a problem about God. If God was all-powerful and all good, how does He let all the awfulness and evil happen? Either he is not all good, or not all powerful. What about my brother?

I grappled with Kevin's position that the Roman Catholic Church was the only true Christian church. He quoted scripture to support this premise: Jesus said, "Upon this rock, I will build my church," meaning the disciple Peter. At this point, the scripture mattered, as well as history. I was also beginning to think about the meaning and power of Catholic sacraments. I was earnest in my quest, as maybe only an adolescent can be, talked to two Protestant ministers who took my questions seriously. I wrote a paper based on *Here I Stand: A Life of Martin Luther* by Roland H. Bainton. Luther started the Protestant Reformation after he wrote the Ninety-Five Theses and tacked it to the cathedral door.

Martin Luther was a protestor-activist, who found he had to do what he did because of his faith and his character, which is echoed by his words: "Here I stand, I can do no other," an intensely feeling statement. His outrage grew over time. He enumerated the reasons first to himself, and then in public when he no longer could remain silent. People who respond as Luther did use feeling as an assessing function, which is often linked with intuition. He did not write a dispassionate evaluation of the corruption of the Church, which would be the response of someone who observes and thinks about it.

When I was an adolescent, I knew nothing about Jungian typology which helps explain who we are, and how we respond to what is going on around us or in us. Maybe most of us who are activists are feeling types, who learn to do it better over time. The capacity to be outraged when people, animals, environment, or principles are treated unfairly or dismissed as inconsequential was my innate response then and still is. My experience with the forced evacuation is a factor when it comes to social justice, but my typology leads the way. Three years of high school debate required that we be able to argue both sides of the question. We wrote significant statistics or quotes on index cards to support the issues we argued. Information helped develop my thinking to balance or to support where my feelings would otherwise take me, or overtake me.

I did not have a name for my all-too-automatic response to unfairness and lack of ethics until I was a Jungian analyst. I called it my "Dalmatian dog syndrome," after the firehouse dog that responds to the alarm by jumping on the firetruck. I still do hear this metaphoric bell, and I especially did during the Trump presidency, when the alarm rang often. In situations closer to home, when something comes up—or in the vernacular, "goes down,"—I now pause to think rather than act. It means that I have to acknowledge that "silence is consent," which is a phrase that I confront myself with before I either do something or do nothing. This arises in very ordinary situations, when something derogatory is said that is sexist, racist, or just plain ignorant, just as it did when I was entering high school and saw hypocrisy clearly. Will I respond? Do I have choice, or is this a compulsion? These days it clearly is choice, including choice about the company I keep, as well as the cause I will take on, or the whistle I will blow. My time and energy are limited resources that now more than ever.

It was the summer after graduation and before college that I had my moment of certainty about God, which was totally subjective, and therefore not debatable. By then, I had been admitted to the freshman class at UCLA. I had also applied to Pomona College, after their freshman class had already been selected, and was high on the waitlist if a space became available. That summer, I went to Forest Home, a Christian evangelical camp. One afternoon, there was a speaker, whose name didn't seem important even at the time, and what he said did not stir me. I have no recollection that there was something in particular that affected me, but affected I was: I had a profound experience of clarity that humbled and brought me to my knees metaphorically. I had been full of myself and my achievements, it was why I had only applied to Stanford, assuming I'd be admitted.

In that moment of clarity, I realized that I could not claim any of my accomplishments, when every single one was due to good fortune and not of my own doing. Intelligence, appearance, personality, health, opportunities, affluence, good role models, parents, they all made this possible for me and I had the hubris to feel I did it all myself. While I had trouble accepting the theology of predestination and a Calvinistic view of the haves and have-nots, I had done the same, and taken for granted that I was among the deserving "elect."

That moment of clarity included contrasting of my life of good fortune with that of my brother Stephen. I would see him once in a while when he came home on some weekends. My parents had found a place for him to stay in a private group home that was founded by a man who was dedicated to his "kids." Sometimes I would be in the car when they picked him up or brought him back. I remember my parents saying that these kids who never grew up had taken a toll on their parents, that they were the only intact couple among the parents. Stephen was healthy, his behavior autistic (though that word was not used then), and he was well cared for.

The contrast between his life and mine, and the clarity with which I realized that I was the beneficiary of undeserved good fortune, humbled me and brought to mind the familiar aphorism, "there but for the Grace of God go I." Thinking this way soon became another problem, but this time about God.

That evening, shortly after dusk, I went by myself to a small chapel on the Forest Home grounds and there I got on my knees and prayed to God. "Something" happened in prayer that was a turning point in my life. I had a felt-sense of the presence of divinity, of a loving energy. I was filled with gratitude. I felt the gravity of asking a big question that went with what I now felt. With all my heart, I asked, “How can I thank you?” The answer which came was: “Help others, be a doctor.” I prayed, “Thy will, not mine, be done.”

I made a promise to God in that mountain chapel that I would become a doctor. This may not seem a tall order, given that my mother, my grandfather, two aunts, and two uncles were physicians. However, I would never have decided to be a doctor on my own. I wasn’t interested or good at science or math, and took the minimum that was needed for a pre-college curriculum in high school. It would not be easy to fulfil this promise.

I took after my father. All the subjects he was good at, I was, too. I loved debate, writing, history, and the humanities in general—which are not pre-med subjects. He had intended to be a lawyer, and instead entered his family business when he was needed, after the unexpected early death of an older brother. Like many children do, consciously or unconsciously, I was on track to live out my father’s unlived life. In so many ways including psychological typology, I was “my father’s daughter.”

It wasn’t easy to do pre-med. I took Chemistry 1A at UCLA with several hundred others, Chemistry 1B with about 30 others at Pomona College, where I had transferred mid-semester of my freshman year. Math through calculus, German, and Zoology were required. I remember crying in frustration at the academic load and difficulties I was having with my pre-med courses at Pomona. Math was hard for me. Zoology required memorizing classifications and details from insects to mammals. I wasn’t interested and didn’t see the point, then I got a “cinch notice” that meant that my grade had dropped at the midterm. Whether I saw the point of learning Zoology or not, it was a pre-med requirement. I had to raise my grade. I buckled down and managed to change the D into a final B. Doing as well as I could in these courses was fulfilling my promise to God, and I kept at it, even when it was hard and not a labor of love.

At UCLA and at Pomona, freshmen took History of Western Civilization, which interested me and was an easy A, as were other courses in the humanities. I took a double-major at Pomona, pre-med and history, and managed to study what interested me. That included the study of both the Old and New Testament, a semester of each, which included new analyses of the writing styles of each book and the historical circumstances of the time. This was an academic, non-religious study of the bible.

The summer between my sophomore and junior years, I enrolled at UC Berkeley. I went to Cal, as it was called, to take a double summer session to fulfill the physics requirement for pre-med. Cal had a pre-professional course that was intermediate between the two courses offered at Pomona. One would have been with the physics majors and math majors, the other was an introduction to physics that we called “movie physics” where principles were taught, no laboratory—and didn’t count for pre-med.

Surprisingly, I was inspired by the courses and loved being at UC Berkeley. The teaching assistants talked about their research projects occurring in the big building above the campus that housed the cyclotron. They were searching for “particles that had to exist because the universe was symmetrical.” If there are protons, there had to be anti-protons. My imagination was stirred by this. I came back to Pomona and signed up for a nuclear physics course. My enthusiasm was short-lived. Nuclear physics was not philosophical. It required advanced calculus. Nonetheless, I took in the beauty of symmetry in creation at the atomic level, which touched my soul.

I loved being in the San Francisco Bay Area. I lived at Stern Hall, which was on the hill between the cyclotron and the campus. From my dorm room, I looked out over the bay, a panorama that included the city of San Francisco and the Golden Gate Bridge. There were glorious sunsets and sparkling lights at night. I was also drawn to the size and range of the University, which I was ready for. I transferred from Pomona to UC Berkeley mid-academic year and joined the UC Class of ’58 as a junior. One of my friends at Cal was Sally Willetts. When she was Governor at Girls’

State, I had been Lt . Governor. Now she was a Representative-at-Large on the Executive Committee of ASUC. Sally urged me to run for office, for Rep-at-Large, which I did, speaking at mealtimes at sororities, fraternities, student housing, co-ops. There were four Rep-at-Large positions, the one with the most votes became the head Rep-at-Large, which I became. The "Ex Com" met regularly, with, as it turned out, some very long meetings. The campus was being politicized by student advocates for national issues. Sandbox or big world? The athletic department, with its national teams and huge expenditures, was under the Associated Students. We rubber-stamped their budgets. This must be what members of Congress do when they are expected to approve the budget for the Department of Defense. Campus politics were in transition. Within the next few years, demonstrations would lead to having the National Guard on campus.

When it came time to apply to medical school, I did so not knowing whether or not I would be accepted. My grades were not straight As, except in the humanities. The sciences and math were mixed, As and Bs, which for medical school are not impressive grades. In a conversation with myself and God, I thought out loud, "Maybe I misunderstood the message that I was to be a doctor. If I made a mistake, when I apply, I'll not be accepted into medical school."

I had the advantage of having been a pre-med at Pomona College. There was a faculty pre-med committee that took the responsibility of writing letters of recommendation based upon personal knowledge of applicants. Pomona came through with this, even though I had transferred to UC Berkeley. Of the medical schools I applied to, my hope was to be accepted at UCSF. I wanted to live in San Francisco.

I was interviewed as part of the application process by two professors at UCSF and came away thinking I would not be accepted. The first interview was with a professor of medicine, who looked at my application, noting all the humanities courses I had taken, and seemed to sniff, as if to say, "You really like all this stuff?" He was a tall, distinguished man, who didn't seem to relate to me or to what I was interested in. The second interview was, from my standpoint, even worse. This was with a psychologist, a clinical professor who got me to talk about my brother, which made me get tearful and cry. So much for getting into UCSF, I thought—which was a wrong assumption. I was accepted.

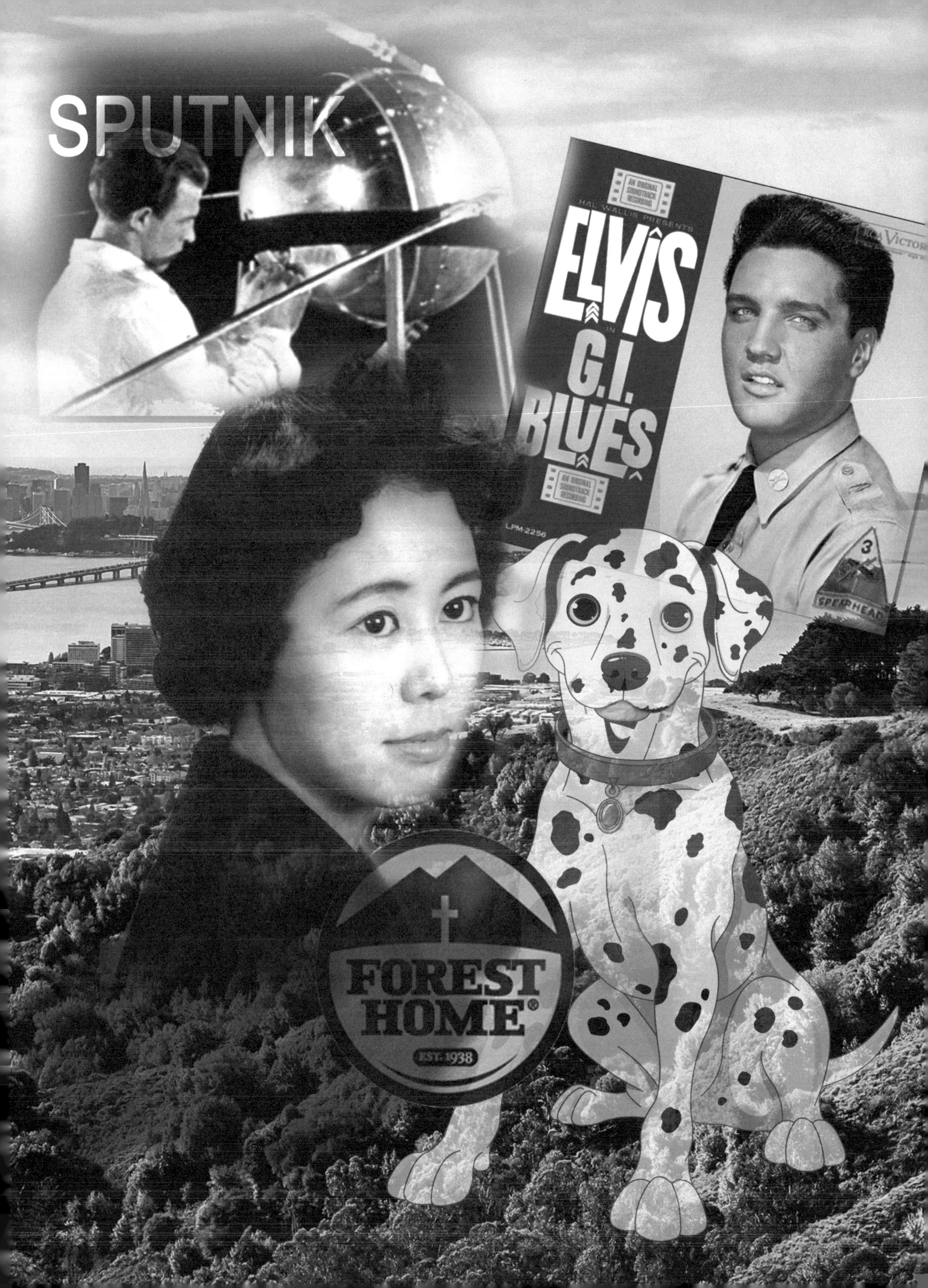
SPUTNIK
AN ORIGINAL SOUNDTRACK RECORDING
HAL WALLIS PRESENTS
ELVIS
IN
G.I. BLUES
AN ORIGINAL SOUNDTRACK RECORDING
LPM-2256
RCA VICTOR
SPEARHEAD
FOREST HOME®
EST. 1938

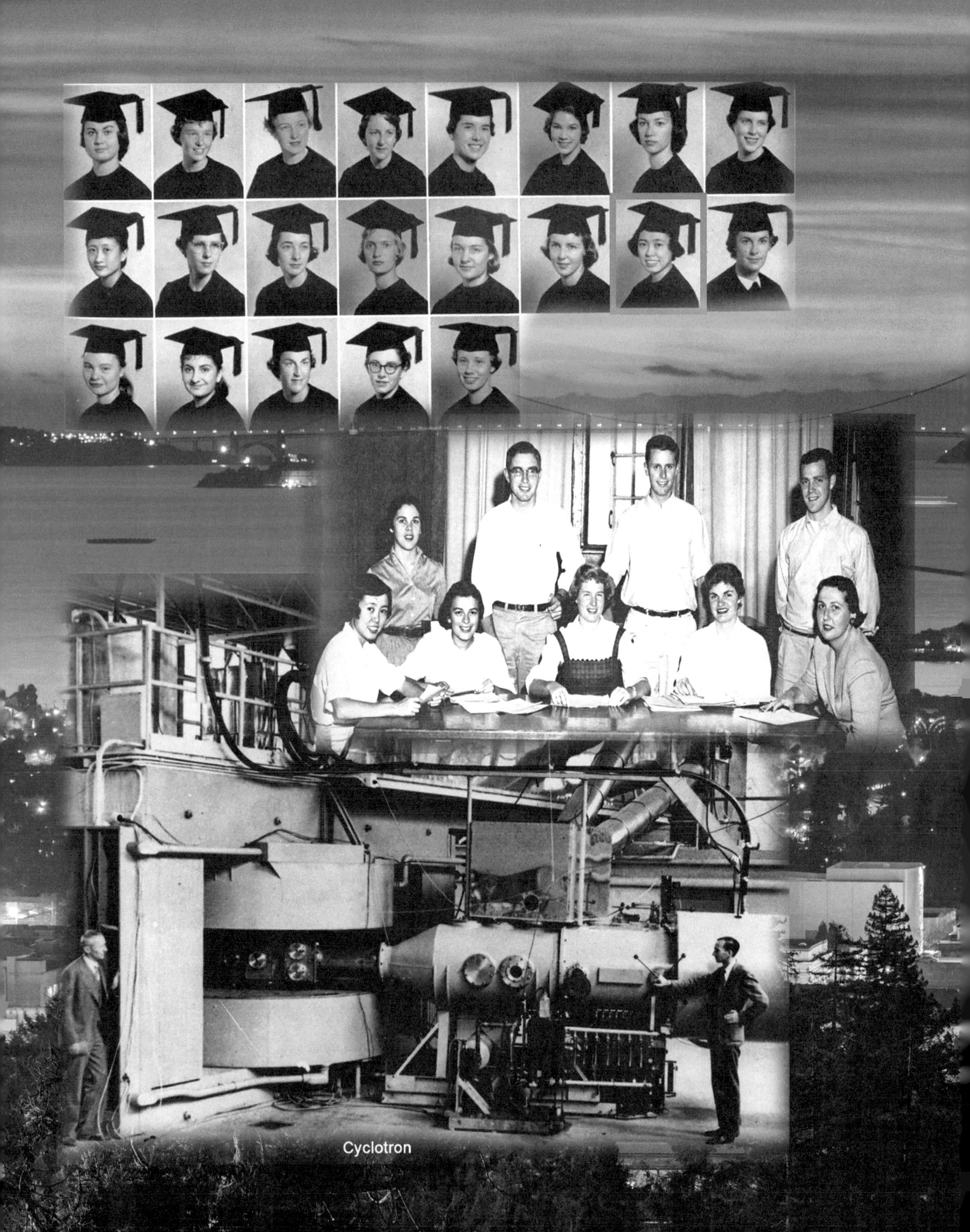

Cyclotron

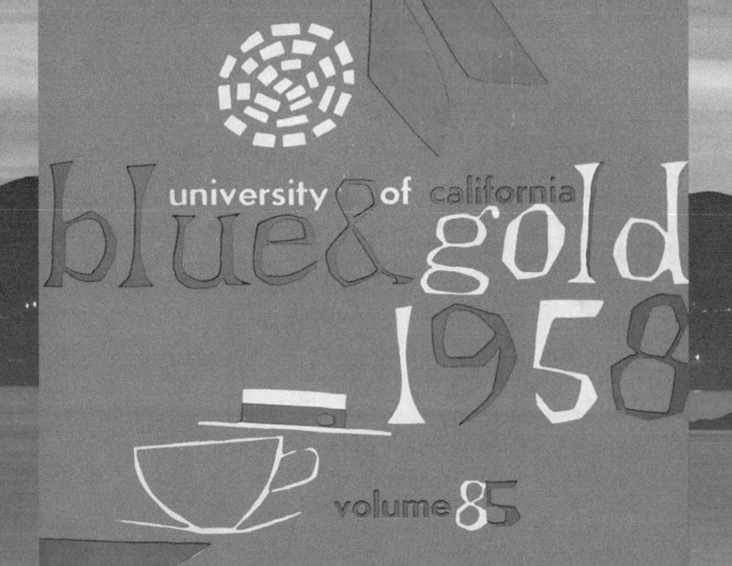
university of california
blue & gold
1958
volume 85

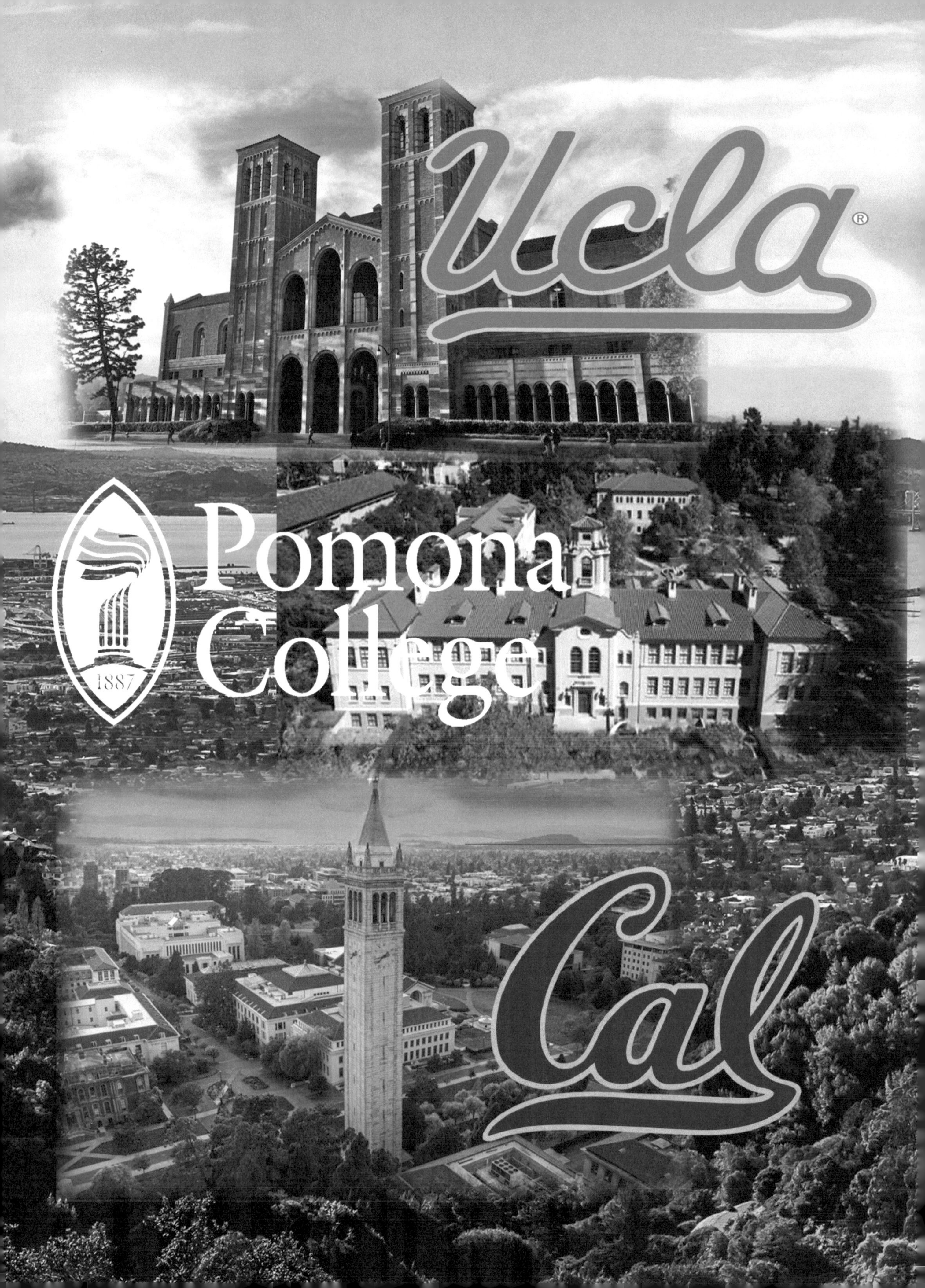

UCLA®

Pomona College

1887

Cal

Section 2

Medical School, Finding My Calling, Family Crisis, Grief

Chapter 10

Medical School

When I graduated from Cal in the summer of 1958, medical school was on the horizon. Not just figuratively. It was visible across the bay from Berkeley. UCSF's tall white buildings stood out against the trees and hilltop behind them. It was on Parnassus Street, named for Mt. Parnassus in Greece. The mountain towers above Delphi, which is associated with the Delphic oracle, and Apollo, the god of the Sun. Apollo is associated with healing, and its opposite, disease. He fathered Asclepius, the physician god of medicine.

Rare and difficult cases are sent to UCSF for diagnosis and treatment. Medical students saw uncommon cases at Moffitt, the teaching hospital; the saying was that if you hear the sounds of hooves on Parnassus Street, expect a zebra, not a horse. To see ordinary diseases or learn physical diagnosis, we went to San Francisco General Hospital and Laguna Honda Hospital.

My medical class had 100 students as we began, and ten percent were women, which was a large percentage back then. There also was racial diversity, mostly Asian, one African-American, and a couple of Hispanics, but it was predominately white and male. At the time, American medical schools were likely to have no women, or a handful at most. The Women's Medical College of Pennsylvania was the exception. It was founded in 1850 to train female MDs. In 1970, it began admitting men, and is now the Medical College of Pennsylvania. Morehouse School of Medicine in Atlanta, founded to train African-American MDs, began in 1975, and became accredited in 1985. In the East, there had been a Jewish quota in my mother's time. I did not feel any personal discrimination based either on my gender or race. Our class was small enough that over time, I knew everyone, as we all did. Mostly, everyone was an individual. Race and gender were what was visible on the surface, though once we knew one another, those factors didn't make a difference. We all felt oppressed by the enormity of what we had to learn.

We were in the medical school trenches together, and our outside friends were civilians. Many of our classes and then our clinical rotations were in small groups, beginning in our freshman year with human anatomy. It was an initiatory experience to pull the sheet off our cadaver. My classmates Terry Horner, John Harris, Richard Maurer and I called ours "Granny." We carefully dissected skin, muscles, vessels, nerves, and organs, learning form and function as we went along. Our hours were long and many an evening before an exam we would be there, huddled around our cadaver, going over what we would have to identify and answer questions about.

The anatomy exam was stressful, to say the least. Every cadaver in the room was part of the exam. There would be a string around some part, usually something very small, for us to identify and answer a question about. It was tense, something like waiting for the music to stop in musical chairs, only the opposite. The bell would ring and we'd quickly move on to the next anatomy table, look for the tag as fast as possible, which could be deep inside, each numbered to correspond to the numbers on our clipboards. In microbiology or histology we'd also go from one station to another, physically moving ourselves from one microscope to another looking at slides. We learned what healthy and sick blood looked like in hematology, and how each organ of the body worked in physiology. Laboratory classes required us to do experiments, recording each step and noting each result. There was an enormous amount to learn and memorize: the layers of the skin, the names of all the muscles, large and smaller blood vessels, names and parts of organs brain, heart, lungs, kidneys, bladder, sexual organs, and so on and on. First, we learned what normal was and then, in pathology, we learned what dysfunction and diseases did to the body.

When I was accepted into medical school, I didn't know what to expect. I was concerned that it would be like pre-med. It was a surprise to me that what I was studying had my attention. I was memorizing a lot of names which zoology had also required. Only now, what I was learning mattered. It was relevant information that I needed to know to be a doctor to help people, and not just to get a good grade for a required course.

I have a feeling that the difference and relevancy also had a mystical "something" to it, which began in anatomy working on and learning from a cadaver. While we called her "Granny," we treated her with respect. I think that this can be either sacred work or a sacrilege to work on a dead human body—depending on how we do it. Many cadavers were the bodies of people who designated that their body or organs would go to the medical school at their death. Granny helped us to become doctors. Some of the cadavers may have been unclaimed bodies, but still, there is something about dead human bodies that I felt when I walked into the anatomy room. I think of this as the beginning initiation into medicine as a sacred group—like a priestly order.

Then came physical diagnosis, which we would learn by examining living human beings, who, knowing we were students, let us learn on their bodies. We practiced on them, after we had learned on each other, to recognize what we were hearing through the stethoscope, took blood pressures with a blood pressure cuff, looked at the back of eyes with an ophthalmoscope, and into ears with an otoscope, used the reflex hammer, hitting below the kneecap to watch the leg react, and a tuning fork to check bone conduction. We got small black bags and now had our own equipment. We got white coats and name tags, which had our first and last name, followed by the initials, J.C., for "Junior Clinician."

We practiced on patients at Laguna Honda, who were mostly old people and people with chronic disabilities. Examining them in the hospital setting was entering a special space. Having another human being willing to let us listen, palpate, touch their body sets us apart. It is a rite, and the right, of the medical profession. It was natural for me to treat each person I examined with respect and to appreciate that they allowed me. I was treating them, to use Martin Buber's terms, as an "I – Thou," rather than an "I –It," which I do with patients. I would introduce myself and ask, "How are you?" and really listen to how they answered.

San Francisco was a wonderful city in which to be a medical student. Most of us had come directly out of college, and were young and single. (Some classmates were married, some had children, a few were easily a decade older, and one was balding and had grown kids.) I studied hard, should have gotten more sleep, and I also had fun. I had a convertible, and in sunny top-down weather, my friends and I would take a study break on weekends. We'd drive up to see the view from Twin Peaks, then over the other side and down to the Great Highway at the edge of the ocean, past the Amusement Park to the Cliff House and Sutro Baths, and circle back through Baker beach and the Presidio. Or we'd cross the Golden Gate Bridge to Marin to find sun when the city had its summer fog. We went to the Red Garter in North Beach on an occasional night when Terry Horner was invited to play the gut bucket with the band, and we anatomy partners went along for the fun. There were Irish coffees at the Buena Vista Cafe, or cracked crab and French bread picked up at Fisherman's Wharf, and the parking area around Coit Tower was a great place to enjoy the meal and the view.

These pleasant recollections are from my pre-clinical years of medical school while we were on an academic semester calendar, with exams, mid-terms, finals, holiday, and summer breaks. We had begun classes in the fall of 1958 after a formal welcome and orientation to medical school, with a reception that followed. At this reception, a mutual attraction started up between Jim Cornelius, a classmate from Sacramento, and me. As we got to know each other, we found that we were both entering medicine for altruistic and idealistic reasons. His hero was Dr. Thomas Dooley, a former U.S. Navy physician, a devout Catholic who was a famous anti-Communist humanitarian in Southeast Asia, whose book *Deliver Us From Evil* (1956) was an inspirational best-seller. Dooley founded MEDICO (Medical International Cooperation Organization) which built medical clinics in Laos.

As we spent time together, the connection between us grew. We talked about marriage, and told our parents. When we did, his mother got very upset—she would not have her son marry me, a Jap. My father did not want me to marry a Catholic—his prejudice was based upon the Catholic men he had known through business. I had not met his parents, my parents had not meet him. We had considered ourselves adults who could decide for ourselves and had announced our intentions, not asked permission. Religion was, however, important to us both. I was willing to take instructions to consider converting or promising our children would be raised Catholic, but would need to really believe that this was right for me to do in the end. We talked with a priest I knew and also checked out what might be involved at St. Anne's Church, the parish close to the medical center. Time was a problem, as we were on different schedules in the clinical years and on many rotations. There just wouldn't be time for this. Marriage got put on hold.

In the third and fourth years of medical school, we rotated through departments and services, both inpatient and outpatient, and had a lot of hands-on experience under supervision. I drew blood, did several spinal taps, held retractors in surgery and sewed up skin, delivered babies, did psychotherapy, wrote up the process notes for each session, took histories with a review of systems, and did physical exams noting my findings, tentative diagnosis or possible diagnoses, and suggested further tests. We made rounds with the attending physician (clinical faculty) and residents, saw wounds and lesions, listened with stethoscopes to what various diseases of the heart or lungs sounded like, palpated tumors, took notes, got blood, urine, and stool specimens, and made out laboratory forms. We would come back later to see the patients, check on them, and on the lab or x-ray reports that had come back. I'd never considered myself dexterous, so that surgery of any kind held no appeal. Women were not encouraged at all to go into surgery, though it did seem to me that some women would have made excellent surgeons, with their smaller hands, and a lot of experience in cutting and sewing.

In teaching hospitals, patients are sometimes referred to as "teaching material." One attending's bedside manner might be better than another's, but usually, we were making rounds on "the gallbladder," or organ that was diseased or on the post-op site. Our attention would be on it, not on the patient. On rounds, teaching is through questions: coming up with a right answer, or describing the finding, mattered most. The human being who was at that moment exposed, handled, talked about as if not there, and yet still hanging on every word was reduced to "teaching material." When the patient is dehumanized in the interaction with the doctor, it dehumanizes them both.

The one-up/one-down position is male-speak, which linguist Deborah Tannen describes in her books. This makes rounds a competitive event, the point being to not be humiliated by saying, "I don't know." This explained the psychology of "why men don't ask for directions" because doing so automatically puts him one-down. Men may have also learned from experience that if the other man doesn't have the answer, he might make up a wrong one to avoid saying, "I don't know." Medical students "aced" rounds with answers that began with showing off familiarity with the literature, "according to the New England Journal . . ." Medicine was a male profession when I was a medical student. At the time, obstetrics and gynecology, a surgical specialty in which all the patients were women, was notably misogynist. Since feminism has become more mainstream, this changed, at least it did so at UCSF when I last heard about this.

Internship

Internship came next, preceded by another round of decisions and applications, but this time the process was organized by the internship matching program. We applied for several different internships. We ranked them in the order of preference. Medical centers and hospitals that had internship programs received our applications, and they in turn matched us by ranking applicants in order of preference and technology. On match day, we got the result and knew where we would go next.

My first choice was a rotating internship at Los Angeles General Hospital, and I got it. It was one of the four big city-county hospitals in the United States with reputations that made them testing grounds for doctors-in-training, due to the large numbers of patients and responsibilities. I wanted to be challenged, to be on the front lines, to know that I could do this. That was my beforehand idea. I was being heroic, thinking like an archetype: Artemis in competition with her Apollo brothers. I soon found that "heroic" concept was forgotten in the midst of being weary and sleep-deprived, doing my best and often in over my head. Fortunately, interns are part of a team.

When I began the internship, I had asked that my first rotations be on internal medicine, because this was the specialty I thought I would go into. At LA County Hospital, the acute admissions I was seeing and treating were mostly uncontrolled chronic conditions, like the complications of alcoholism or diabetes. Once discharged from the hospital, patients were followed into the resident-run outpatient clinic. The clinic was disparagingly referred to as the "crock clinic," meaning the patients came to complain. Considering that we interns and residents were able-bodied, overworked young adults, we wanted patients to get to the point and have a problem that could be fixed by a prescription or "punted" (referred) to another service. When poverty, poor nutrition, poor medical care, lack of transportation and aging contributed to the medical problem, both doctor and patient felt dissatisfied. Calling it a "crock clinic" put the blame on the patient. With my typology, empathy for suffering came easily, which at least made me a sympathetic listener, who took time to explain something; both can help a patient feel better

All admissions to LA County Hospital came through emergency services, where triage was done. Someone who needed to be seen right away—suffering a heart attack, bleeding, or unconscious, was a "red blanket." The gurney with the patient draped with a bright red cloth, sent non-stop up the elevator to the admitting medicine or surgical floor, and was assessed and treated immediately. After Marilyn Monroe died from an overdose, "red blanket" admissions came one after another to the medicine floor. These were women who had overdosed with a variety of drugs and were in states ranging from hysteria to coma. There were work-ups to do, IVs to put in, vomiting to be induced or a naso-gastric tube put in and used with suction as a stomach pump—extra work beyond what already was a busy night. I remember two things about this night. The anger and hostility at the women expressed by a resident, who told them to do it right the next time (a male resident—though all of the residents I had in my internship were men). The second was my own effort to understand why they had copied Marilyn Monroe in wanting to die. I came to the conclusion that if she, with all that she had compared to them, found no reason to go on living, they with their misery found in her suicide a imitable way out.

Within months after starting the internship and while on an internal medicine rotation, I unexpectedly received a telegram from UCSF Langley Porter Neuropsychiatric Institute, the teaching hospital of the Department of Psychiatry of the University of California Medical Center in San Francisco. It was short and to the point. It said that I was accepted into this residency, and please respond by return telegram. It was unexpected because, in my mind, I hadn't completed the application. I had made out the application, signed and sent it in, but it was supposed to have included names of references, which I did not follow up and include. I said yes by return telegram because I wanted to go back to San Francisco and I rationalized that whatever I ended up doing, a year of psychiatry wouldn't hurt.

As my life turned out, I suppose I could say it was "meant to be," and fate had a hand in it. The likely practical explanation is that psychiatry must have used my medical school evaluations from supervisors in the psychiatric clinic, where I saw a couple of patients, wrote process notes and discussed my work with them. I had had a mixed experience with psychiatry. The lectures had not impressed or intrigued me. I was, however, engaged with my patients in the clinic, and it was gratifying to realize that their sessions with me had been helpful. I was ambivalent about applying for the residency, which was why I started but didn't complete the application.

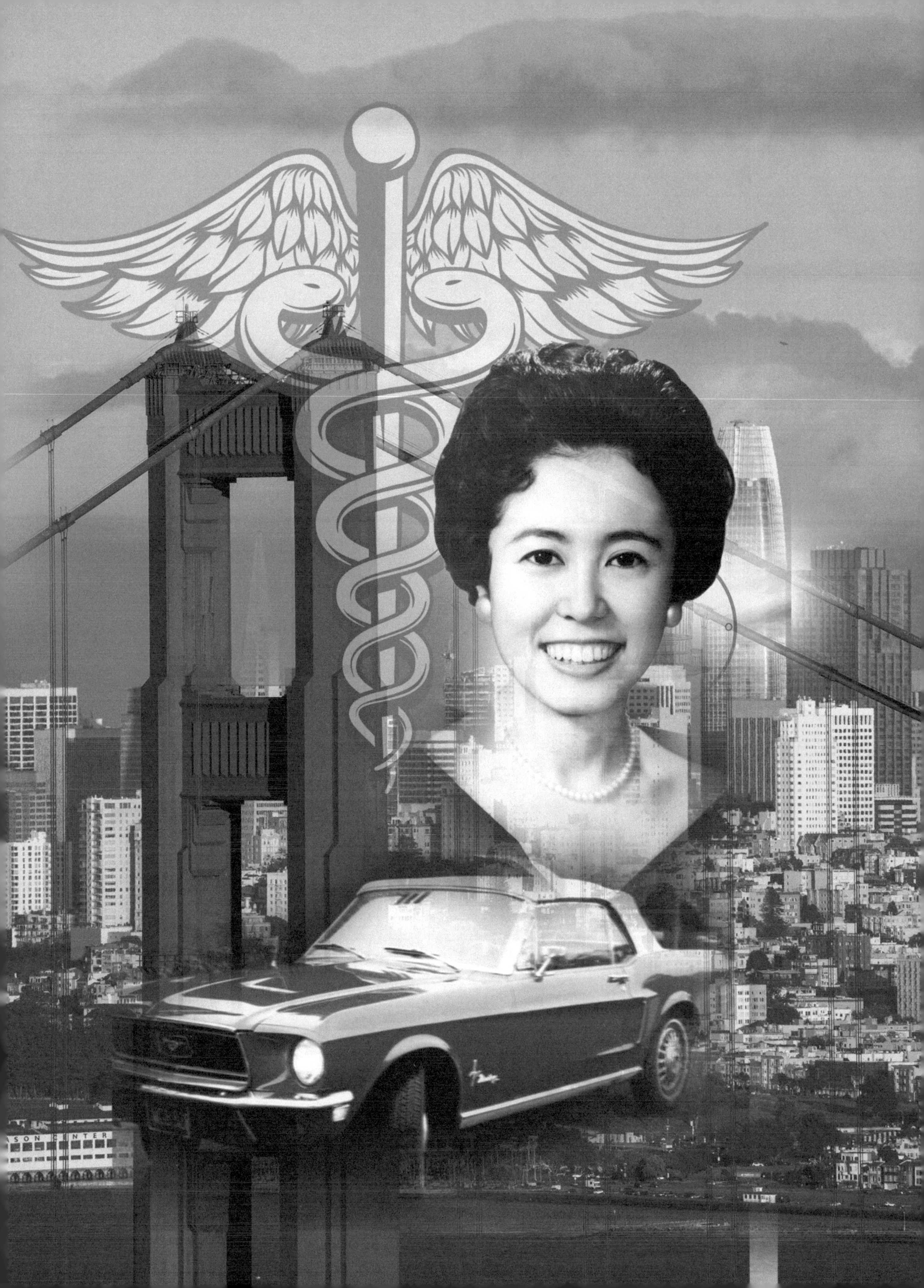

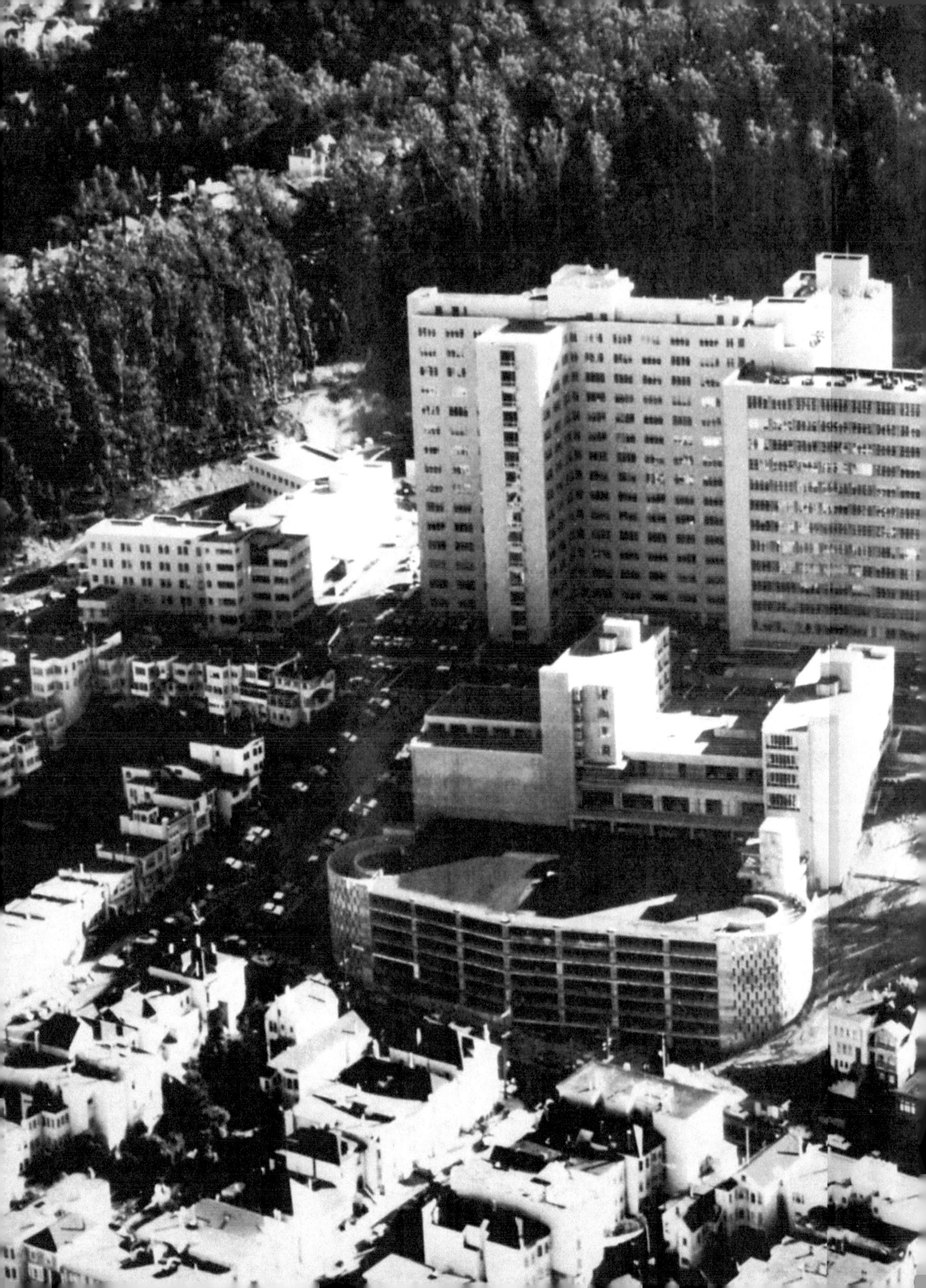

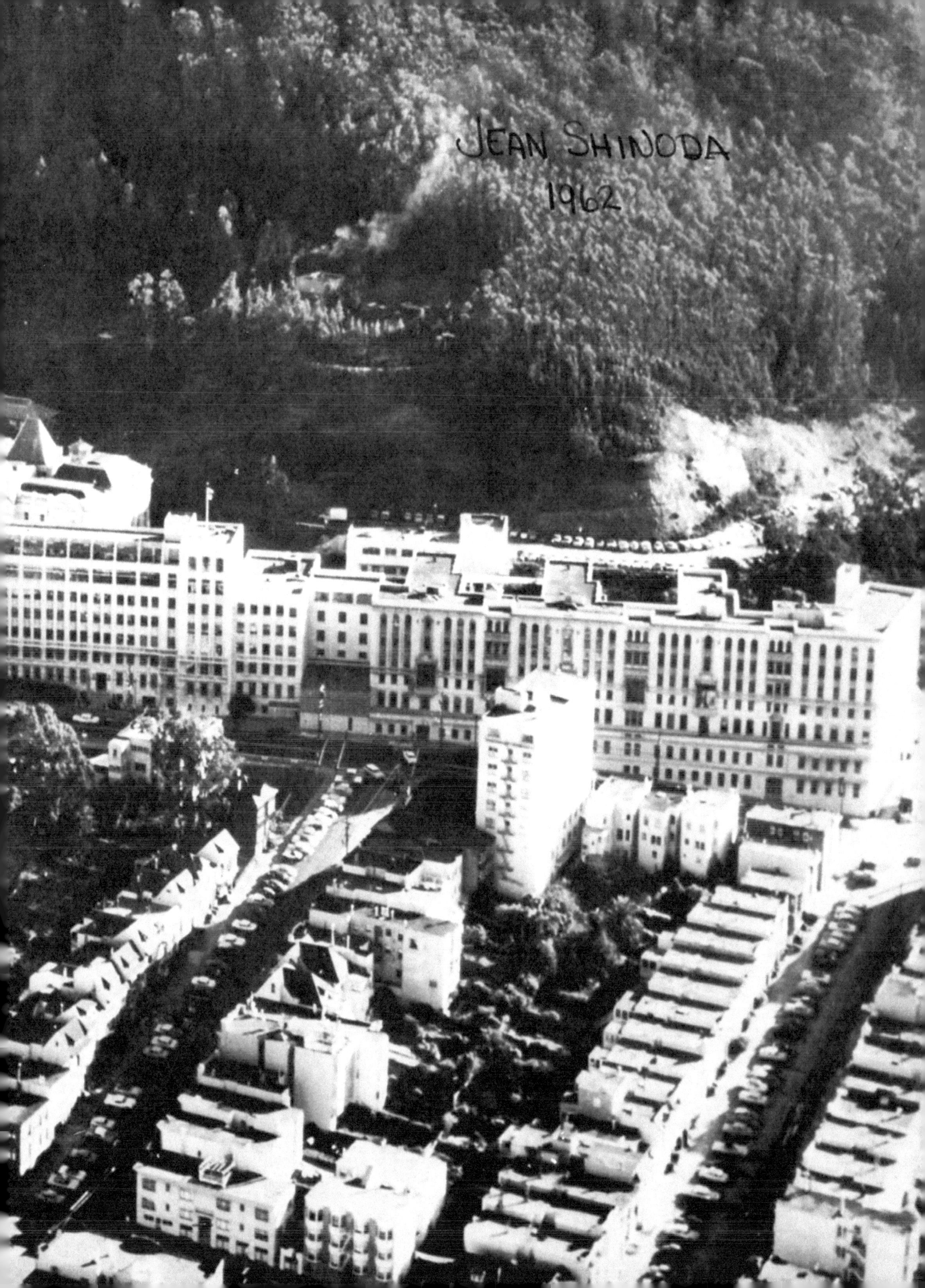
JEAN SHINODA
1962

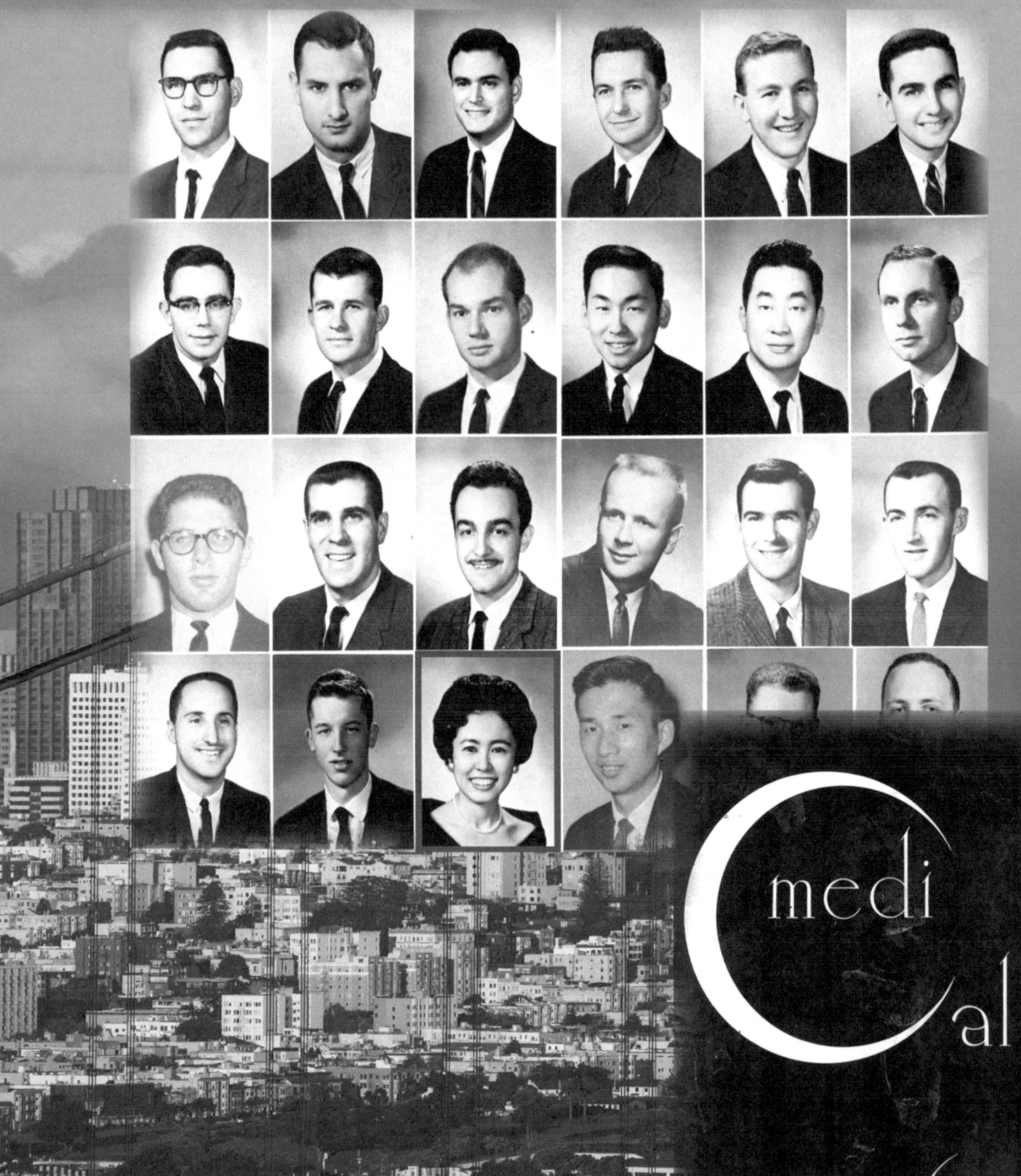
mediCal
1962

Chapter 11

Began Residency – Found My Calling

On July 1, 1963, I began my residency in psychiatry at Langley Porter Neuro-psychiatric Institute (LPNI, which later became LPPI when "Neuro" was dropped). It was a set-apart building next to Moffitt Hospital and the adjoined Life Sciences Building where most of my medical classes had been held. I was assigned to a locked, acute inpatient ward. At the time, Langley Porter was a teaching hospital with selected admissions. Patients could stay until they were discharged. Some of my patients had come through the emergency room at UCSF or SF General Hospital and referred directly for admission at Langley Porter. Some had been referred by a psychiatrist, others had been seen in the LPNI outpatient clinic, brought in by relatives who had become alarmed when they realized that the patient was hallucinating, acting bizarrely, or had suicidal thoughts and delusions. Most were young adults who had not been treated by a psychiatrist before.

I found it was easy for me to feel a connection with my patients, to relate to and draw out the person underneath the symptoms who had been taken over and

was overwhelmed. I wasn't afraid of the psychotic world into which they had descended. I was finding that I had a talent or a gift for this work, something similar perhaps to what "horse whisperers" are able to do to with horses. After I felt the connection, I would wonder if there had been some triggering event that tipped a fragile psyche into psychosis, thinking that whatever it was would make sense once I knew more about the patient.

I thought that each of them must have held themselves together until she or he couldn't do it anymore. I responded to them with care and authenticity, using feeling-intuition at times to say what I thought they could be experiencing, and I would ask them to let me know if I was on the right track. I could imagine how it would feel to hear voices that said negative things to them about them or about others, or urged them to do something hostile to themselves or others. It was natural for me to relate with each of my patients as I-Thou rather than I-It.

No matter how out of touch my patients were from reality, or if they had seemed threatening to someone else, when I sat with them, I listened to what they were feeling from my heart and not just my mind. I was interested in their delusions. I inquired about who the voices were and what they were saying. I listened to this "crazy talk" as condensed, disguised, or metaphoric language, in the way that I would try to understand a complex poem (T.S. Eliot's poems, *Four Quartets* and *The Wasteland* come to mind). I used my intuition to translate as much as I could from what I knew of their family history and events prior to the psychosis or suicide effort. I wanted to understand, not to pigeonhole them with a diagnosis or a formulation, but to know them. In doing so, something like magic—or trust and love—happened between us. Using usual terminology, I'd write of forming a therapeutic alliance or establishing rapport in my notes.

They were in the "underworld," a world we all normally enter in dreams. My patients needed help to get out of their waking nightmares. Their discerning, decision-making, waking egos were submerged and needed an ally. Beginning with an intuition that I had (which was not a point of view that I was being taught), I listened to what their "voices" were saying. By asking questions, I was learning what was disturbing or meaningful to them, and sense emerged in what otherwise made none at all. It was the beginning of what I now do as a Jungian analyst who works with dreams. Dreams are not like logical thought. They are often symbolic metaphors or commentaries on what is going on in the waking life of the dreamer. Or they are the opposite, as if serving as a reminder of better times to compensate for the bleakness in the dreamer's current waking life.

The underworld in mythology is associated with the maiden Persephone. She had been gathering flowers in the meadow, It was a sunny day, the sky was blue, and all was well. And then, everything changed. Hades came for her in his black chariot and black horses. He grabbed the terrified maiden who screamed in fear as Hades took her into the chariot and plunged down into the underworld. In this myth, which corresponds to the shock of rape or molestation, betrayal, or sudden physical trauma, innocence is abducted. When this too much to bear, psychosis can result in some who are susceptible. I tell the story of Persephone who became Queen of the Underworld in *Goddesses in Everywoman*, which corresponds to the person who, with help, emerges to become a guide for others.

I was treating my patients and their hallucinations with respect. In response, their trust in me grew. They also left each session usually feeling calmer and better because I really listened, which is itself healing medicine. And as I tried to unravel the connections, some of it began to make sense to them, too. There is something in most people, once they let their guard down and are not hiding behind the acceptable social face or persona they put on, that makes them able to sense or feel another human's "realness" or authenticity. I think dogs and young children instinctively know this and hence who to trust. Psychiatric patients may have learned not to trust through betrayals and loss. It takes time and constancy to build trust.

Trust was essential when "voices" said one thing, and a psychiatrist was saying something else, or didn't say anything much at all. This was often especially true about medication. Doctors in hospitals wrote medication orders: which ones, what dosage, when given, and what to do if patient refused them. With psychiatric patients and anti-psychotic drugs, I learned that a therapeutic alliance was especially important. For one thing, dosages are hit-or-miss when the doctor and patient are not allies, and powerful drugs have powerful effects, both good and not. To "titrate" drug and symptoms as analogy was a way for doctor and patient to work together, and helped a patient strengthen the ego that got taken over by the psychosis. I think of chemistry lab experiments in which one chemical was in the beaker. In solution form, it is colorless, looks like water, then an indicator was added, also colorless, and then drop-by-drop-by-drop, the second colorless chemical was added, until suddenly, the solution in the beaker turned pink. To reach the desired effect, we had to titrate how much was needed. Care with the dosage depended on the patient's involvement in observing. I preferred to start with a lower dose and increase it as the patient got used to it, while watching for side effects and for the efficacy of the medication to diminish symptoms that it was for.

Effective anti-psychotic drugs (phenothiazines) were developed in the 1950s and had become available by the time I was a psychiatric resident. I could prescribe Thorazine, Stelazine, Prolixin, or Mellaril, each related chemically but slightly different in dosage and effects. This was a breakthrough. In many ways it was as momentous in the treatment of psychosis as antibiotics were for infectious disease. It would lead to the emptying of California's state mental hospital system within the next decade. These drugs could silence hallucinations and reduce paranoia. They had side effects such as tremors, a mask-like face, cog-like movements (which an anti-Parkinson's drug helped), and most commonly, a dry mouth, some dizziness, fainting if you stood up quickly, and an uncomfortable feeling of being drugged.

Voices often were accusatory, demeaning, and repeated negative things about the patient that had been said to them in childhood. The voices could also be warning the patient about others. But also, in some lonely individuals, they were voices or personalities that kept them company. Patients were often paranoid. I learned they often had reasons to be once I learned their personal history. Mistrust of doctors and authorities who said that they were doing what was best for them led to such treatments as pre-frontal lobotomies, forced sterilization, and use in experiments. Given the treatment of mental patients in the past, being suspicious or paranoid of psychiatrists was not exactly crazy, especially when the drugs they prescribed had scary side effects.

A relevant aside here: Two psychiatrists, Price M. Cobbs, MD and William H. Grier, MD, wrote *Black Rage* in the mid-1960s. Price was on the clinical faculty at Langley Porter where I heard him speak about Black rage and, given the history since slavery, that there is something wrong with a Black person who isn't on guard or paranoid about white authority.

When does it makes sense to consider if someone is trustworthy and on your side? Or if "we" are on the same side? As a new psychiatric resident, I needed to be on the same "side" as my patients in order for us to have a therapeutic relationship. This was the opportunity I was given on the inpatient service at Langley Porter. I had been a medical student and an intern on the psychiatric units at San Francisco General Hospital and Los Angeles General Hospital, where people were brought for observation, often by police. Some were brought in for floridly psychotic behavior, many drug related, and all were initially on three-day involuntary holds. This was an entirely different patient population. At Langley Porter, I had the opportunity and time to get to know and help my patients.

I became a psychiatric resident shortly after effective antipsychotic medications became available—which I came to think of in my idiosyncratic way as "ego glue." No one functions well when overwhelmed by fears and voices. Medication helps a fragile ego hold itself together. This plus the time it takes in therapy for trust to develop is needed by patients. The ability to discern reality, think straight, make good decisions, and feel centered are signs of a well-functioning ego—which the therapist needs to have as well to teach and model for her or his patients.

In my psychotherapy and analytic work since, most people I worked with often appeared to others as normal functioning adults. But, they were individuals who came to work with me beset by anxieties, depression, lack of meaning, psychosomatic symptoms, low self-esteem, and mid- or late-life problems. I was fortunate to begin my psychiatric training as I did on an acute hospital service at a teaching hospital that admitted people who were first admissions, many of whom were schizophrenics. Once they no longer hallucinated or were delusional, I could help them to see themselves and their choices, and to become discerning about obstacles and bad patterns.

It seems to me that almost everyone has stress points that can become too much for an ego to hold or handle. I was learning about breaking points that brought my patients to the hospital. In the years since, I've seen how strong people can reach psychological and spiritual breaking points, and observed how overwhelming stress, depression, major losses, or lack of meaning can be expressed through a breakdown in functioning by any bodily organ, not just the mind. I think each of us has an Achilles heel. Remember him? Achilles was the Greek Hero who had only one point of vulnerability. When he was an infant, his mother Thetis dipped him into the river Styx, which protected him against all weapons, but she was holding him by the heel—which left this part unprotected. This is where the arrow struck, and how he died.

I Found My Calling

I had taken a zig-zag course to become a psychiatry resident. I had gone to three colleges, and had four years of medical school and one year of internship before I came to Langley Porter. I hadn't wanted to be a psychiatrist and had begun this residency as a means to return to San Francisco, rationalizing that a year of psychiatry would be useful to whatever I ended up doing. I had begun this journey in a conversation with God at Forest Home, in which the promise that I would be a doctor had come spontaneously as a means of saying "thank you." Gratitude brought me here, where I found that I had a gift for this work, and that I could connect with my psychiatric patients. I had found my calling and I knew it.

FOUND MY CALLING

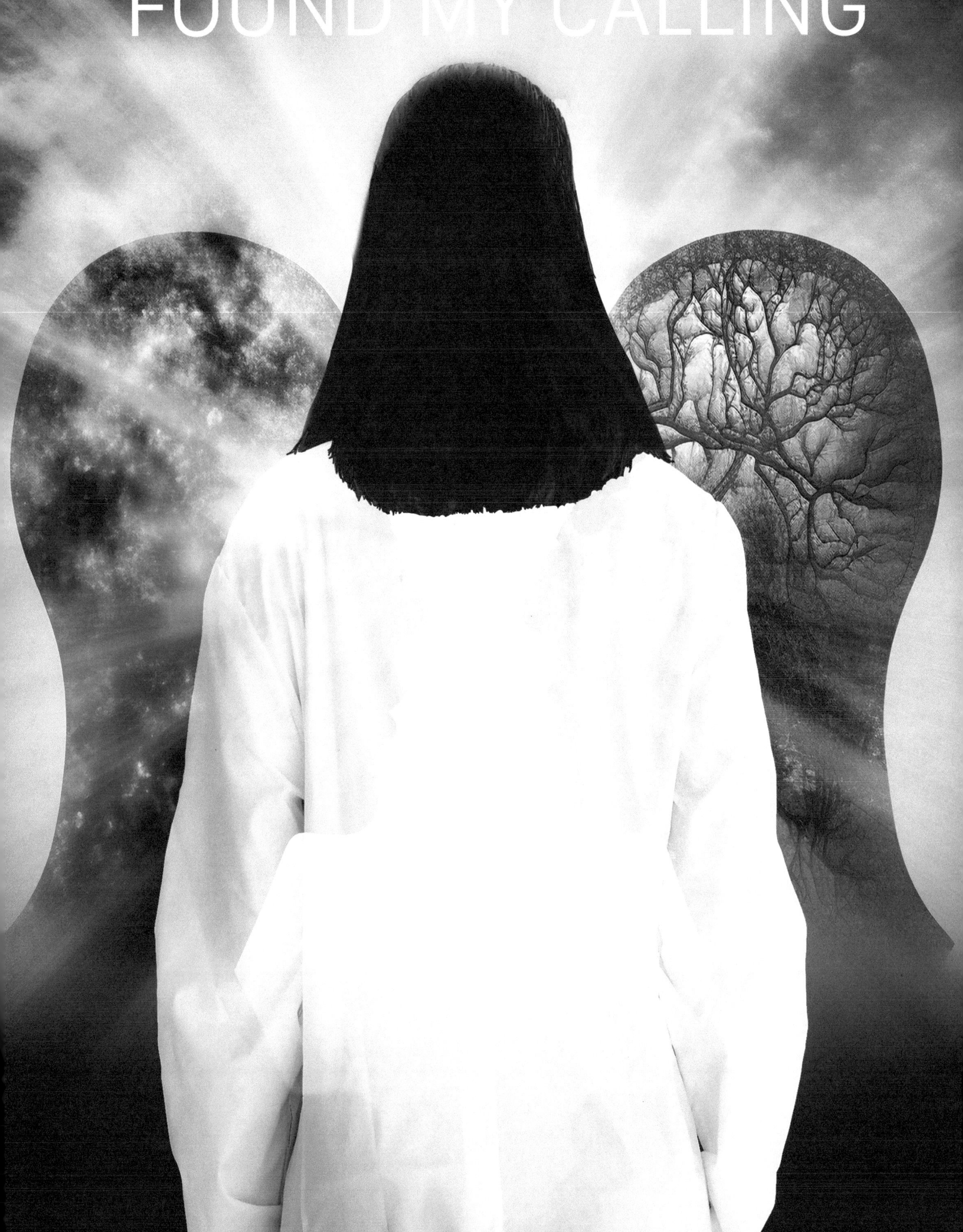

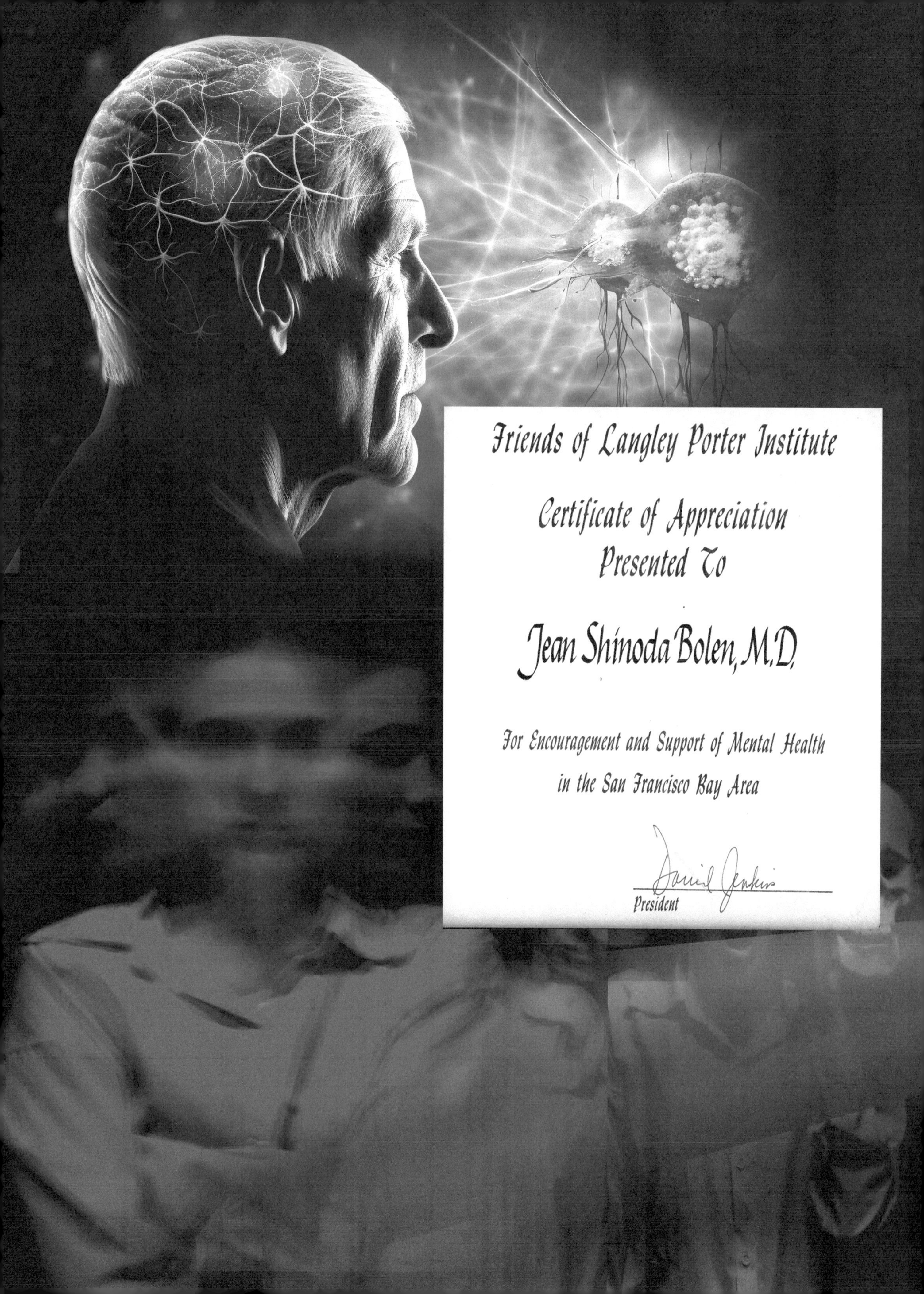
Friends of Langley Porter Institute
Certificate of Appreciation
Presented To
Jean Shinoda Bolen, M.D.
For Encouragement and Support of Mental Health
in the San Francisco Bay Area
President

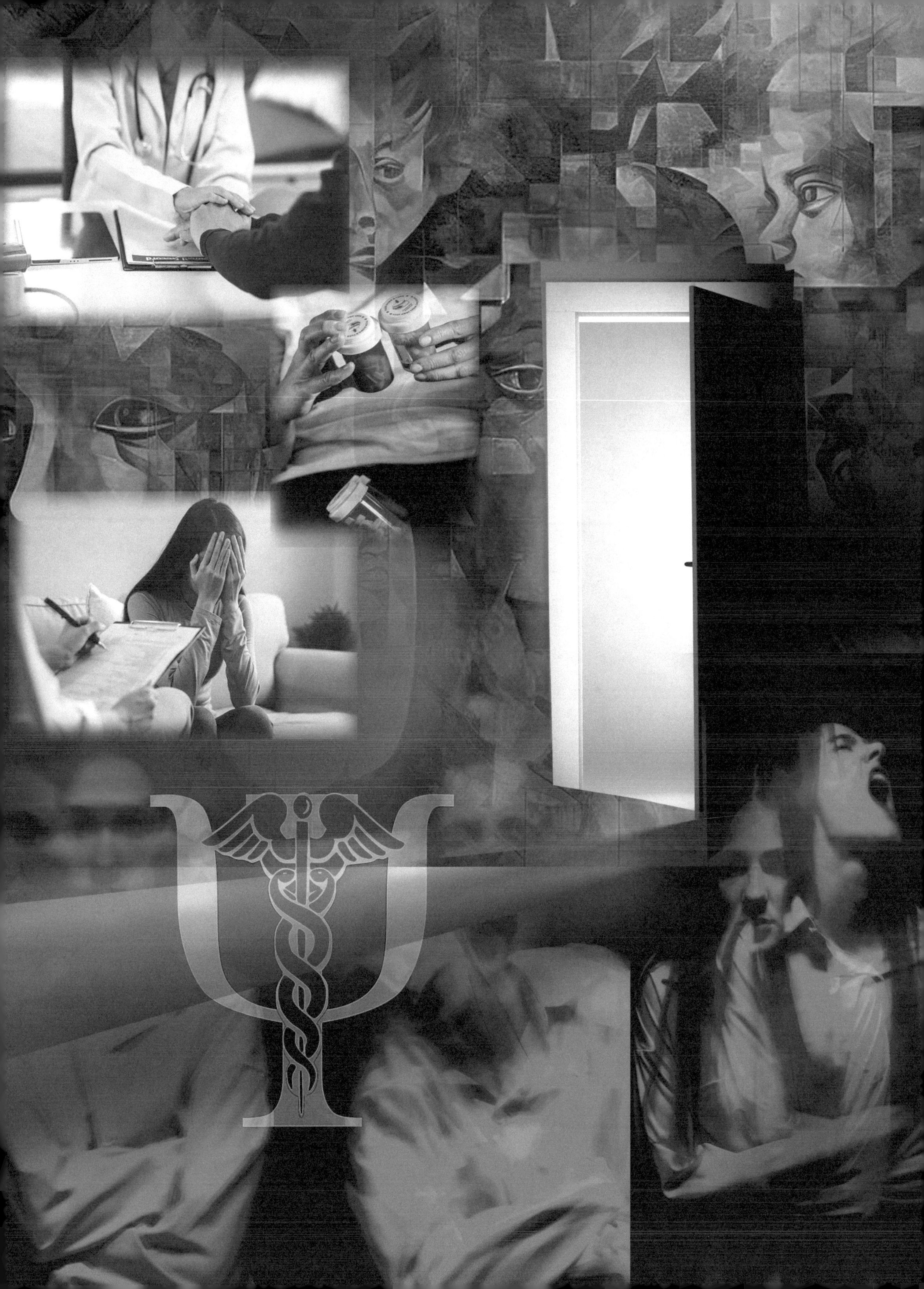

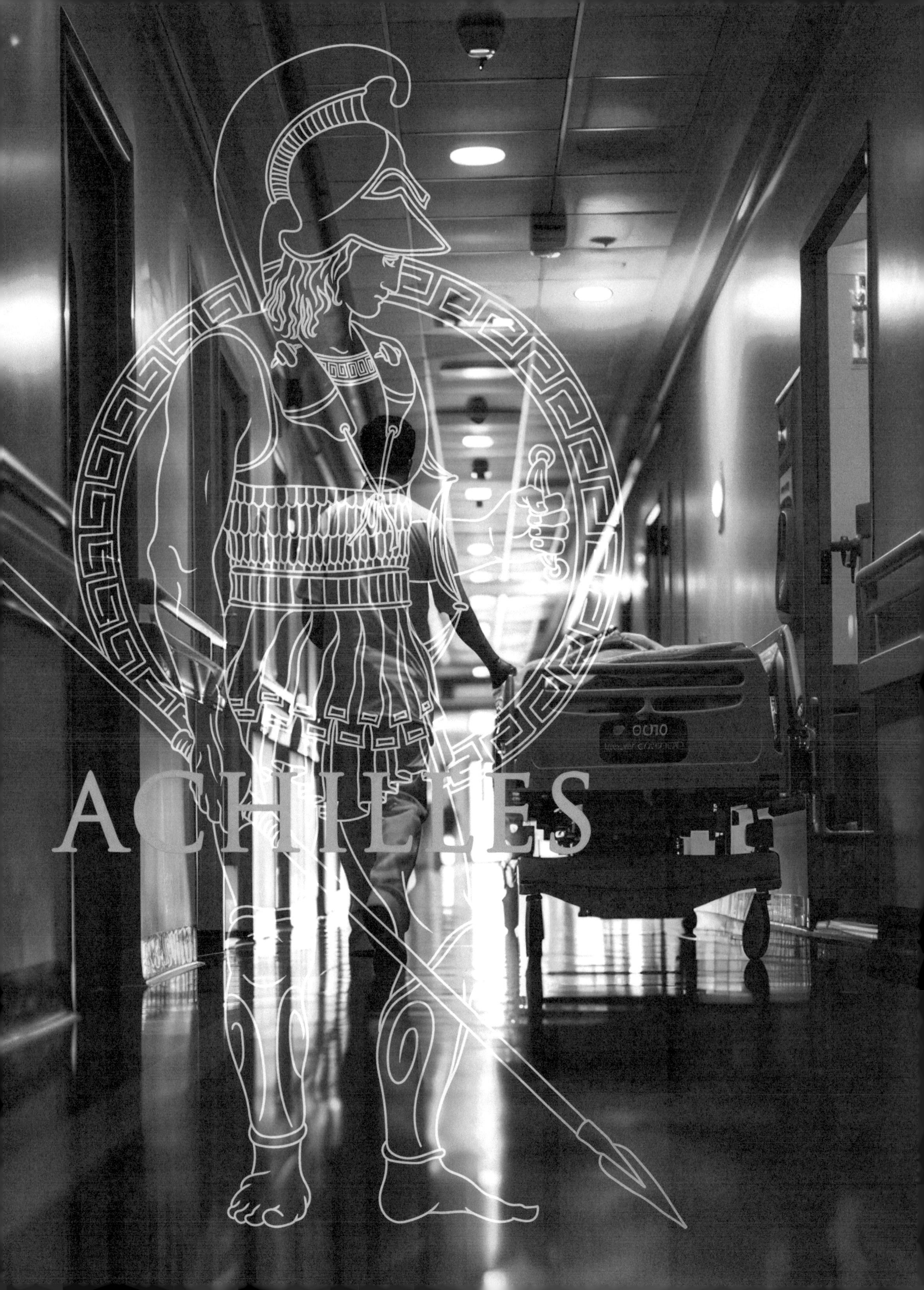
ACHILLES

Chapter 12

Family Crisis

I had settled into my residency and was happy to be back in the Bay Area when my mother called to tell me my father had been readmitted to the hospital and would be discharged the next day. My father had developed cancer in the lining of his mouth that had spread, and he had undergone major disfiguring surgery to remove his jaw, lymph nodes, a salivary gland, and muscles on one side of his neck. He had also undergone a series of radiation treatments at UCSF, flying to San Francisco from Los Angeles regularly. It had been a heroic effort of hope and stamina over several years. Now, there was nothing further that could be done, which meant he was being sent home to die. In response to a sense of urgency I felt from her, I made the necessary calls and made arrangements to be with them as soon as I could be there.

When I got to the hospital, my father was dressed and ready to leave. He had on his usual business suit, shirt and tie, and appeared to be comfortable. My mother was quiet. Nothing seemed amiss—other than the gravity of the situation, which we did not discuss. I brought them home from the hospital, as usual entering the house through the kitchen where we could sit down around the table and feel glad to be there. My mother went into their bedroom. After a while, when she hadn't returned, I went to see why, and found her just standing there. The only words she said were "I have nothing to wear." I led her back to the kitchen, where she continued to stand, and she did not say anything to either my father or me. When I asked what was the matter, she repeated, "I have nothing to wear." It was as if she had become catatonic. Reality was too much to face, and all her concern was focused on "I have nothing to wear," which she said without emotion.

In dreams, when the dreamer finds herself naked or poorly dressed in a social situation, this often is a statement about loss of a usual or former role or persona, of feeling inadequate or "not up to" a new situation. This is a fairly common dream. It reveals the dreamer's anxious reaction to what is expected of her. My mother was not dreaming. She was out of touch with reality and profoundly depressed. Her focus on having "nothing to wear," under the circumstances, was "crazy." She had reached her breaking point.

My mother was my father's support until there was nothing more that could be done except send him home. Now his care would be up to her—and from her psyche's response, this was more than she could do. I also knew she blamed herself for not insisting that a biopsy be done after the doctor they consulted looked at the area on the inner side of my father's cheek and was sure it was a benign condition. He said that it wouldn't be necessary to put my father through an unnecessary biopsy and expressed this as if it doing her a professional courtesy, doctor to doctor.

That evening, John and Miki Fukushima, friends of my parents whom I had known most of my life, came to the house in response to my call for help. Miki helped my mother get ready for bed and said she'd help her with her wardrobe in the morning. I reached out to a psychiatrist who was the director of a private psychiatric hospital nearby, through his daughter, a former classmate, and told him the circumstances. The next day—in what seemed surreal then and now—the three of us went to the hospital, and my father, who had terminal cancer, signed my mother into a mental hospital for evaluation and treatment. She was mute and passive, without emotion. I felt that she was cocooned in a thick invisible blanket of sadness that we could not penetrate. The whole situation was bleak.

My mother was started on medication that would take time to tell if it was helping her profound depression. The hospital program was designed to engage patients in activities and encourage expression of feelings. While this didn't seem to do much, the hospital did mobilize her into its daily routine, like getting out of bed, dressing, meals, sitting in community meetings, and going to therapy sessions including art therapy. I know I could not have managed to do this alone.

Meanwhile, I had taken an indefinite leave from my residency and organized our family home around my father's needs, but also in preparation for my mother coming home so she would not have to do anything. I had arranged for some help and had temporary power of attorney. We had daily visits from Miki and John, my Uncle Mits (Mitsuya Yamaguchi, MD), and my mother's youngest sibling. I spoke regularly to my mother on the phone, though I avoided talking about the two elephants in the room: my concern about the progression of my father's cancer, and the reason she was in a mental hospital. Somewhere underneath her defensive armor of numbness and depression, I knew that she needed to know about him, though I feared it could make her worse.

When I learned that my father was to go back to the hospital again, this time for palliative surgery to remove as much of the cancer as safely possible, I told her. It was as if my mother's mind and agency, her will and determination, woke up and got directed at me. She told me that I must call Dr. Milton Erickson in Arizona and get him to come to see my father. She and my uncle Mits had learned medical hypnosis with Dr. Erickson, a psychiatrist and founding president of the American Society of Clinical Hypnosis. She was insistent. I managed to do as she directed.

I picked Dr. Erickson up at the airport. Other than my mother's faith that he could help my father somehow, I had no expectations, and had not heard of him other than from my mother. When I brought him to my father's bedside, a surreal situation only got more so. My father had had the palliative surgery that morning while I was at the airport. He now had a tracheotomy, which made talking difficult to impossible, and he was seeing things. His visual hallucinations were side effects of the anesthetic and analgesic meds he had received for the surgery and post-op. He was cheerful and excited as he pointed at whatever he was seeing that we could not. His gestures and facial expression were as if he were saying "Just look at that! It's amazing! It's gorgeous!"

Dr. Erickson talked to my father in a conversational tone, calling him Joe. He spoke to him for what could have been twenty or thirty minutes, while my father continued hallucinating and didn't seem to be paying attention. I recall Dr. Erickson spoke about roses and how they grow, and how a bud opens up into a beautiful full bloom, describing the petals opening step by step and yet while we don't see this happening or know how it happens, it does. He talked in this same way about how a baby grows from newborn to three times its birth weight in the first year. I think that he may have been preparing the ground for the idea of that my mother believed was possible and wanted Dr. Erickson to do, which was to plant seeds of healing and remission. I had only been half-listening because it felt to me that I was the audience at a tragicomedy: my father hallucinating and pointing to things I couldn't see, Dr. Erikson in a storytelling mode, calling him Joe as if Joe was listening, and me, the daughter who had gone on what felt like a fool's errand.

My father's hallucinations stopped and he came home on pain medications. Shortly after, Dr. Erickson visited us at the house. My father knew from my mother's interest in hypnosis about Dr. Erikson (who was and is famous in this field). A conversation between them took place in the living room. Dr. Erickson was an engaging personality who easily established rapport. Never once did Dr. Erickson verbally suggest that my father close his eyes or do any usual induction into hypnosis. This time I did pay attention. He must have planted a suggestion in the hospital—now that I know something about such things, it could have been a particular phrase or touch—which had this effect. Once again

Dr. Erickson spoke to Joe about how roses and babies grow and how just as imperceptibly, my father's need for pain medications would become less and less. He also suggested that his body knew how to heal itself. While he had not directed my father to close his eyes, at some point as he listened, he did. Dr. Erickson told him that when he opened his eyes, he would feel peaceful and rested. This was all he did and said. By the next day, my father's need for pain medication dropped to a third of what he had been taking. I was amazed and becoming a believer. I kept my mother informed.

Meanwhile, Mom was still a patient in the psychiatric hospital. The brief intensity and insistence that she had focused on me about Dr. Erickson passed, and she was again passive and depressed. She was not as depressed as she had been on admission, when "catatonic" best described her, but she was not okay. My father's nursing needs had increased with the need for more post-surgical care. We now had two shifts of nurses; one stayed all night.

During the day, when my father and I spent time together in the living room, we often watched television. That's where we were when news came that President John F. Kennedy had been shot while in a motorcade in Dallas. From the first reports and then the replays and breaking news and commentaries, all eyes were focused on this. This was November 22, 1963. JFK had been assassinated, followed by more events which we followed closely, one report after another, the swearing in of Lyndon Johnson, the return with the body to Washington, John-John, the memorial service and procession, and the interment at Arlington Cemetery. I wondered what my father was thinking as he watched, knowing that he didn't have much time left in the world and that soon, we would be at his funeral. These were my thoughts.

My mother's psychiatrist called from the hospital to say that the therapy and medications were not working. He was recommending ECT—electroconvulsive therapy—and needed my permission. I knew that my mother would not want it (I was right about this) and I also knew that if my father were to die while my mother was still in the hospital, this would be sad for both of them. She blamed herself for not insisting that a biopsy be done after the doctor-expert said it was unnecessary. Her polite response had been a thank you for his consideration and courtesy; I think the family Samurai culture made being polite and deferring to his expertise her only acceptable response. Hindsight and self-blame are not fair. It also could be that it had not yet become malignant. Or it could be that she had an intuition that was correct and overrode it. Rather than be rude, polite women suffer the consequences.

I gave my permission for my mother to undergo a series of ECT treatments. She responded to the treatments and was no longer depressed. She could leave the hospital for brief visits to us. She was not herself. I could tell this in her voice when we talked on the phone before she came home. Before ECT, she was depressed. Now she felt fine, but in some way that people like me tune into people and know each other, she wasn't the person I knew as my mother. Later, I read reports about ECT. I could relate to the woman who described her post-ECT husband as cheerful and able to work, but she said, "It's as if his soul is missing," which is what I was feeling. (This was what the wife of a lobotomized husband also said). This phase of response to ECT also passed, as did one outburst of anger at me for giving permission for ECT. Gradually, she returned. I could talk to her about what had been happening since she was in the hospital.

I had several conversations with my father after my mother was hospitalized, which was before he had the palliative surgery, and needed round-the-clock nursing. Then just he and I were in the house. This was when he talked to me about my brother and the decision for Stephen's lobotomy, which he had pushed for, over my mother's doubts. He said it was the one thing he had done that he regretted. I could tell him that it may turn out to have protected Stephen—the lobotomy cuts him off from being anxious or fearful, no matter what. Stephen was in a good situation where he was, but if he needed to someday be institutionalized, it could matter.

Then that "someday" happened. I already felt the responsibility for my mother and father when news came that the private place where my brother had been living was to be closed down. The patients were under the care of a physician-psychiatrist who couldn't continue and now, suddenly, Stephen and all the others were to be sent back to their parents. I had last seen Stephen in the hospital when I was in junior high school and he was four years younger than me. I had ever again seen him again after his surgery and anti-convulsion medication. I always remembered him as he was back then. It felt as if it were a very long time ago.

In the process of going through hundreds of archival family photos and memorabilia with Lynda Carré, as source material for the photo booklets she was creating for my autobiography, I was more than a little surprised when she uncovered a small old envelope from my mother's things. In it contained a special group photograph accompanied by a loving handwritten note about Stephen from a caregiver in the place he lived. At the time that photo was taken, I was twenty-seven and had just begun my psychiatric residency and taken a leave of absence when my father was dying. The old photograph included young adults and staff members at the private care facility where Stephen lived but which I never visited. In the photograph, I could see how Stephen grew into a tall adult man, the only Asian person in the photograph, with friends leaning on and around him. He was twenty-three years old then. All these many years, until I read that note and saw that photograph, I held an old image of Stephen as a young child, I would not have recognized him. It was a revelation to me that he looked very fine.

After my father died, my mother eventually recovered and later reopened her medical-psychiatric office. She continued in practice for several decades into her late eighties and died a decade later. I was sent Stephen's ashes which are buried with our parents.

My mom did come home and was herself before my father died and after my brother had settled into his institutionalized life. She was home by Christmas. My father was mostly in his bed. He had round-the-clock nursing, was well cared for and comfortable, and it seemed to me that he was himself. I'd sit awhile or talk with him in brief one-sided conversation; with the tracheotomy, he could be heard only by putting his hand over the opening.

We had a signal system set up with the nurses. If my mother and I were needed, we could be notified without the nurse leaving his side. In the early morning on January 21, 1964, we were awakened by the signal. When I got to his bedside, he was awake, his head was up, he was looking intensely at something to my left where there was nothing that I could see. I was looking at him when I saw his eyes grow wide, and his face light up—it literally seemed to be infused with joy, and then in the next nanosecond, he was gone. The body he left behind, after the cancer, the surgeries, the weight loss was not him, it was like discarded, worn-out old clothes. It had been animated a nanosecond before and then he—his soul left it, and he went toward something that I couldn't see. But from what I saw in his face, and my own soul to soul recognition and trust in this experience, I knew this was a profound message. There is something to go towards after we die—on the other side of physical reality. He was 54 years old when he crossed to the "other side."

For me, my father's memorial service at Hollywood Presbyterian Church and interment at Evergreen Cemetery were ceremonies of closure and respect, shared by the community of people to whom he mattered. He had fulfilled the words from Micah 6:8 I chose to have engraved on the headstone: "What does the Lord require of you but to do justice, love mercy, and walk humbly with your God?"

My father often said, "Life is short," and it was for him. When I turned fifty-four myself, I realized how young he was when he died and how short his life turned out to be.

My father's cancer in the lining of his mouth was the kind that develops in patients who have been long-time smokers. The heat, smoke, and carcinogens in the cigarette irritates the mucosa cells and until they became malignant. In his father's eyes (my grandfather, the fundamentalist Christian), smoking, drinking and breaking any of the Ten Commandments were all sins. My father had tried to keep his occasional smoking from me and succeeded for years. Eventually I found out, but even then, I never saw him smoking. My mother told me that it was a secret he kept from his brothers, and via this indirect communication, the inference was clear that I was not to mention this. It was something he did out of sight, in the basement.

After I had heard radiation oncologist O. Carl Simonton, MD, speak about his approach to the treatment of cancer nine years later, I wondered if my father's sorrow and guilt at having championed my brother's pre-frontal lobotomy contributed to the cancer he developed in the "smokers" area. His smoking was also a secret source of guilt. Dr. Simonton placed an emphasis on mind-body immune system connections, linking the development of a cancer to the psychology and susceptibility of the person who gets cancer. I also think that my mother blamed herself for not insisting that a biopsy be done. How much, I wonder, did my parents carry unnecessary burdens of guilt and responsibility that contributed to her hospitalization for depression, and his development of cancer?

At the time of his death, my father was ready to leave. He was now mostly in bed and peaceful. He had hung on until my mother recovered and could come home, and she had. His last gift to me came a nanosecond before he died, when I saw his face light up with joy at what he was seeing. What I saw in his eyes and face told me not to fear dying, there is something wonderful that comes next. This was an unforgettable moment and a transmission that touched my soul.

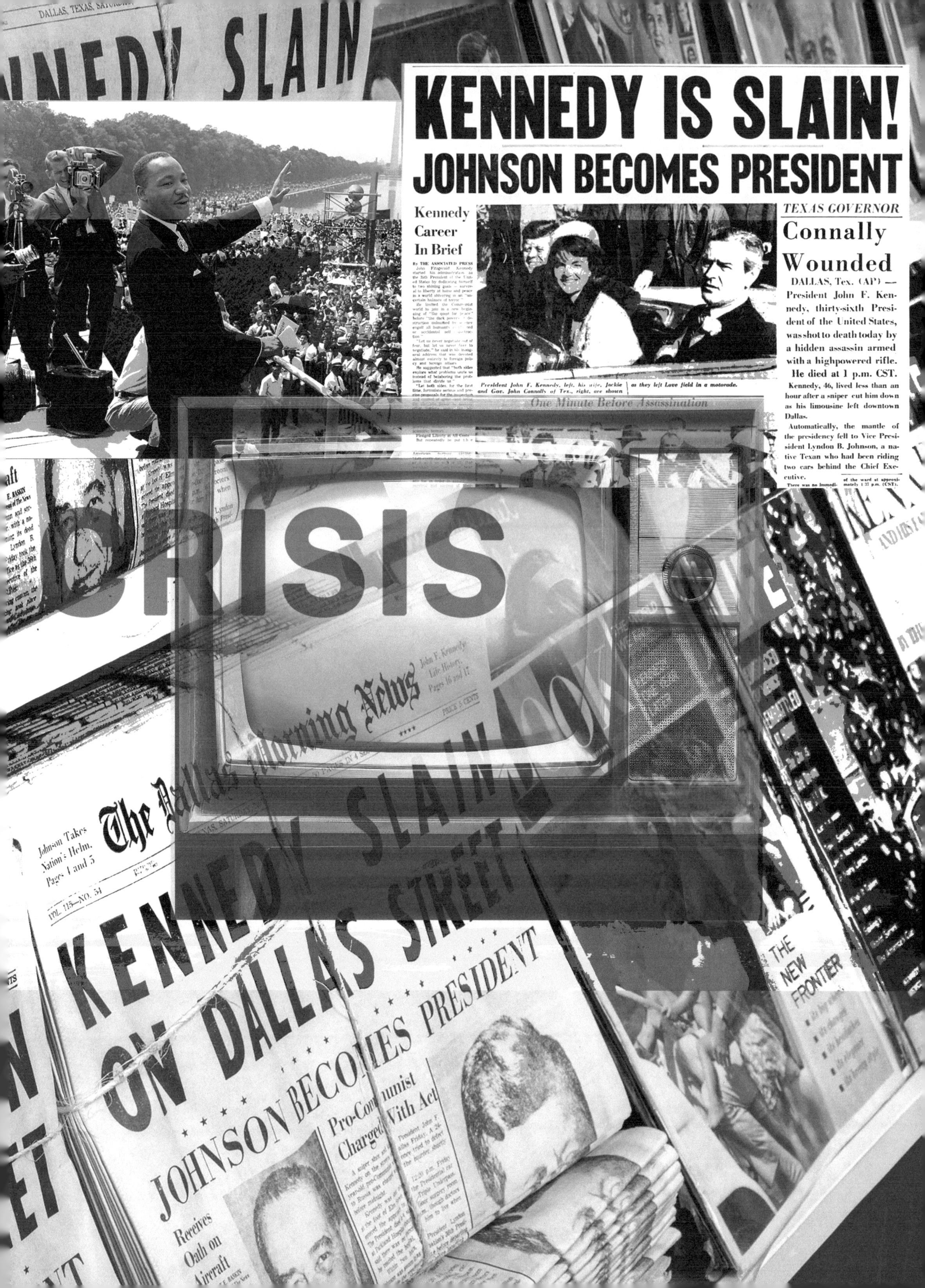

KENNEDY SLAIN
KENNEDY IS SLAIN!
JOHNSON BECOMES PRESIDENT
Kennedy Career In Brief
TEXAS GOVERNOR
Connally Wounded
DALLAS, Tex. (AP) — President John F. Kennedy, thirty-sixth President of the United States, was shot to death today by a hidden assassin armed with a highpowered rifle.
He died at 1 p.m. CST.
Kennedy, 46, lived less than an hour after a sniper cut him down as his limousine left downtown Dallas.
Automatically, the mantle of the presidency fell to Vice President Lyndon B. Johnson, a native Texan who had been riding two cars behind the Chief Executive.
President John F. Kennedy, left, his wife, Jackie and Gov. John Connally of Tex., right, are shown as they left Love field in a motorcade.
One Minute Before Assassination
CRISIS
The Dallas Morning News
John F. Kennedy Life History, Pages 16 and 17
Johnson Takes Nation's Helm, Pages 4 and 5
KENNEDY SLAIN
KENNEDY SLAIN ON DALLAS STREET
JOHNSON BECOMES PRESIDENT
Pro-Communist Charged With Act
Receives Oath on Aircraft
THE NEW FRONTIER

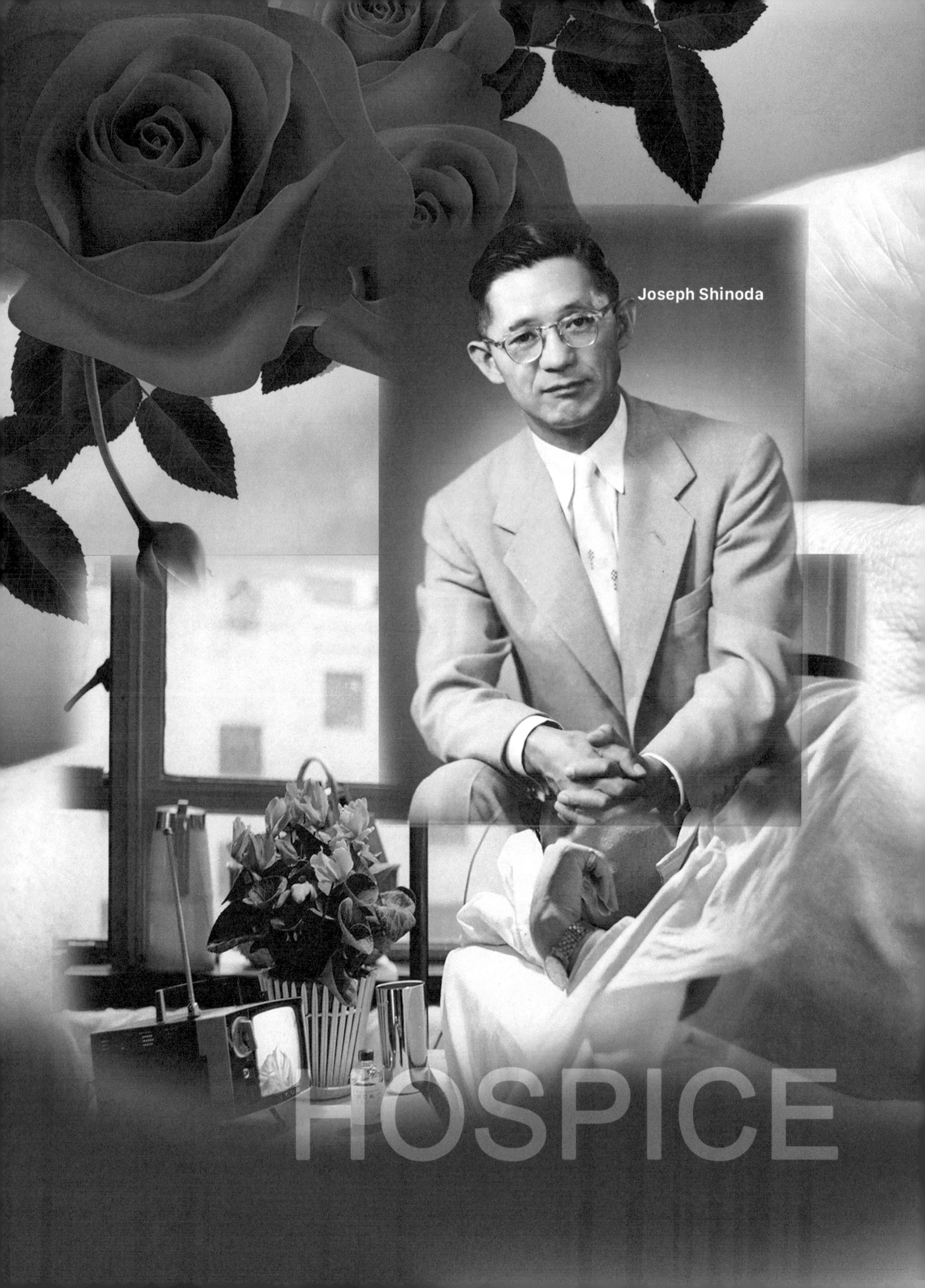

Joseph Shinoda

HOSPICE

Milton H. Erickson, M.D.

PSYCHIATRIC

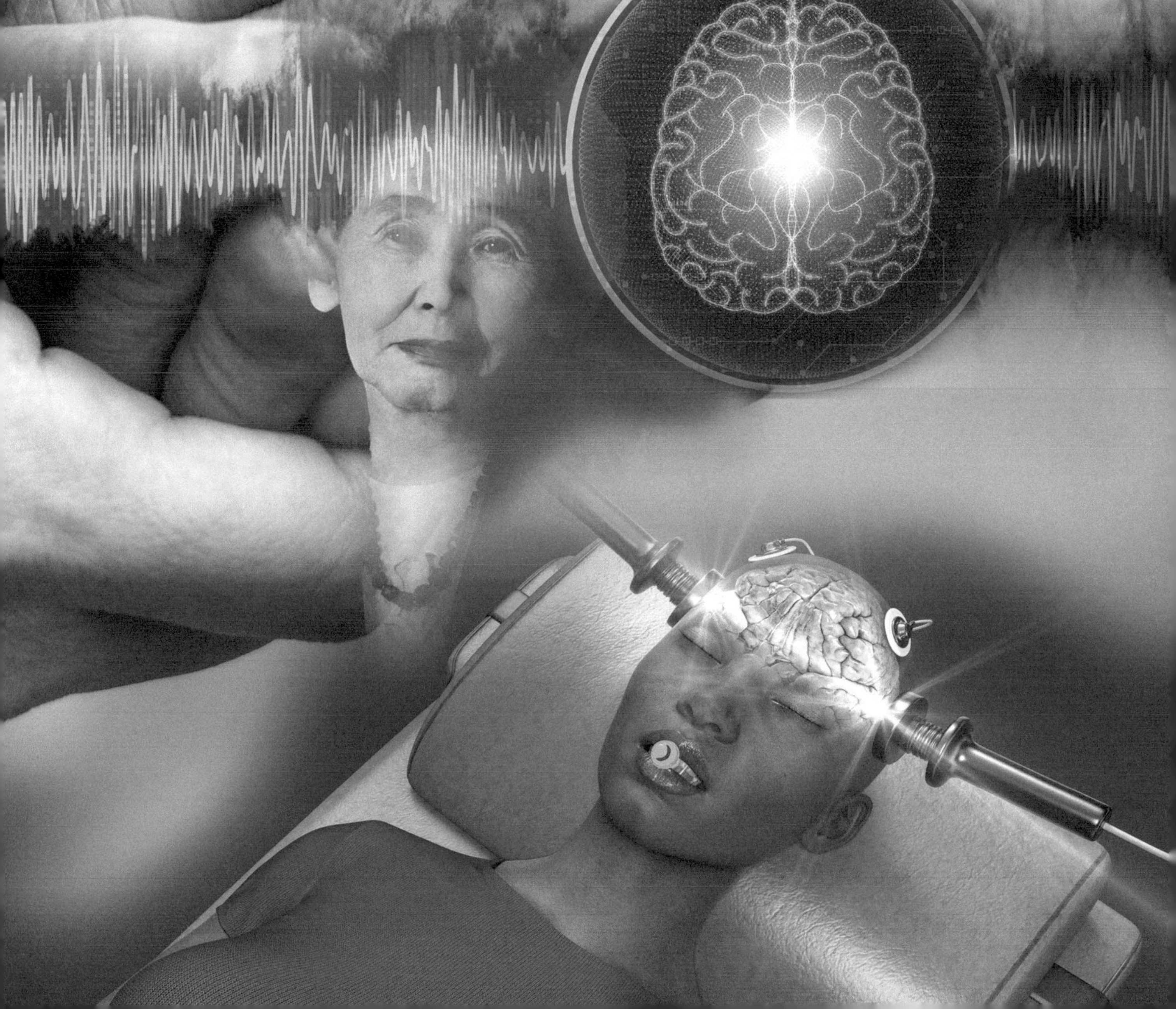

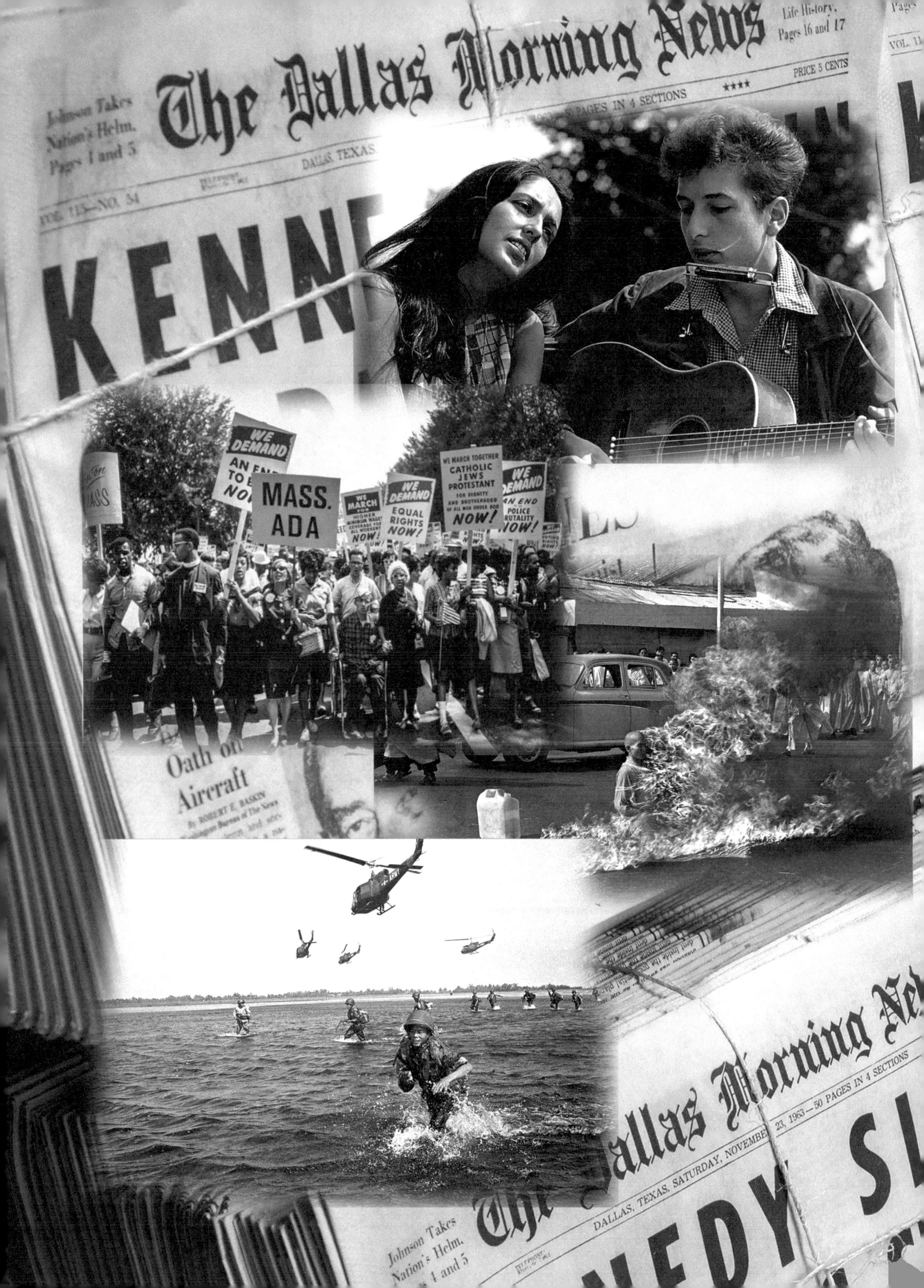

The Dallas Morning News
Life History, Pages 16 and 17
PRICE 5 CENTS
50 PAGES IN 4 SECTIONS
Johnson Takes Nation's Helm, Pages 1 and 5
DALLAS, TEXAS
KENNE
WE DEMAND
MASS. ADA
WE DEMAND EQUAL RIGHTS NOW!
WE MARCH TOGETHER CATHOLIC JEWS PROTESTANT FOR DIGNITY AND BROTHERHOOD OF ALL MEN UNDER GOD NOW!
WE DEMAND AN END POLICE BRUTALITY NOW!
Oath on Aircraft
By ROBERT E. BASKIN
DALLAS, TEXAS, SATURDAY, NOVEMBER 23, 1963—50 PAGES IN 4 SECTIONS
NEDY SL
Johnson Takes Nation's Helm,

Chapter 13

Back to Residency – Bottled Up Grief

I came back to San Francisco to resume my residency six months after I had taken a leave of absence. I was assigned to a different inpatient service, where ECT was administered on weekday mornings, and I observed electroconvulsive therapy for the first time. To be effective, a series of treatments is given, and soon I'd be expected to provide the treatment myself. It disturbed me to see an induced grand mal seizure, even under the best of conditions. I thought of my mother, knowing that this is what she endured against her will, and that I had given permission for it to be done. She had seen it done, and unlike other patients, would have suffered the anticipation of what was coming. Yet, it did work when nothing else had, and she was herself and with my father before he died.

That evening, I came back to the large, spacious flat in Sausalito, which I shared with Elaine Fedors and Carol Halpern. Elaine was there, and over a glass of wine, I began telling her about watching ECT, about the circumstances that led to it, and as I spoke I began to cry. Soon, I was sobbing and sobbing and sobbing. It felt as if the tears were coming up from the soles of my feet, as if a lid was taken off of a huge reservoir of tears. It was exhausting. I was wrung out and I went to bed, spent. Sleep put me back together again. The next morning, I woke up, went to work, functioned, and came back. My tears began again, though less deep than before. I had held myself together as long as I had been in Los Angles, and I was the responsible one. I had unexpressed grief that I didn't know that I carried until it began to pour out.

I think back to when I was the girl who cried at the "Lassie" movies or on watching "Bambi," or when I couldn't help but cry when I expressed myself, especially when I was hurt or angry and said so. How did I become the person who hadn't shed tears at my father's funeral, and didn't even know that I had bottled up all my grief, until it came pouring out? I think that this was a consequence of the education and training to be a woman doctor, and that it probably happens to most women who enter "alpha male professions." We learn what little boys are taught by expectations, by observation, by bullying and ridicule very early. "Boys don't cry." Women who work as doctors, officers, judges, politicians, and in other male-dominated roles aren't supposed to either. This is downside of having authority.

Since I learned firsthand about bottled up tears and sobbing them out, I could tell patients who feared that if they started crying, they'd never stop, that this is not what happens. When it is safe to do, walled off emotions do pour out. Afterwards you do feel that you are wrung out, but after that, there is more of you available—your psyche no longer expends energy keeping the lid on. I also was surprised at how fresh the tears are when they do come. It is as if the loss just happened. From my patients, I knew that unexpressed grief can be held in for years.

I also learned firsthand about anniversary reactions. I had made no effort to keep January 21, the day my Dad died, in my mind and the date was not one I consciously observed as it is in some religious or family traditions. However, I learned that an unconscious part of me kept track, when I found myself feeling sad for "no reason" in January the year following his death. The first time, I had to do some psychological detective work on myself to check out what this could be about. After which whenever I found myself in a sad mood in January, and checked the date, it usually was this anniversary reaction.

This delayed grief reaction that came up months later when it was safe, and anniversary recollections are experiences I can draw on as examples of "nothing goes to waste," which I have said about the practice of depth psychotherapy. Anything I have experienced or felt or even vividly imagined may someday help my empathic understanding of another person's psyche or situation.

Sustaining Friendships

Sometimes I hear myself humming a tune or a line from a song, or a poem comes into my mind. I welcome them like dreams, as comments from another part of myself. I caught myself doing this early one morning as I walked among the redwoods in Muir Woods. I had finished writing the previous chapter, ending it with my father's death and mention of the services that followed. I had the next chapter, this one, on my mind and was thinking about what to include. These thoughts soon disappeared from my mind in the presence of the trees that towered over me and sounds of water in the creek alongside of the path as it went through and over small stones and logs. In this meandering mode, the refrain from The Beatles song, "I get by with a little help from my friends" came to me. It got me thinking.

I have said nothing about what had sustained me through the perfect storm of crashing events, my father dying, my mother's breakdown, and my incapacitated brother to be sent home. I had the support of my good friend, Myrna Cramer. In her company, I took "time outs" which temporarily liberated my free spirit as we took to the road, drove to places, talked and laughed. This was sustenance I needed, a restorative respite from the front lines of family disaster. And then, afterward, the outpouring of held-in grief emerged in the sanctuary of coming back to the shared flat that was home and to my housemate-friend Elaine, with whom I could talk honestly and cry.

From my early teens on, friends have been there for me through summer camps, hard times, adventures, spiritual epiphanies, troubles I got into by speaking truth to power, medical school, internship, residency and later on, pilgrimages or advocacy. For all that I am independent and self-sufficient, can go off on my own to explore, write a book, or take on a cause which can get me in difficulties or bring recognition, I have been sustained by friendships, which I know on several different levels.

Most significant and precious are the few soul-depth friendships in which a bond was formed by deeply personal and meaningful conversation and experiences with one another over time. And, always when I thought back, there were many good friends with whom I shared a phase of life, like school days, summer camps, and college. In medical school and internship, my friends and I shared the stressful and rewarding experience of being a member of a tight group that learned together, saw life and death, and were initiated into a different life than our peers outside of medical training. In my mid-adult years after this, friendships took a backseat to the demands of this phase of life, and became significant once again in the last third of life.

Invisible (Mystical-Spiritual) Assistance

In this sad time for my father, mother and brother, I was the only one in the family still standing, so to speak. I had important decisions for them on my shoulders, but I didn't feel alone. I had invisible help. There was a mystical-spiritual something that kept me together. The words of Rodgers and Hammerstein's "You'll Never Walk Alone" song describe it:

> When you walk through a storm
> Keep your chin up high
> And don't be afraid of the dark. . .
> Walk on, walk on, with hope in your heart
> And you'll never walk alone!

This song reminds me of my connection to the invisible, to a soul sense that I am not alone that I first got as a Girl Scout in the mountains under the Milky Way, and later, when I felt a sense of profound gratitude and made the promise to become a doctor.

This spiritual certainty that I am not alone is a theme that was strengthened in medical school when the going was tough. I found my own private chapel, and while it was open twenty-four hours a day to everyone, I always found it empty. This was in the late 1950s into the early 1960s, when San Francisco felt safe, and there weren't homeless people on the streets or encampments under freeway ramps. Driving home late at night from San Francisco General, or taking a study break late at night, I'd sometimes go to sit or kneel in this small wooden chapel that was between the sidewalk and sidewall of Grace Cathedral. I pray when I need invisible help to stay true, to keep on keeping on, to have courage, and trust. There is something deeply sustaining about prayer or meditation as a communication with the invisible realms outside and inside of our small ego self. I know that when I notice myself singing "You'll never walk alone," that it has a very positive effect. I am amused and happy to get the message. I also have consciously sung the song to myself when I needed a little boost from the invisible world.

Training to be a Psychiatrist

I was in my psychiatric residency from 1963-1966, which was a creative time for new psychotherapies and the use and abuse of psychedelics. Haight-Ashbury, the intersection and a neighborhood made famous by hippies, was within walking distance of UCSF Medical Center and overlooked Golden Gate Park, where the Summer of Love events were held in 1967. LSD had not been outlawed and research was being done with it, and it was being used recreationally. The community mental health movement and the first generation of anti-psychotic drugs (the phenothiazines of which Thorazine was best known) were emptying institutions that had warehoused and kept psychotic people off the streets. With medications, patients could be treated in clinics close to their homes.

There were new and exciting treatments introduced to us at Langley Porter. Fritz Perls, the founder of Gestalt Therapy came and described what it was and its effectiveness in an auditorium talk, and then he did a demonstration group with residents, of which I was one. Virginia Satir, a hands-on founder of Family Therapy who lived with the family when she did therapy with them, came and talked. Thomas Forrest Main, the psychiatrist who had introduced therapeutic communities in mental hospitals in Scotland, came and influenced us to do them on wards at Langley Porter. We observed and learned about psychodrama from its founder. It was a new era and an exciting time to be in psychiatry, with innovative therapies and new effective medication.

In the course of the residency, I trained at San Francisco General Hospital, where I rotated through emergency, and the inpatient observation, and treatment wards. I was on the private practice service at UCSF, and at Langley Porter for inpatient, day treatment, and outpatient clinic. I had remarkably good training experiences in psychotherapy on the outpatient service where I saw patients for two years either part-time or fulltime. I had two continuous cases, outpatients that I saw twice a week in long term therapy with clinical supervision from analysts in private practice, each once a week, as well as having a caseload supervisor for the other patients I had, some on medications.

I was gravitating toward doing psychotherapy in a way that fit me. I was able to "try on" ways of working with patients and learned what worked for me by doing. The preeminent psychoanalytic Freudian model was to be a blank slate on which the patient could project and work through problems—often negative feelings toward parental figures, who had abandoned, belittled, or abused the patient. I'm not very good at being inexpressive. I also felt that being a blank slate, withholding positive responsiveness (such as mirroring or compassion or information) and emphasizing interpretations invited negative transferences, which could result in patients leaving therapy in anger, or giving up therapy entirely.

The Jungian premise was that a therapy relationship was like a chemical reaction between two elements, the patient and the doctor. Both were to be affected by the work. I found this to be true.

Every experience I had or felt through an empathic connection or identification—from reading fiction or biography, seeing films or documentaries, and certainly from every patient—added to my field of understanding, through listening with an open mind and heart. That I do this makes it possible for me to feel what someone whose gender, life experiences, sexual orientation, racial background, and age is different from my own. It also fits an aphorism from the Latin poet, Terrence, who said, "Nothing human is foreign to me." We humans share a collective unconscious, and we can tap into the shadow and the light of generic human experience. As a consequence, in all of us, feelings and thoughts can arise unbidden and come from beyond personal experience. It then is up to us whether we choose to tend and feed them with our attention or not. Therapy is a way of focusing, of examining, of helping people become compassionate toward themselves and others, and learning. In learning by doing, I was doing the same. Both doctor and patient are together in this "chemical" reaction.

I learned a lot from my patients, from clinical supervision, and in seminars. Most of the required clinical seminars were developmental and Freudian. Jungian analyst Joseph Wheelwright, MD, held a seminar once a week at lunchtime for anyone at LPPI interested in attending, which I did over three years, when I could. Once he brought his friend Erik Erickson, whose thoughts about the tasks of the stages of life made a major contribution to psychology and to my own thinking. Donald Sandner, MD, another Jungian analyst, was chief psychiatrist on one of the treatment wards that I rotated through at SF General. I met with David Allen, MD, a psychoanalyst, and John Talley, MD, a Jungian analyst, weekly for clinical supervision, to discuss my twice-a-week continuous cases, I was doing the work and seeing the psychology of each of my two patients, one as a Freudian would, the other as a Jungian. I was one of several residents who went with Harry Wilmer, MD, a Freudian psychoanalyst who was becoming a Jungian, to San Quentin Rehabilitation Center (then known as San Quention State Prison) to do group work with the incarcerated men who lived in a unit outside the walls of the prison itself in the year before they were released.

My introduction to C. G. Jung's ideas about the psyche became the foundation of my own work with patients, my writing and teaching. UCSF was the

only medical center in the United States at the time where I could have gotten supervision from Jungian analysts in a psychiatric residency. The C. G. Jung Institute of San Francisco was unique among American institutes in being founded by MDs, some of whom had analyzed with Jung. There were several on the clinical faculty at Langley Porter who volunteered time to supervise residents and were assigned randomly to new residents. I had found my way to a psychiatric residency at UCSF and once here, via more serendipity, synchronicity and grace, or so it felt, was introduced to Jungians and Jung, a psychology which valued spirituality, creativity and wholeness.

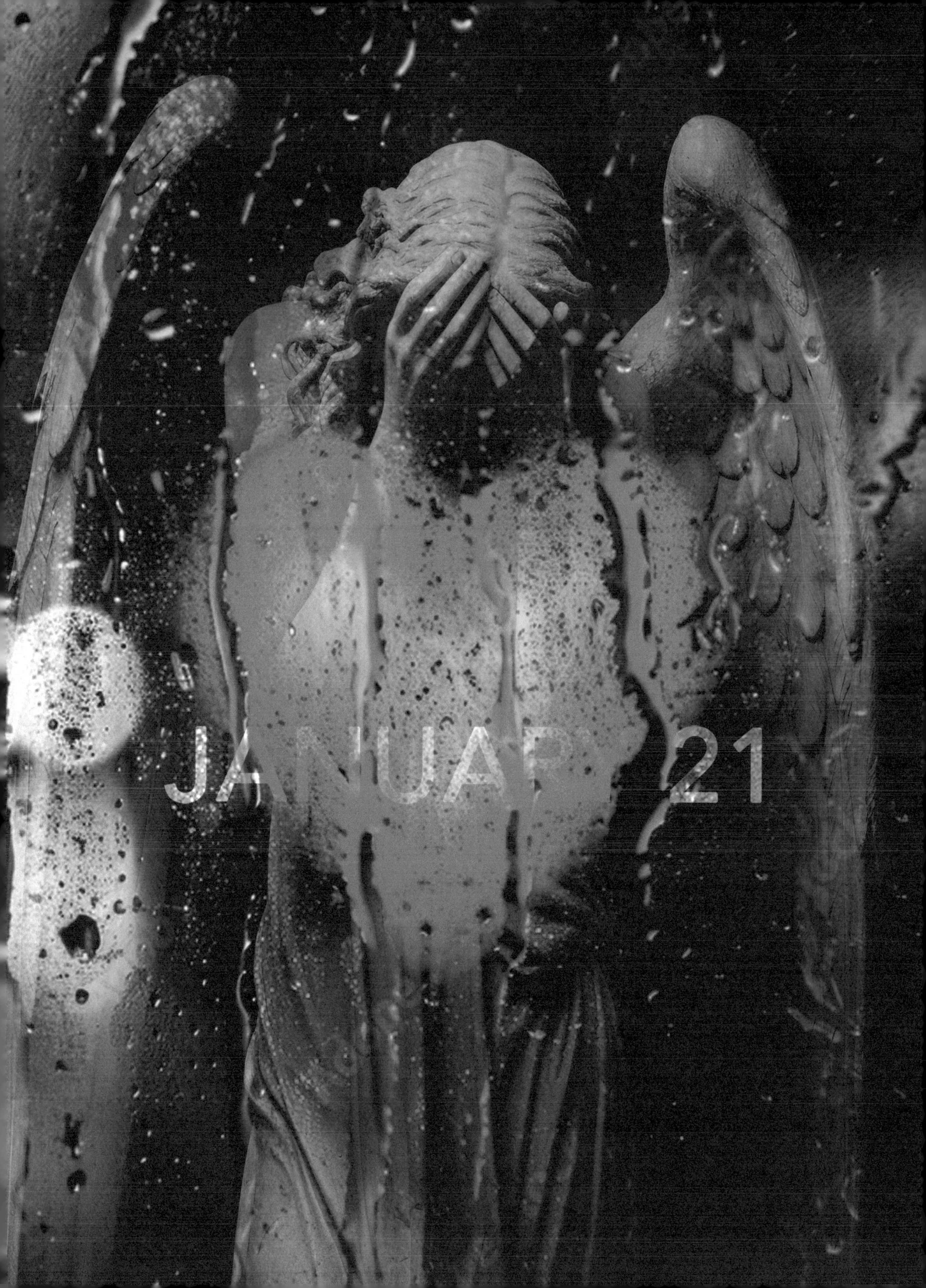
JANUAR
21

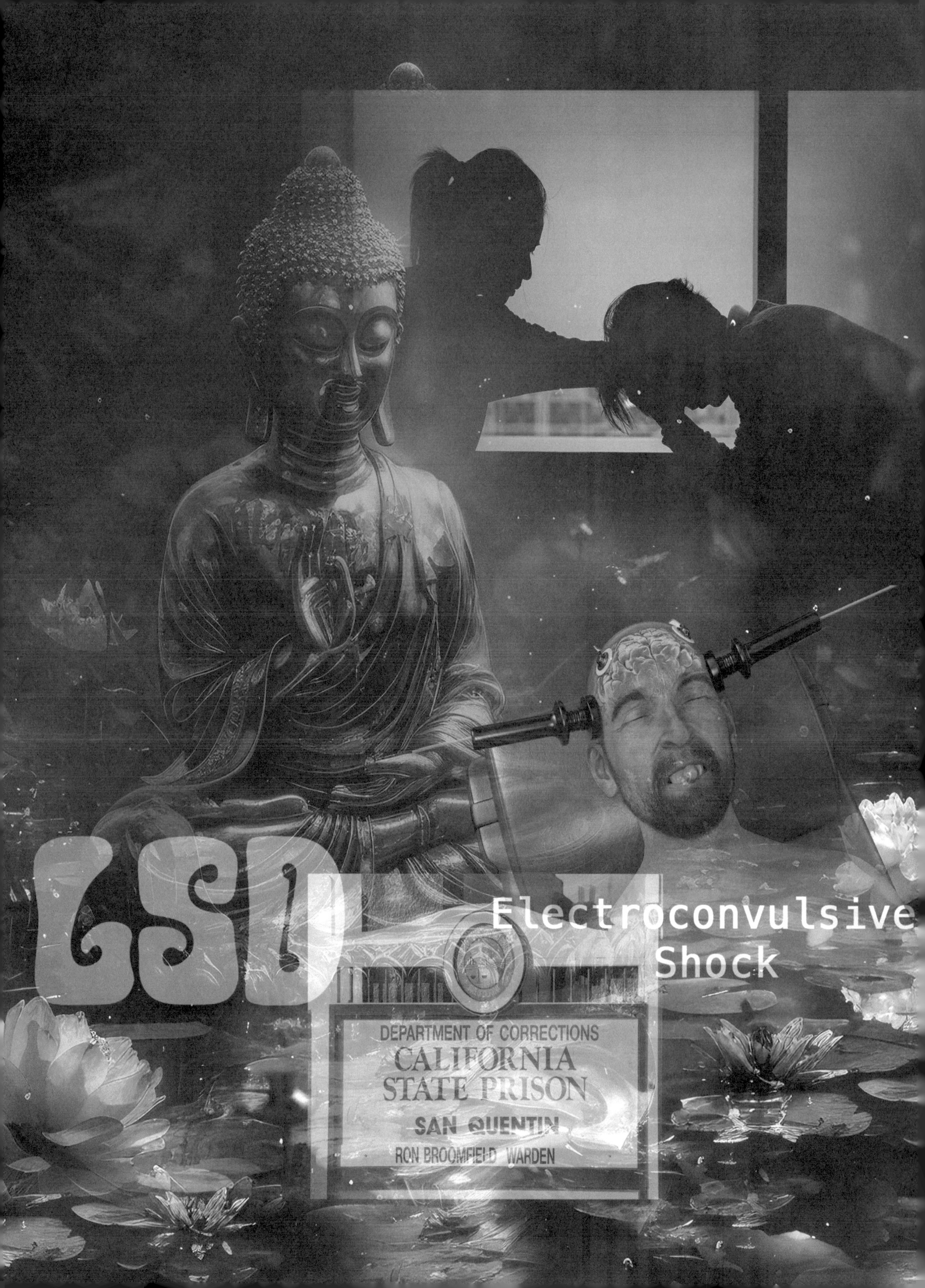

LSD

Electroconvulsive
Shock

DEPARTMENT OF CORRECTIONS
CALIFORNIA
STATE PRISON
SAN QUENTIN
RON BROOMFIELD WARDEN

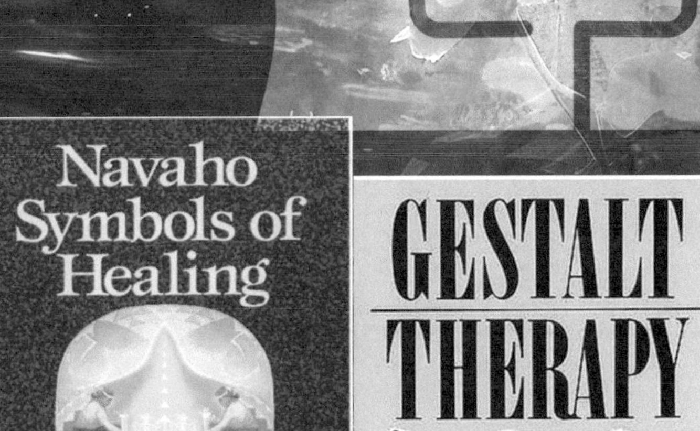
Navaho Symbols of Healing
A Jungian Exploration of Ritual, Image, & Medicine
DONALD SANDNER, M.D.
GESTALT THERAPY
Excitement and Growth in the Human Personality
FREDERICK PERLS
RALPH F. HEFFERLINE
PAUL GOODMAN
VIRGINIA SATIR
YOUR MANY FACES
THE FIRST STEP TO BEING LOVED
New Foreword by Mary Ann Norfleet, PhD

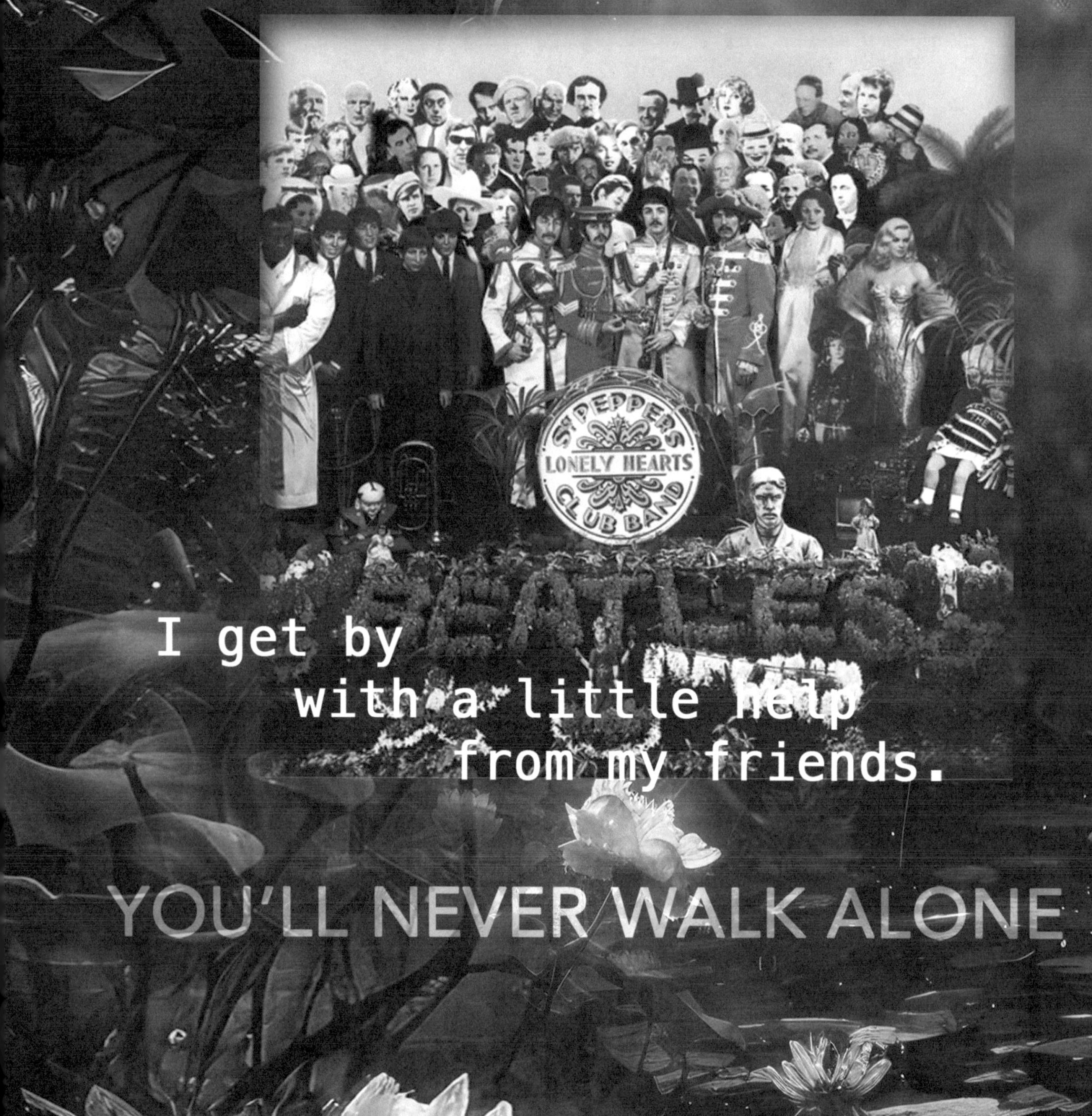

LONELY HEARTS
CLUB BAND
I get by
with a little help
from my friends.
YOU'LL NEVER WALK ALONE

Section 3

Marriage, Private Practice, Magazine, Motherhood, Jungian Institute

Chapter 14
Thanksgiving – Marriage – Feminism

Thanksgiving 1965 turned out to be a very special occasion at our stunning-view apartment in Sausalito. The idea for the Thanksgiving dinner was hatched by Dick Rawson to introduce his friend Arthur Viseltear to Elaine Fedors, my friend and housemate. Dick was a psychiatric resident, Elaine was an occupational therapist, and both were at UC Langley Porter. I had plans to be in Los Angeles for Thanksgiving until I found out the week before that I was on call on Friday after Thanksgiving. Shortly after this change in my plans, Dick ran into Jim Bolen. They had been Air Force buddies. Both had enlisted after high school and had lost track of each other after they left the service. Jim went from the Air Force to college and then into the business world, where he was an account executive with a PR firm in San Francisco. Dick went to college and then on to medical school and then into his current residency. Dick invited Jim to come for Thanksgiving to round out the party, which was where we met.

Arthur and Elaine were married early the next year. Jim and I married several months following their wedding. Even though Dick didn't marry his date, there was laughter and speculation later about how two weddings could have resulted: what was in the turkey? Synchronicity must have played a part. Jim had also planned to travel out of the area over the Thanksgiving weekend when work for a client required him to stay.

The dinner was festive and fun. Following our initial Thanksgiving get-together, Jim and I spent time that weekend with lots of conversation and spontaneity. We learned a lot about each other. Besides the mutual attraction, as we got to know about our respective journeys to where we now were, and our appreciation for each other grew. I liked that he was not intimidated by my MD. It was what I did, and it was interesting to him, which was a relief, since this was not always the case with men outside of medicine. Jim had signed up for the Air Force after graduating from high school and had been stationed in California. With the GI bill and his own efforts, he had graduated from San Jose State University, took a year of traveling in Europe before going to work for the PR firm. His grandparents on both sides had immigrated from Croatia to Iowa. The Croatians in Iowa, like the Japanese in California, kept their ethnic identity. His father was killed in an accident when he was about four, leaving his mother a widow with four children.

Jim had an ear for languages and music, which he had picked up on his own. It was an ability that made him able to say words in other languages and sound like a native. When he traveled in Europe he was often assumed to be a European, not an American. While on the Spanish island of Ibiza on the Mediterranean he impressed a famous flamenco guitarist who offered to be his teacher if he stayed to learn from him for a year, which Jim didn't take up. My musical tin ear (I can sound pretty good only by singing next to someone carrying the tune, otherwise I'm likely to go off-key) made me appreciate what came so naturally to him.

Though we had known each other for only about four months, the evening he proposed, I intuitively knew he would. Tradition has it that the man proposes, and we women of the silent generation were very traditional and waited for him to do so. The man has had time to think about it, get a ring, and arrive at the decision. The woman is on the receiving end—sometimes the proposal is a surprise, sometimes it never comes. The asking and the response, when the answer is yes,, is a moment of commitment. Jim asked, and even though I had anticipated it, I paused. I felt a sense of gravity—it was in retrospect, an archetypal moment. It brings Hecate the ancient Greek Goddess of the Crossroad to mind. *Yes or no?* It's not that

I thought with my mind where a yes or a no would take me. It was a significant pause before saying yes because it felt momentous to me.

In ancient Greece, when a traveler arrived at a major fork in the road, he might find a statue or pillar with three faces. One faced the road that brought him here, and the other two looked down separate paths. Which path to choose? Hecate was a pre-Olympian deity, who was at the threshold between day and night, between upper world and underworld. She could see past, present, and future. She is also considered the archetype of the midwife who attends births and deaths. A marriage proposal can be considered a Hecate moment as well. Saying yes to marriage means an end to a phase of life and the birth of a new identity.

The summer before the fateful Thanksgiving dinner, I had been accepted to finish my psychiatric residency at the Payne Whitney Clinic in New York City. In the works was an application for a fellowship at St. Bartholomew's in London to follow. I didn't weigh this option at all after the knowledge (gnosis) came to me that Jim was going to propose. By saying yes, I was taking the road where marriage would lead me, to where an inner compass directed me. Retrospectively, I wonder if my biological clock was subliminally ticking. I know that it was not a conscious consideration. I wasn't baby oriented.

James Bolen was thirty-one and I was twenty-nine when we married on May 21, 1966, at Grace Cathedral. We met with the Canon of the Cathedral who would marry us. Neither of us were Episcopalians: I had been baptized in the Presbyterian Church, and Jim was raised Catholic. We didn't have religious issues, it was a relief to not have to rehash the Reformation again (while I was in medical school, marriage had come up with another Jim, also a Catholic, and religion was the issue). Jim teased that the Episcopalian Church recognized his confirmation, but not mine. My baptism counted as one of two sacraments recognized by Protestants. The other is the Eucharist or Holy Communion. These for Episcopalians are the two great sacraments, with five lesser sacramental rites. Marriage was a sacramental rite. In this Episcopalian ceremony, our mutual vows were to "love, honor, and cherish." "Cherish" replaced the once usual "obey" which was said by the woman, not the man.

My mother was happy to come and not be involved in planning either the wedding or the reception. She helped out with the one hitch that came up. Daniel Shinoda, my father's youngest brother, and a minister in the Holiness church, objected to having champagne served at the reception. My physician mother ran interference, talked with him, and he came to the wedding anyway. My uncle Mits walked me down the aisle. He is the uncle who had been an intern in NYC at the time of the forced evacuation and had gotten papers from Mayor LaGuardia's office so we could leave California, avoiding the concentration-relocation camps— Mitsuya Yamaguchi, MD. My attendants were Elaine Fedors Viseltear, my now married former housemate, Kay Hessen Hensley, my friend from high school who was with me at Forest Home when I made the decision to become a doctor, and Liz Hutchinson, from my medical school days. Ours was a big wedding in the main sanctuary. I remember feeling the solemnity of walking down the aisle on my uncle's arm to Jim, and then smiling and practically skipping as we held hands and went out.

The ceremony itself was witnessed by everyone there, but something invisible, subjective, and numinous happened in or to me as Canon of the Cathedral, who was officiating, performed it. Marriage is a sacrament in the Episcopalian church as it is in the Catholic church. I had not expected to feel what I did; it was energy-divinity-grace, a blessing-whump, "ineffable" is the proper word. I expected to be married for life, but not for religious reasons. It just was what marriage meant and had meant for generations. I was the first person on either side of my family to marry someone who was not Japanese.

We inherited the apartment in Sausalito. Elaine had moved to Los Angeles. Our third housemate, Myrna Cramer, who became Marriam Ring after she chose the name Marriam and then married Al Ring, and who was my best friend in high school, left for New York. My psychiatric residency was extended through December 1966 because of the six month leave of absence that I had taken in my first year.

I was now thirty, married, and expected that children would come next. At the time, marriage and children went together. Choice had to do with when, rather than if. Given my age, "soon" would not be too far off. This was when I had the opportunity to take pure Sandoz LSD (Lysergic Acid Diethylamide) under the best of circumstances—mellow surroundings, music, and a handful of friends. I was cautious about its effects on my chromosomes that might affect being a birth mother and so I declined the opportunity.

I knew that LSD could have positive effects in the treatment of alcoholism and on the fears of people who were dying. I knew from what I had read, and from people at Langley Porter and San Francisco General who told me that LSD could bring about mystical and beautiful experiences. But I also saw many who had experienced "bad trips," and needed anti-psychotic meds, sometimes long after the effects of the drug would have worn off. I also knew that people who had positive experiences often seemed to forget them, much as many people do who don't remember their dreams.

Digression re LSD
LSD and its Effects between 1943-1968 until it became Illegal

In April 1943, Albert Hofmann, a chemist working for Sandoz in Basel, Switzerland, synthesized LSD and accidentally experienced "an uninterrupted stream of fantastic pictures, extraordinary shapes with intense, kaleidoscope play of colors," which lasted two hours. Research began in Switzerland and Harvard. Between 1950-1960, hundreds of papers were published discussing LSD, which included its use in treatment for alcoholism, Humphrey Osmund's work, Aldous Huxley's experience of taking LSD for the first time in 1955, and reports from the First International Conference on LSD Therapy (April 1959) held at Princeton, NJ. In 1960, Timothy Leary established the Psychedelic Research Project at Harvard. LSD began to appear on the streets on sugar cubes in 1963. Timothy Leary and Richard Alpert were then later fired by Harvard. The Second International Conference on the Use of LSD in Psychotherapy and Alcoholism was held at South Oaks Hospital, Amityville, NY, in May 1963.

In October 1966, possession of LSD became illegal in California. Sandoz Pharmaceutical recalled LSD in April 1966 and withdrew sponsorship of research. The Summer of Love (1967) was held in San Francisco. In October 1968, possession became a federal crime. In October 1970, most known hallucinogens (LSD, psilocybin, psilocin, mescaline, peyote, cannabis, & MDA) were criminalized under the Comprehensive Drug Abuse and Control Act.

Since then, I've heard many people speak about their extraordinary moments, experiences while awake or in dreams, or through hallucinogens, music, or shamanic experiences that did or did not affect them afterwards. I had my own profound non-drug-induced extraordinary state of consciousness initially at summer camp in my adolescence, after which I knew I was not alone in a meaningless universe. Later, I felt in communion with whatever God is and unaware of the divinity of gender. These and later subjectively felt profound soul experiences were major events in my life. They stuck with me. I knew them to be soul experiences.

Sometimes, people in analysis recall such events in the past or have current dreams that convey the depth and mystery of such events. I am aware how some especially meaningful words are inadequate, are more like symbols themselves than simple definitions, such as *soul, archetype, mystery, mystical* or *numinous*. Yet I also know from experience, that once there is a vocabulary, it's possible to retrieve past events for which there was otherwise no vocabulary. These come from beyond our previous or personal experience, drawing information that is transpersonal from the collective unconsciousness.

I think that the collective unconscious can be compared to the internet, which holds everything put into it. Or to the ocean from which moisture rises, becomes clouds, rains, then via lakes, streams, and rivers gathers everything that erodes into or falls into or is thrown into water and flows back to the sea. Whether in bytes, bits or molecules, everything that ever was may then be a latent possibility that can come up in a dream or in the imagination when something stimulates the collective memory of our species. Maybe this works like a browser that finds more than we think we are searching for, taking us back to a much earlier source.

The personal unconscious, mine for example, might hold whatever has come into my mind, much as this happens on a computer screen and been even momentarily on the desktop, like something seen but not consciously saved by me. The personal and the collective unconscious overlap one another. As a result, archetypal images come up in personal dreams beyond the personal experience of the dreamer. Or, a dream remembered from the past may now provide the symbols with which a current situation can be grasped.

My friend Valerie Andrews had a dream in her childhood that she had not forgotten. In the dream, a lion pinned her down, scaring her but not harming her. It was a lion that could not roar. Five decades later, she developed a throat problem and recalled the dream again. She thought about the meaning of a lion that cannot roar, as a metaphor. She thought of having words stuck in her throat, of not expressing a difference of opinion or when how often she swallowed her anger. Might the lion who could not roar be her unexpressed power of expression or a symbol of her latent power?

Feminism: I am a Woman. Hear Me Roar!

The lion in Valerie's dream led me to recall an aphorism from the early days of Feminism, "I am a Woman, Hear Me Roar!" Being silenced is the plight of women in traditional patriarchal cultures and relationships, which means that anger and power are then only expressed by men.

Feminism is a movement to liberate women's voices, feelings, talents, intelligence and observations, which began fairly recently in the United States when women sought the right to vote. Gaining suffrage brought about political equality at the ballot box after close to seventy years of effort (1848-1920). Equality in the workplace and in relationships were goals sought in the second wave of feminism which began in the mid-1960s. "The problem with no name" was described by Betty Friedan in *The Feminine Mystique* (1963) and struck a nerve. Women were supposed to be fulfilled by marriage and children, and while there were women who were content with being "Mrs. Him" and "the mother of," there were many others with all the advantages of suburbia who were depressed, and felt guilty for not being happy when they "had it all." At the same time, the first National Commission on the Status of Women (1963) published its findings: women were paid less than men for doing the same work, were not promoted, and were discriminated against entering many fields.

It does seem that women now can and do enter professions and roles that most couldn't before. While efforts toward gender equality have been growing, there is a greater lack of racial equality that is being brought into consciousness and culture, as well as the right to same-sex relationships and marriages. It did seem that the American culture was moving toward equality for men and women, with women increasingly entering leadership positions in the twenty-first and second decade. Then, in 2022, the Supreme Court of the United States overturned Roe v. Wade, which for fifty years was the legal principle for women to decide for themselves whether to bear children or not. While the opposition intends to keep women down—in their inferior place—efforts to do so have had the opposite effect in the United States with increasing gender education, equality, and choice.

While I was a psychiatry resident (1963-1966) the women's movement was entering my consciousness mostly through the news, reading, and sometimes through a woman patient. Women's movement events were not taking place in San Francisco, or weren't considered newsworthy until later. We were the center of the hippie movement which incorporated the sexual revolution/free love, rock and roll, drugs, and the Peace Movement, with the ever-present peace symbol on flags and Volkswagen buses.

The 1960s in the United States was a time of social unrest, protest, and growth of infectious ideas. Significant historical events took place: the assassination of JFK (1964), the Civil Rights Movement with the march from Montgomery to Selma (1965), the assassination of Martin Luther King, Jr. and Robert Kennedy (1968), and the Vietnam War protests (which began in 1964 and didn't end until the US withdrew troops in 1973).

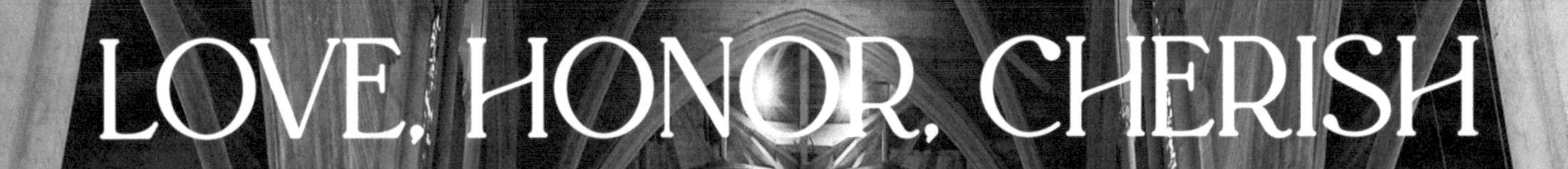
LOVE, HONOR, CHERISH
DELL
75c
THE YEAR'S MOST CONTROVERSIAL BESTSELLER
The Feminine Mystique
BETTY FRIEDAN
"The book we have been waiting for ... the wisest, sanest, soundest, most understanding and compassionate treatment of contemporary American woman's greatest problem...a triumph."
—ASHLEY MONTAGU

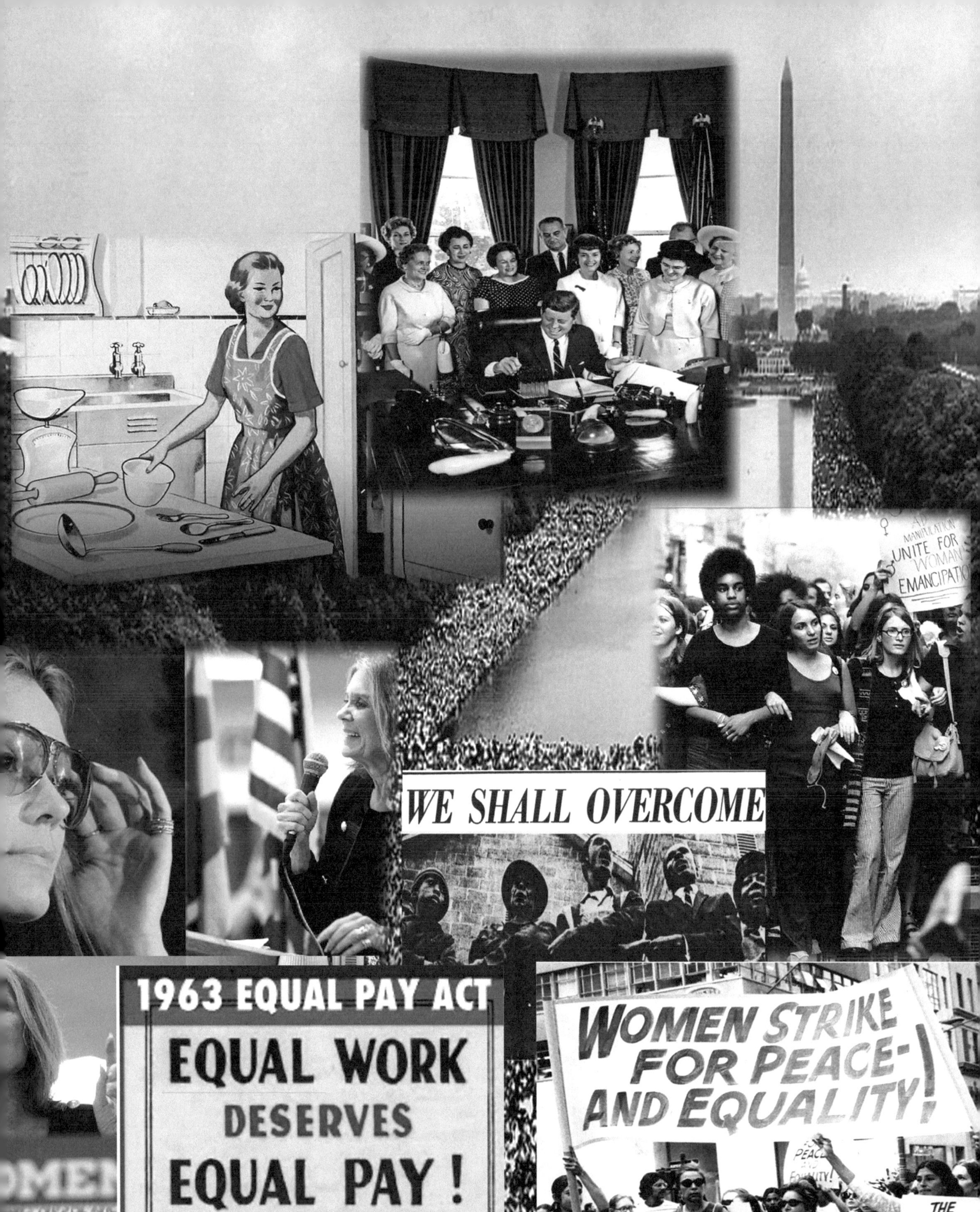
AD
MANIPULATION
UNITE FOR
WOMAN
EMANCIPATIO
WE SHALL OVERCOME
1963 EQUAL PAY ACT
EQUAL WORK
DESERVES
EQUAL PAY !
1963
WOMEN STRIKE
FOR PEACE-
AND EQUALITY!
I'M NO
BREEDEF
FOR THE
MAN'S WA
SISTERHOOD
IS POWERFUL-
END THE WAR!
THE
WOMEN O
VIETNAM
ARE OUR
SISTERS

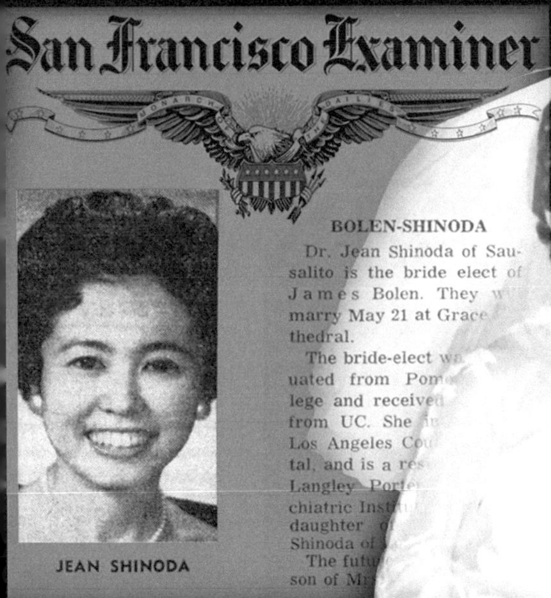

San Francisco Examiner

BOLEN-SHINODA

Dr. Jean Shinoda of Sausalito is the bride elect of James Bolen. They w marry May 21 at Grace thedral.

The bride-elect wa uated from Pom lege and received from UC. She Los Angeles Co tal, and is a res Langley Porte chiatric Insti daughter o Shinoda of

The futu son of M

JEAN SHINODA

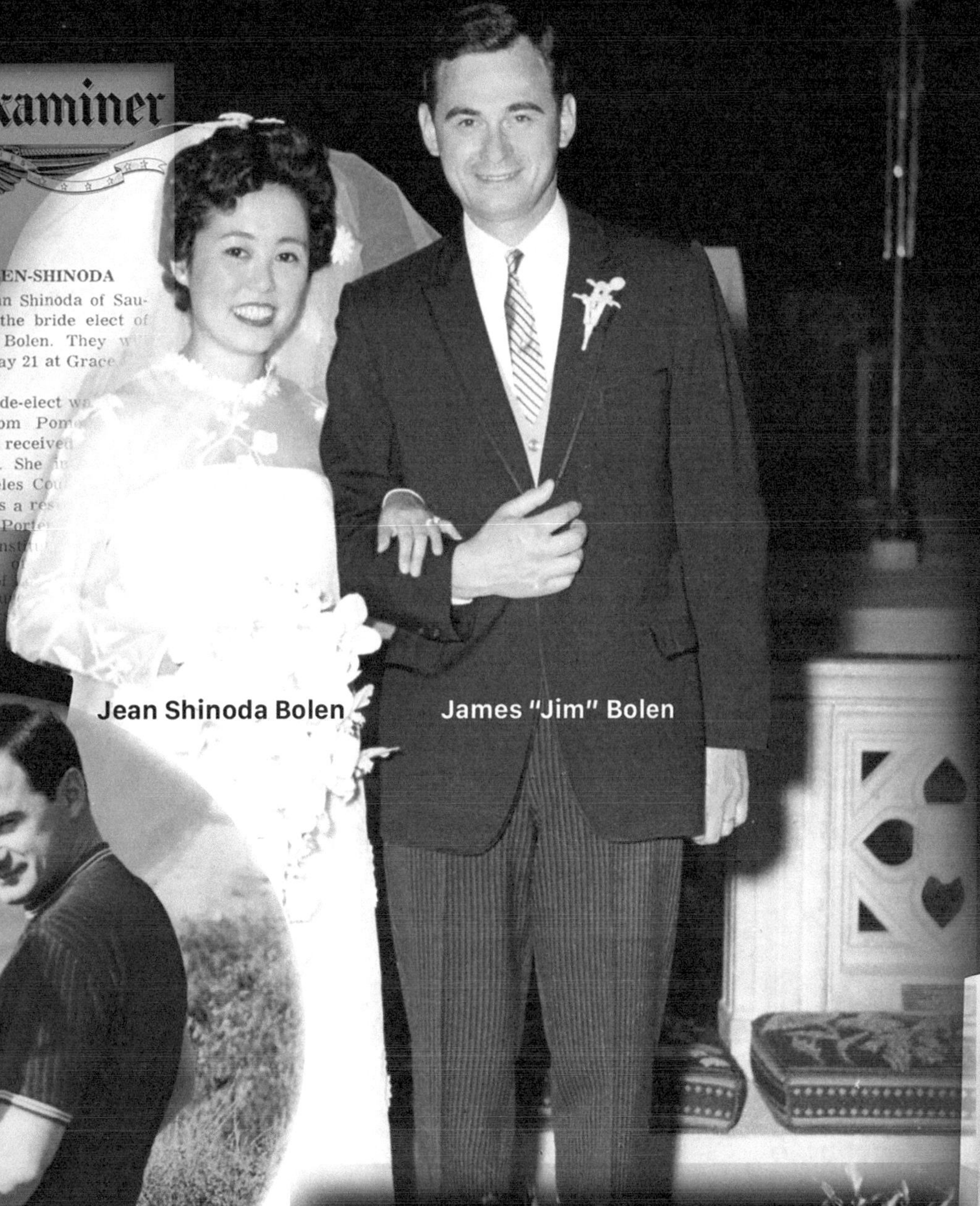

Jean Shinoda Bolen

James "Jim" Bolen

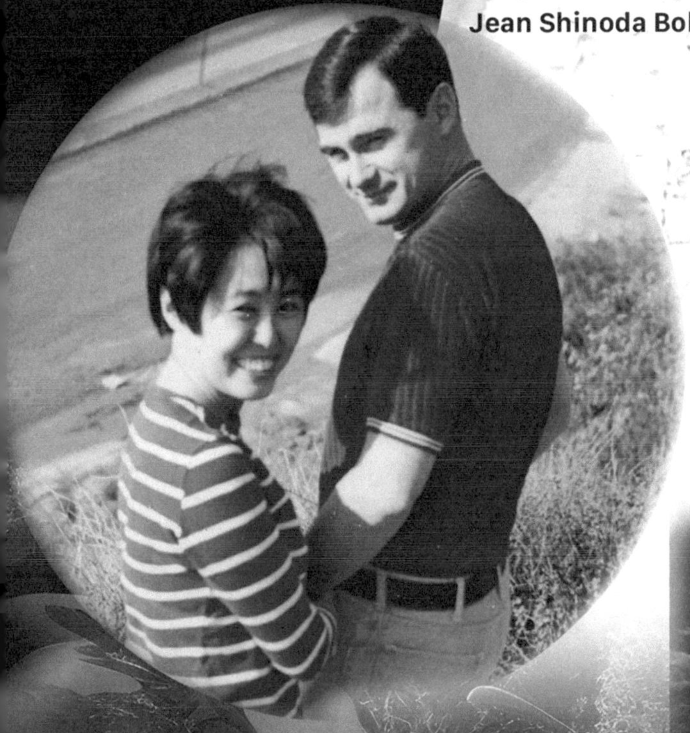

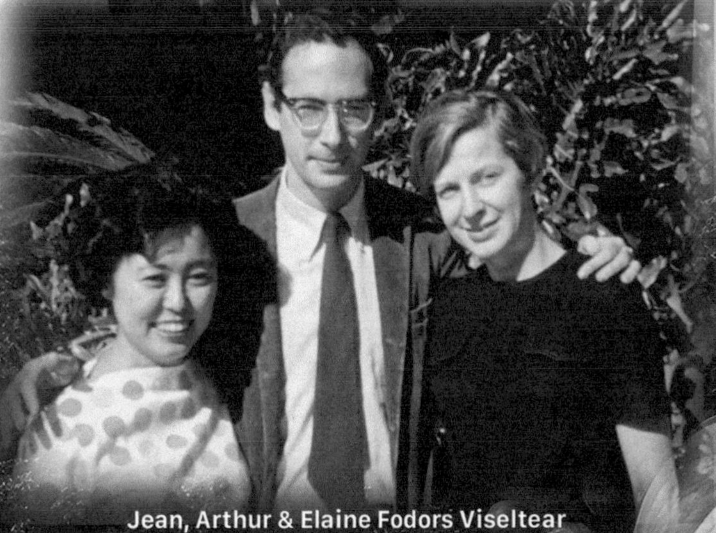

Jean, Arthur & Elaine Fodors Viseltear

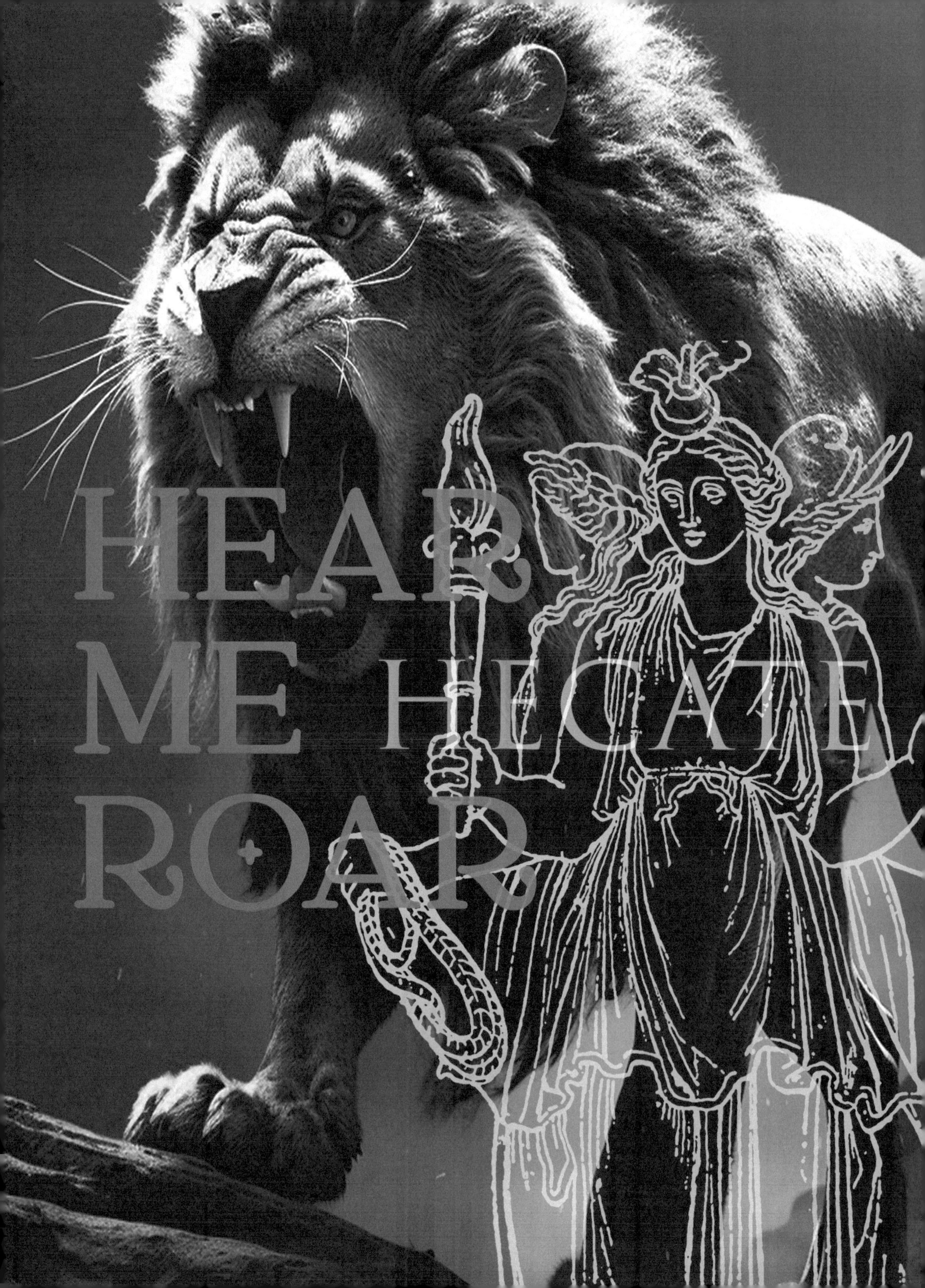
HEAR
ME
ROAR
HECATE

Chapter 15

Psychic Magazine - Psychic People

Before we had children, Jim and I used to say that *Psychic Magazine* was our first child. It had been conceived in conversations in the first years of our marriage, after I had graduated from my residency, began private practice, and was doing work I loved. Jim was not happy writing for clients of the Public Relations firm he worked for, especially when the latest and most important client wanted to fill more of San Francisco Bay to build on. He liked what he did, he just didn't like to put his writing and ideas to use for people or causes he didn't believe in. It was something I fully could understand. After conversations about what he would like to write about and promote, the subject became psychic phenomena, a long-time interest of his, and a field where there were no quality publications. On one of our first dates, he took me to see a stage performer who mixed psychic phenomena with hypnosis. It reminded me of some of my own family history.

As the nineteenth century was turning into the twentieth century, before my grandfather (Minosuke Yamaguchi) married, started a family and went to medical school in Cleveland, Ohio, he had drawn large audience to his lectures and demonstrations of hypnosis in Japan. He was interested in the new field of psychology that had beginnings in hypnosis. He attended the 1909 Clark University lectures at which both Freud and Jung spoke. The two had travelled by ship together to introduce psychoanalysis to America. My grandfather was psychic himself. My mother told me about the dream he would have when someone he knew in Japan had died. The person would come to him in a dream carrying a suitcase. At breakfast, grandpa would tell the family that so and so had died—he had the dream. Weeks later, mail would come via ship from Japan with the confirmatory news. This was a family story and was apparently indisputably true.

My father had created a trust to take care of my brother as long as he lived. I could draw a percentage of it from it annually, which I did, and let it accumulate, since the residency had paid enough for rent and other expenses. This could be needed capital. Plus, I was working and believed in Jim and his vision and ambition to start a magazine. With his skills and hard work, I believed he could make it happen. In the beginning exploration phase, we often went together to meet the prominent people in the field, the psychics and the researchers, to build relationships and credibility. Jim met and engaged a publication consultant, opened an office, found writers in the field, and worked with an artist to design the magazine. It would be the first high-quality, slick paper, four-color publication in the world on this subject. It would be a magazine called *Psychic*. The logo had an image of a dove above the name. The first issue came out in 1969.

The magazine was being envisioned and then established about the same time as I entered the Jungian institute as a candidate to become an analyst. The two interests—psychic and psychological—were compatible in Jungian thought. Jung's first writing and research was about his mediumistic cousin. Volume 1 of C. G. Jung's *Collected Works* opens with Jung's dissertation for the medical degree: "On the Psychology and Pathology of So-called Occult Phenomena" (1902). "Synchronicity: An Acausal Connecting Principle" (1952) was based on what he had observed for thirty years before writing this definitive work. He had coined the word "synchronicity" in 1930 for coincidences that were connected by their meaning and could not be explained by cause and effect.

Many synchronicities can be considered psychic phenomena and have parapsychological names. Dreams, such as those my grandfather would get when someone he knew had died, were events that happened at a distance and later verified, was a form of *telepathy.* Knowledge of something that is happening at that very moment is *clairvoyance.* Knowledge of what will happen in the future is *precognition,* and hearing a voice that informs or warns about something that is true is *clairaudience.* What makes any of these events a synchronicity is that the message is meaningful, affirms a connection, or feels like a divine intervention. Sometimes, the receiver feels like a beneficiary of grace.

There are numerous anecdotes about such things that science dismisses because such events are not replicable under observation. They are spontaneous examples of Extrasensory Perception (ESP), words coined by J. B. Rhine to describe the apparent ability of some people to acquire information without the use of the known (five) senses. He also adopted the term "parapsychology" to distinguish his interests from mainstream psychology. His experimental research done at Duke University established a scientific basis for the existence of ESP. I went to Durham to interview J.B. Rhine for *Psychic Magazine* at Rhine's insistence that the interview be conducted by someone with professional credentials. This is how I met him and his co-researcher wife, Dr. Louisa E. Rhine.

Rhine's experimental work in Durham, North Carolina on ESP, and that done at Stanford Research Center (SRI) on psychokinesis (PK)—the ability to move objects with mental effort—means that skeptics can't dismiss claims as impossible. I like that ESP and PK have been established scientifically, even though it wasn't an issue for me. More interesting to me were stories about people who had these abilities and how they used them. One source was Shafica Karagulla, MD, a neuropsychiatrist, who wrote *Breakthrough to Creativity* (1940) in which she observed subjects with these parapsychological (or paranormal) abilities, described what and how they got information, checked accuracy when possible.

Psychiatry does seem to accept poltergeist phenomenon as real, in which objects move—not in very small increments which happens in the laboratory but through the air and even through walls, as observed by German parapsychologist Hans Bender in southern Bavaria in the late 1960s. It is inexplicable how it happens, but what is known is that a psychologically disturbed adolescent or child is present when it does.

I witnessed Uri Geller, a noted Israeli psychic and stage performer, take our thick, brass Schlage house key, touch it, and with minimal muscle effort, bend it. Then Jim took the key and traced the angle of the bend on paper. It sat there with no one touching it, and when traced again, it had bent more, as if carrying further Geller's intention that it bend on its own. Geller was a performer who regularly bent spoons. I took what he did with our house key to be an exceptional human ability, a talent or gift that he had honed. I was glad to have my mind expanded to consider that this could be a latent ability in some or in a few humans. Exposure to non-ordinary gifts and realities of people with special gifts expanded my range of thought about what is possible.

I have no problem believing that thought and emotion can have an effect on living things: people, animals, and plants. Healers, horse-whisperers, and green thumb gardeners have talents that are, broadly speaking, also examples of PK (psychokinesis)—of the mind's effect on matter. My intuition, however, is that it is heart rather than mind that is responsible; that it is love that heals, calms, nourishes, and encourages growth in living matter. If it could be measured, I'd wager that psychotherapists who love what they do, and who love the people who are their clients and help them to bloom, would validate this same principle.

I was a candidate at the Jungian Institute and a psychiatrist in private practice when *Psychic Magazine* was launched in 1969. My medical and psychiatric training covered neuroanatomy and neurology, which I first studied as a medical student, then again for the California medical licensing exam, and a third time to become Board certified in Psychiatry and Neurology. I learned about brain structure and nerve systems, its specific functions, connections, neurotransmitters, synapses, the effect of drugs and hormones on them, and the effects of disease, trauma, and aging. I learned about mental illness—that the major psychotic illnesses (manic-depressive psychosis and schizophrenia) often had a genetic component, and that the neuroses usually had its origins in childhood. I learned of inevitable and rare inheritable dementia and dementias caused by diseases or poisons. We studied the brain and the body, which defined a person. Consciousness was a function of the brain, and perception came through the five senses: sight, hearing, smell, taste, and touch, each of which has a specific organ that is connected to a specific part of the brain.

There was no place for metaphysical or spiritual notions (like soul or for the possibility of reincarnation and previous lives, or out-of-body experiences, or ESP) in medicine or psychiatry as I was taught. To consider that there could be truth in these ideas and that the stories people relate about them are true, is a good thing—for a psychiatrist.

The most common challenge for me was how to relate to the voices people hear. I had two perspectives to draw from: the psychiatric and the psychic. With knowledge of both, I don't jump to conclusions. I'm curious and receptive: beginning with "What is the voice saying?" Then, "'Who' is speaking?" Then, "Under what circumstances?" From what I have learned, it's like experiences with real people: You try to get away from those voices that are accusatory or ranting. Other voices are good company that you wouldn't mind hearing from time to time.

Just because you "hear a voice" doesn't make the message true or the listener crazy. It depends. I know psychologically healthy people who hear voices occasionally. One hears her grandmother's voice (she died decades ago), another sometimes has conversations with her brother who died when both of them were in their twenties; she is now approaching seventy. These are voices of specific people who loved them when they were alive, and now are on the other side. Sometimes a voice is a companion. Some children hear the voice of a wise adult when the adults in their lives might be alcoholic, absent, or abusive. Some adults who are alone are not lonely because of the voice that accompanies them.

There also are voices in people's heads that drive them crazy, or vice-versa. Their hallucinations are symptoms of schizophrenia and they are tormented by these voices. Therapy with someone they grow to trust and medications make it possible to get their minds free of these voices. I thought of the phenothiazines as "ego glue" rather than as anti-psychotics, because strengthening the ego's ability to function effectively and not be overwhelmed could then happen. It helps to not pay attention to these hallucinations, because attention makes them grow stronger. Having something else to focus on also helps. I am remembering a woman with schizophrenia who came for help after her usual meds no longer were enough; the tormenting voices overcame her after her television set broke down.

In the psychic realm, there are mediums who claim that they channel distinct personalities, some from the other side, others much more esoteric. Some mediums are awake when this personality comes through, others, like Edgar Cayce (1877-1925), the most famous and recorded of them all, dropped into a trance state when he spoke. He became famous as "The Sleeping Prophet," which was also the title of his biography by Jess Stearn. The Association for Research and Enlightenment (A.R.E.) in Virginia Beach has 14,306 of his transcribed readings which cover a remarkable range of subjects. Cayce was a Christian mystic, yet in trance spoke about reincarnation, astrology, Akashic records, medical diagnosis and treatments, ancient civilizations, meditation, and ESP. His readings have been followed to document retrocognition (knowledge of the ancient past that was not known at the time and discovered to be true) and precognition (or prophecy), with potential that future events could validate more of his readings.

I met Dr. Bill and Dr. Gladys (William McGarey, MD & Gladys McGarey, MD), the two physicians who founded the A.R.E. Clinic in Phoenix, Arizona, around the time they began the clinic in 1970, which had a relationship connection to the Cayce work. They and others co-founded the American Holistic Medical Association.

Allopathic medicine refers to standard medical and surgical approach to diagnosis and treatment of patients and the prescribing of pharmaceuticals. Complementary medicine, or alternative medicine, or integrative medicine, or holistic medicine (the names are somewhat interchangeable) add or differ on treatment, based on differing philosophies about sickness and wellness that I was and have been receptive to learning about. In the usual psychiatric-allopathic medical model of mental illness, a person who hears voices or has visions is schizophrenic or is taking a hallucinogen. A person who dissociates and can't remember what he or she said or did has amnesia, or an alcoholic blackout, or could be a multiple personality, which is a symptom of a very disturbed personality. Edgar Cayce dissociated. He also was an upstanding citizen, husband, and father, whose readings helped and healed and continue to provide information that is used and referred to even now.

We often cannot know the source of psychic or spiritual information, but we can know if the information is helpful and whether tapping into non-ordinary experiences feel like soul experiences. When so, there is an expansion of positive qualities such as a sense of meaning, generosity of spirit, and joy. There is truth in "By their fruits you will know them," as written in Matthew 7:15-20.After speaking to his father's ghost, Hamlet said to Horatio, the model of rationality: "There are more things in heaven and earth, than are dreamt of in your philosophy."

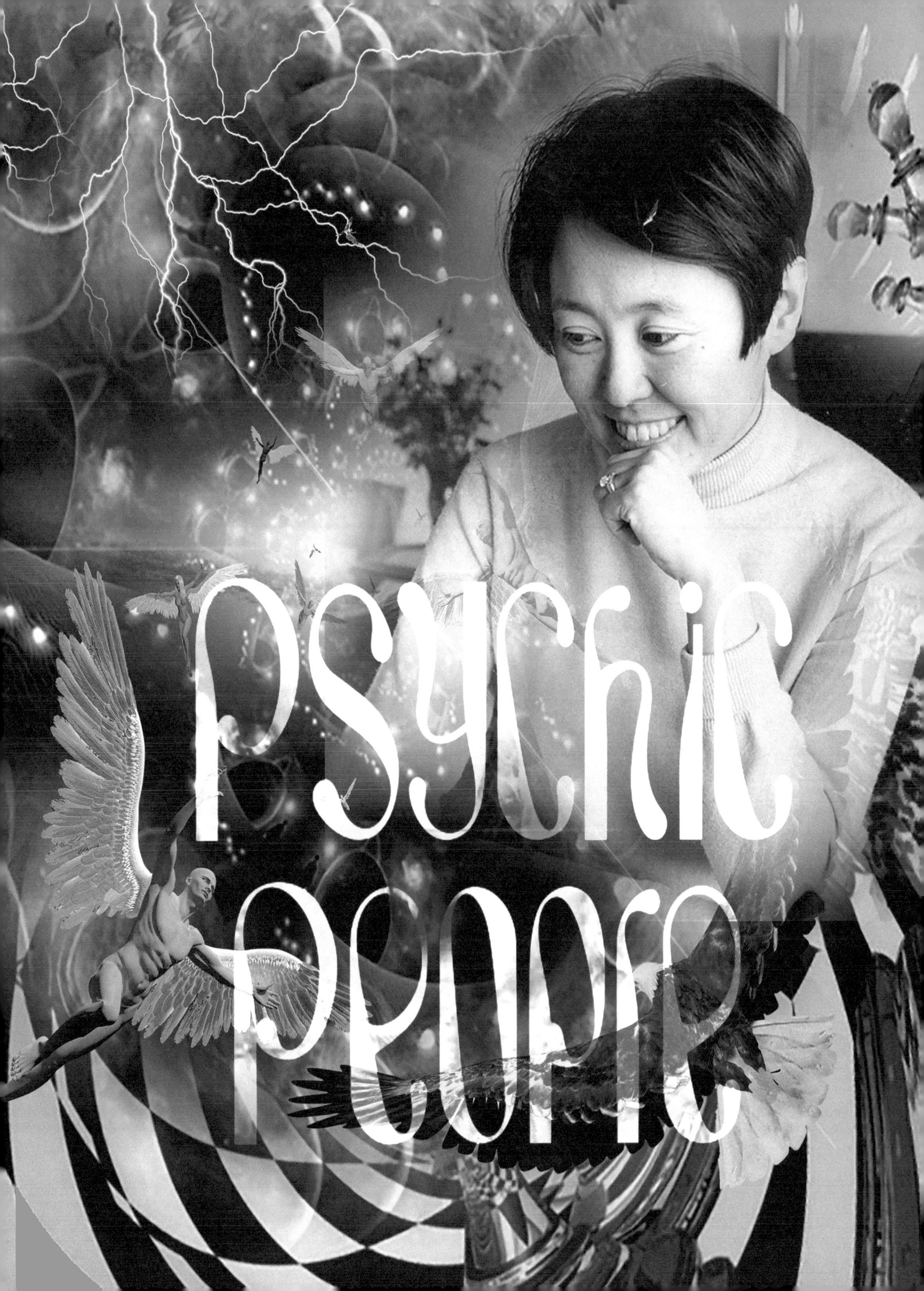
Psychic
People

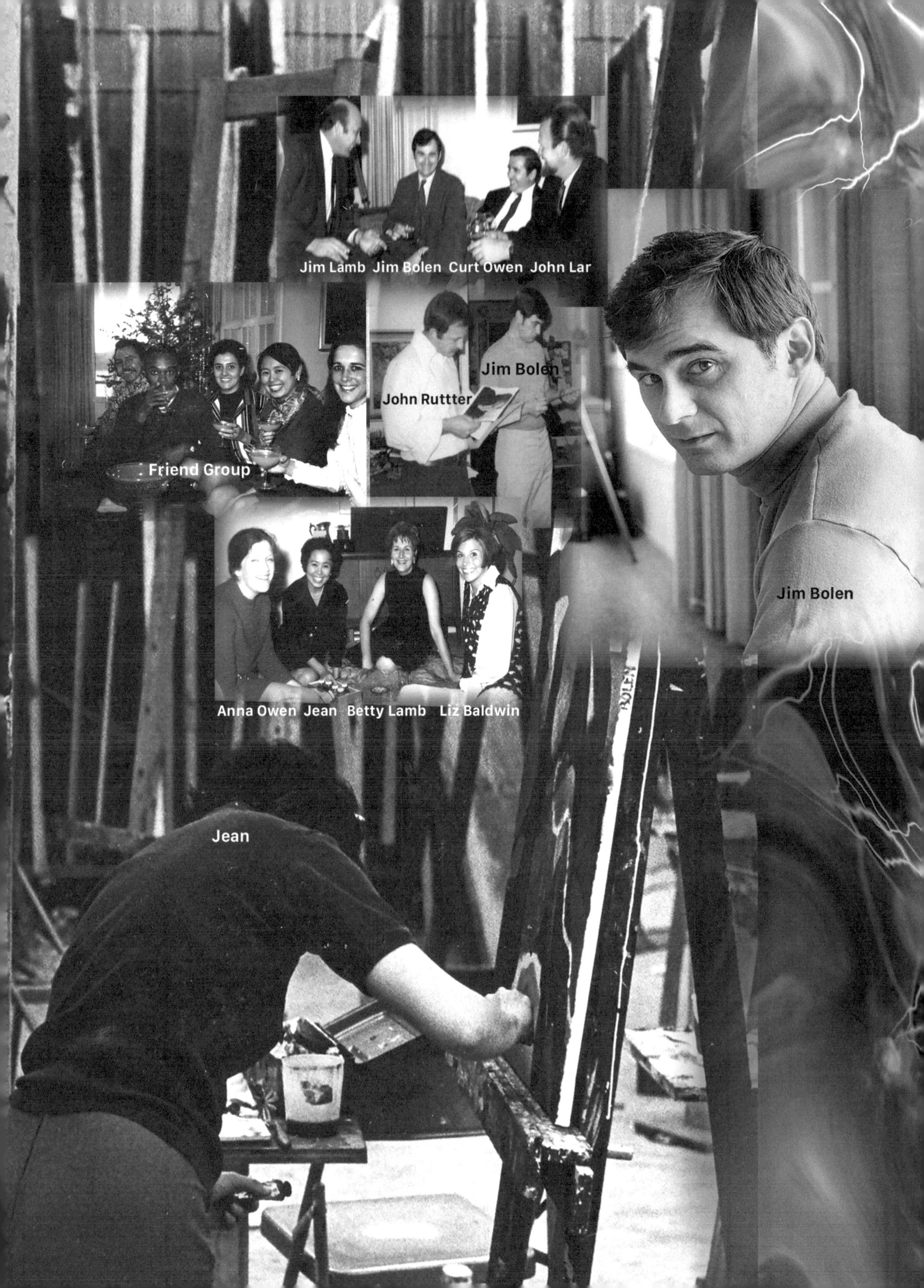

Jim Lamb Jim Bolen Curt Owen John Lar

Friend Group

John Ruttter

Jim Bolen

Jim Bolen

Anna Owen Jean Betty Lamb Liz Baldwin

Jean

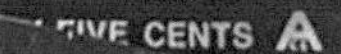
FIVE CENTS
Psychic
JUNE / JULY 1969
JEANE DIXON IN INTERVIEW
ESP IN EASTERN EUROPE AND RUSSI
PARAPSYCHOLOGY, That New Science
ATLANTIS, The Problematical
CRYSTAL SKULL MYSTIQUE,
A Masterpiece of Sculpture
Psychic
A BIMONTHLY MAGAZINE
PETER HURKOS IN INTERVIEW
POLTERGEIST INVESTIGATIONS, GERMANY
VERIFYING PREDICTIONS
The Central Premonitions Registry
THOUGHTOGRAPHY: PHOTOS BY THE MIND
CHARLES FORT, DOUBTER
FEBRUARY 1972/SEVENTY-FIVE CENTS
24518
Psychic
A BIMONTHLY MAGAZINE
DR. GERTRUDE
SCHMEIDLER
IN INTERVIEW
A Psychologist Who Believes In ESP
EUSAPIA PALLADINO
Italian Medium Extraordinaire
ESP THROUGH HYPNOSIS
THE PSYCHIC WORLD
OF JAMES JOYCE
PSYCHIC PHENOMENA
IN LITERATURE

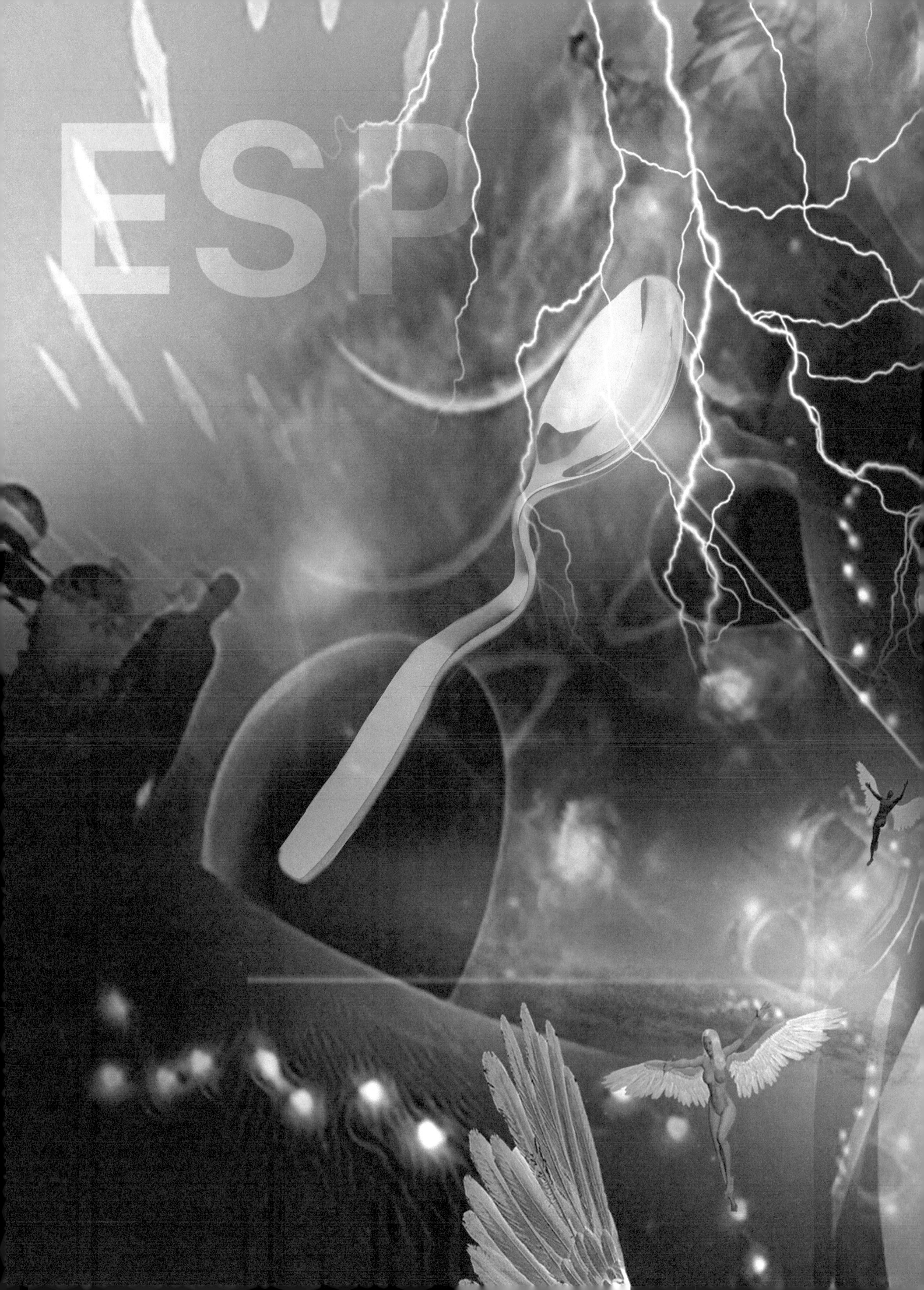
ESP

Chapter 16
Initiation – Giving Birth

I had problems staying pregnant twice. I learned that Nature decides whether I was carrying a viable embryo or not by the end of the third trimester. At three months, the pregnancy either continues, or there is a miscarriage. It was hard on my body and psyche to gear up with hormones and hopes, only to pass blood and some tissue, go to the doctor to be checked, and then have a "D&C" (dilation and curettage—the cervix has to be dilated, or opened, enough for the instrument to then scrape the inside of the uterus, known as curettage). After the second miscarriage, my mother, who had been in general practice delivering babies for several years before World War II and for a while after our return to Los Angeles, suggested that I take desiccated thyroid. It had been prescribed to women back in the day before the pharmaceutical equivalent and thyroid tests, though my thyroid level was normal. Maybe it did work, or maybe as the saying goes, "The third time's the charm."

The third time, I stayed pregnant. When I began having labor pains that were strong enough to be the real thing, Jim drove us to French Hospital in San Francisco, and both of us went into a labor room. Around the time of this pregnancy, fathers who wanted to be involved could be present in the labor and delivery room. We had taken the course for expectant parents who wanted a natural childbirth. He had learned to be a labor coach; I had learned about breathing with each contraction.

I had lots of experience at being at the receiving end of a delivery. I've lost track of the numbers of newborns I had helped come into the world or caught on arrival, first as a medical student rotating through the obstetrical service at San Francisco General and then as an intern at Los Angeles County Hospital. In these hospitals, women in labor arrived at various stages, including those who gave birth on the gurney before they could be wheeled into the delivery. At SFGH, I recall number of women in labor, and the cacophony of groans and moans and screams. For medical students, it was learning on the fly in the "see one, do one, teach one" tradition, this time about how to evaluate the stage of pregnancy by how much the cervix had dilated and thinned.

I also remember the awe I felt at delivering my first baby: with a last big push and groan-cry from the new mother, out came the head of this newborn, and then its shoulders, followed by all the rest of the baby, still attached to a throbbing placental cord, the blood-tinged amniotic fluid making it slippery and messy. During delivery, the new mother's legs and feet are held wide-apart and up in stirrups, her large pregnant body is on the delivery table with the vulva and vaginal walls and cervix stretching thin by the pressure of the baby's head; the opening grows in size as labor progresses, the intervals between labor pains become shorter and the pain more intense until, just before the delivery, the baby "crowns." The top of its head, covered with baby hair, now fills the opening and, if there is no more elasticity, the mother's skin could tear without help from me. There is the last big push.

I'm positioned to catch the baby, to ease it out of a woman's most private anatomy, seated on a stool between the mother's legs. I'm gowned in green surgical scrubs, a mask covers my nose and mouth, my head is covered, and my hands are gloved. It's all to assist and not contaminate either emerging baby or mother. The newborn emerges from the body of its mother after an exhausting effort.

I clear its mouth and nose with gentle suction, and then it takes its first breath and cries. I have helped a new human being enter the world. It's messy and sacred work.

I liked delivering babies and did two more elective obstetrical rotations in my internship at John Wesley hospital, a county hospital and at USC School of Medicine facility, which had the size and feel of a small private hospital. Of all the specialties I did not go into and yet affected me deeply, obstetrics had the biggest impact on my thinking, especially after my own experience with pregnancy, labor, and delivery. (The doctor gets the credit for "delivering" the baby, when in reality, the mother and baby are doing the work.)

I have a number of observations from being the pregnant one, and doing the work of labor, which certainly is a different perspective than being at the other end, helping the baby out if need be, otherwise, catching it as it comes out. From what I remember and from the distance of time as I write this, I know it is time-altering. Labor rooms, even a private one such I was in, might as well be underground since time of day is immaterial. We leave the ordinary world of orderly scheduled time, in which we wake up, dress, have breakfast, and go about whatever our ordinary day. This day began at night when I began going into labor. In a hospital gown, checked by the doctor, who confirmed that yes, this is the real thing. It helps to not be alone in labor, for my husband to be with me. We both act calm. While ordinary clock time does not matter, timing the labor pains (the interval of time in between the contractions), and the intensity when it arrives matters a lot. It's also very different to be the pregnant mother when your uterus has gotten the message that it is time to expel the baby (which is called the fetus until it comes out, and then becomes the newborn or neonate).

The uterus is an expandable muscle-walled container that has grown huge. When not pregnant it is about the size of my fist. Contract and relax, contract and relax, contract harder and relax, contract harder still (pant till it passes) and relax until the contractions grow stronger and stronger with shorter internals between, and build up to a crescendo. The cervix has thinned out completely, and the natural response is to want to push and push hard. Having learned to pant (short quick breaths with each contraction), this can be done until the urge to push passes, which provides time to go from labor room to the delivery room.

The team is there: my doctor, George Winch, MD, a nurse, and an anesthetist in case needed. Now I am the about-to-be mom on the obstetrical table with feet in stirrups, and Jim is gowned and masked and present. When the next strong contraction comes and I hear, "Now push!" I do, with all the strength I can muster, and my about to be newborn's head is out. With the next contraction—"It's a girl!"

If I thought to myself, This hurts!" and as the contractions continued, "This really hurts!" I do not remember. I don't remember the pain itself at all. I also remember that I felt close to giving up on natural childbirth during a particularly strong contraction just before being wheeled into the delivery room. It could also be that in the joy of giving birth to my beautiful new baby, labor pains are forgotten, which would be a useful adaptation for the preservation of the species.

At one point during labor, I lost my sense of being a unique person and had a sense of being "everywoman" who had ever been in labor. What I was experiencing was archetypal—transpersonal. It was hard, painful work. I was amazed that a new human being had grown inside of me and was coming out of me into the world. I was learning through my body what women have been expected to do and be, and felt a sense of sisterhood with all women who had preceded me in this initiation into motherhood.

This was a major initiation, which made me wonder if this could be the basis of male ritual initiations. The initial birth into motherhood begins when the fetus shifts position and contractions begin and continues until the newly pregnant woman becomes a new mother, or dies in childbirth. The contractions grow more intense, last longer, and become more painful as the entry to the uterus is thinning out. The last most painful muscle contraction usually results in "crowning" as the hair of the about to be newborn becomes visible, at this point, often the mother is asked to pant and breathe and then push—and out comes the newborn!

First time motherhood is a physical initiation into becoming a mother, and has been since long before obstetrical medicine. Might exceptional male initiation rituals carry a similar meaning, and could they have been based on observing the physical initiation of the transformation of girls into motherhood? Male rituals signify rebirth into a new status, and often seem to require that the initiate survive an ordeal, and can require shedding some blood, usually in a symbolic act. Just as women occasionally die in childbirth—as in hazing—death happens.

The most intense part of the birth process is called the transition phase, which is the final stage: the cervix is fully dilated and thinned to allow passage, the baby is in the birth canal, and must go under the arch of the pubic bone. This is when the about-to-be new mother hears, "Now push!"

After two miscarriages, the medical recommendation was to give my uterus a rest but not go back on birth control pills. This was an unintentional pregnancy. Melody Jean was born on October 10, 1970, and though I had nursed her and used contraceptive foam, I got pregnant again, and on February 16, 1972, our son Andre Joseph was born. Seems as if there was some intention for both of them to arrive when they did, regardless. And, in Melody's case, to literally hang in there. When her placenta was delivered, part of it was atrophied, as if it had separated from the uterine wall. It was the most miserable-looking placenta I'd seen. After the newborn arrives, the job of the mother and doctor or midwife is not over until the placenta is delivered—a tired uterus must contract again and push it out. Only when all of it is out and the uterus contracts is the danger of hemorrhage over. This was probably the cause of my mother's post-partum hemorrhage after my birth, when my father sounded an alarm barely in time. Otherwise, I'd have been a motherless child.

Melody was put in an incubator briefly because she was a small baby, weighing in at five pounds, five ounces. I have pictures of her in the incubator, eyes open and looking around. From the time she arrived, I had the feeling that she arrived curious at being here. I wondered if she might she be an "old soul." I was introduced to the idea of old souls and young souls prior to having babies, which made me think along these lines, just as it made me think about people in my practice who, in the absence of safe and caring adults, seem to have an innate wisdom that got them through difficult childhoods without becoming like the adults who raised them, even as their siblings did. Ideas of reincarnation, that we may have had many lives or that this one could be our first, is a common belief in many eastern mystical religions. The idea that people have souls seems universal. Issues of abortion have led to debates over when the soul enters the body. The Dalai Lama and his followers take for granted as reality that he is a reincarnated being.

People sometimes talk about such things in their therapy, such as the man who was certain that he was a woman in a previous life. Or the strong déjà-vu certainty of a colleague, who on visiting an obscure village in France for the first time in his (this) life, was certain that he had been here before, so much so that he knew what was around the corner or up the hill from the village. In Jung's psychology, we have access to the collective unconscious, containing archetypal images and experiences of human beings. Sometimes people have dreams in which they keep going back to a place that is known by them only in dreams. In this life, it is a symbolic destination that represents something to them. Jung's collective unconscious might be thought of as just one step away from reincarnation.

Ian Stevenson, MD, a chairman of Psychiatry at the University of Virginia, had an interest in parapsychology and reincarnation which led him to India to investigate children who were convinced that they remembered their immediate past life. The result of the research was published in the monograph "Twenty Cases Suggestive of Reincarnation" in 1966, a classic in reincarnation research. He continued this research and traveled extensively, investigating 3,000 cases of children.

My son Andy was three or four when he startled me as I was driving down the hill. I commented about the way he talked, saying, "Andy, you don't sound like anyone in our family. The way you pronounce words you could be from Boston." His immediate comeback was "I used to be a Boston judge!" He didn't add any details when I tried to learn more, but his statement was so clear and definite that it had a ring of truth about it. Not only was it the way he talked (he could have been a Kennedy kid) but how he spoke with authority. The puzzle was also how he was raised in an egalitarian family and talked like a boss. In time, his Boston accent and boss attitude went away.

Andy was a full-breech delivery, which made his transition into the world difficult for us both. It was a long delivery, which did not require a Caesarian section, but when he came out, he had been through an ordeal and there was concern for him. An ambulance with an incubator was called. Andy, with his Dad, went in the ambulance from French Hospital to Children's Hospital, which had a neonatal nursery. Back at French Hospital, in my hospital room, with my newborn son elsewhere, my instinct was to check out, which I did as soon as I could. I went to Children's Hospital where Andy was doing well on his own. They wanted to keep him for another day because his skin looked slightly jaundiced. I looked at what they were concerned about and wasn't impressed—pointing out that he was half-Japanese. When I said I would sign him out "AMA" (against medical advice) if I had to, he was discharged and we could take him home. In his first months, he wanted to be held almost all the time which, and with three adults (parents and babysitters) there were enough arms for this and time for Melody as well, who was walking, talking, and curious about her baby brother.

Like Melody, Andy was conceived through the barrier of contraceptive foam that was, in both cases, supposed to provide rest for my uterus. Andre Joseph Bolen was born on February 16, 1972, weighing six pounds, four ounces. If, as psychics often say, we choose our parents, it did seem that both of them had to arrive during a very small window of opportunity if they wanted to come when they did and have Jim and me for their parents.

I wonder now, as I look back at their lives, if the ease or difficulty of the birth process and the delivery might have something to do with readiness or resistance to coming into the world. My brother Stephen did not want to come out and was pulled out with forceps. Did he and my parents pay a lifetime of angst because of brain injury caused by an impatient physician—a cause and effect scenario? Or might the soul about to come into the world, aware of what this life would be like, resist being born and what happened be part of the story? I have tried to imagine what it would be like to be him and wonder if as souls, whether we do choose the circumstances into which we are born and what purpose suffering could serve. I thought of Andy's breech position, which made his entry much more difficult. Thinking metaphorically, could there be some resistance to what would be in store for him?

Andy came into the world with what we called his "birth bump" on his forehead. It was small, round and raised, it felt rubbery, and it was just below the hairline. It was like a birthmark, which is why we called it his "birth bump." It was not a concern to his pediatrician. The only reason to have it removed was cosmetic. It resembled a wart, and it could be removed if Andy wanted it taken off, which he did when he was nine. We thought the removal would be a minor office procedure. It turned out to not be so simple, as the bump went deeper and was more rooted than expected. The pathology report said that it was a neurofibroma. It would turn out to be the first sign of a fateful condition that would be a major challenge or cross to bear.

INITIATION:
GIVING BIRTH

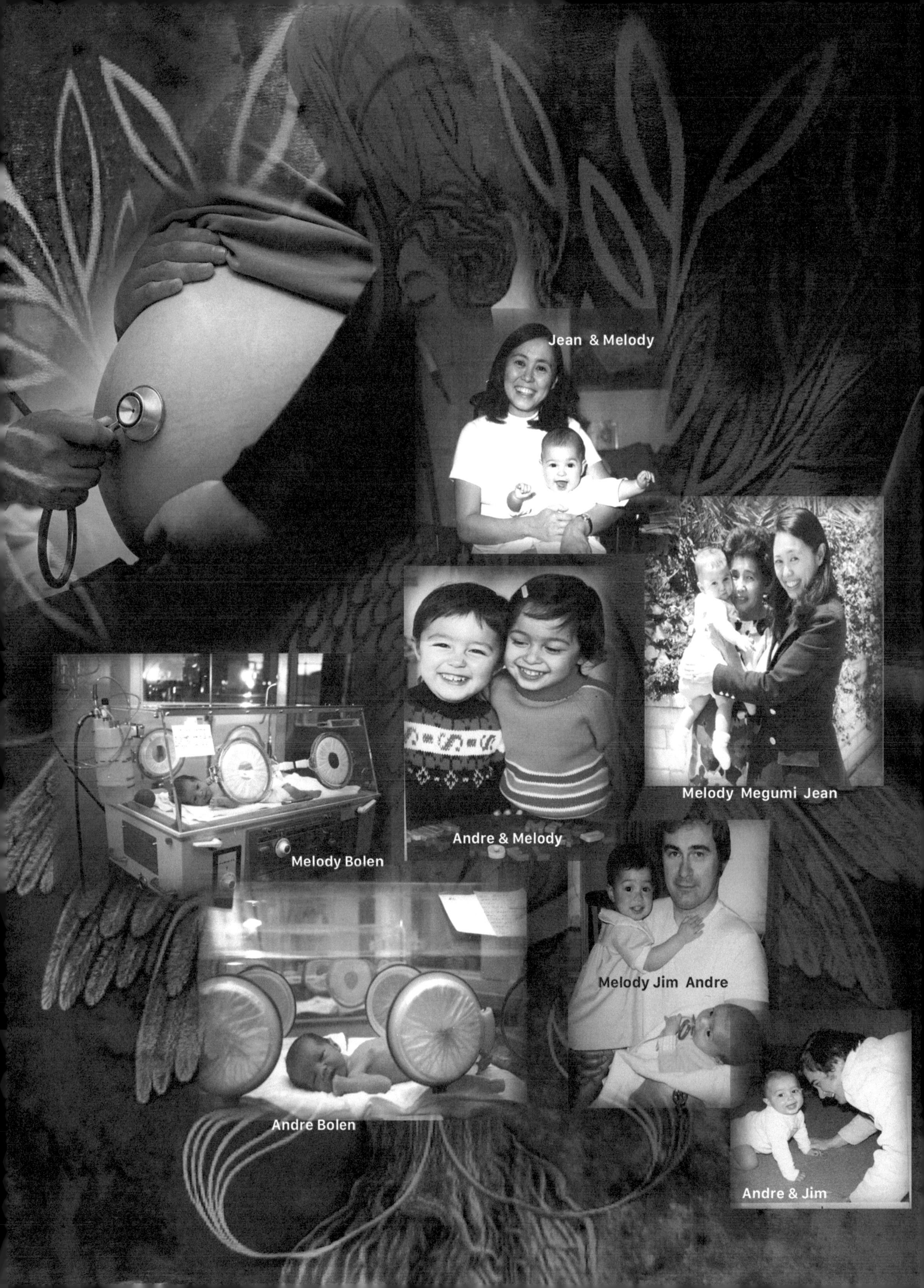

Jean & Melody

Melody Megumi Jean

Andre & Melody

Melody Bolen

Melody Jim Andre

Andre Bolen

Andre & Jim

transpersonal
EVERYWOMAN

"I used to be a Boston judge!"

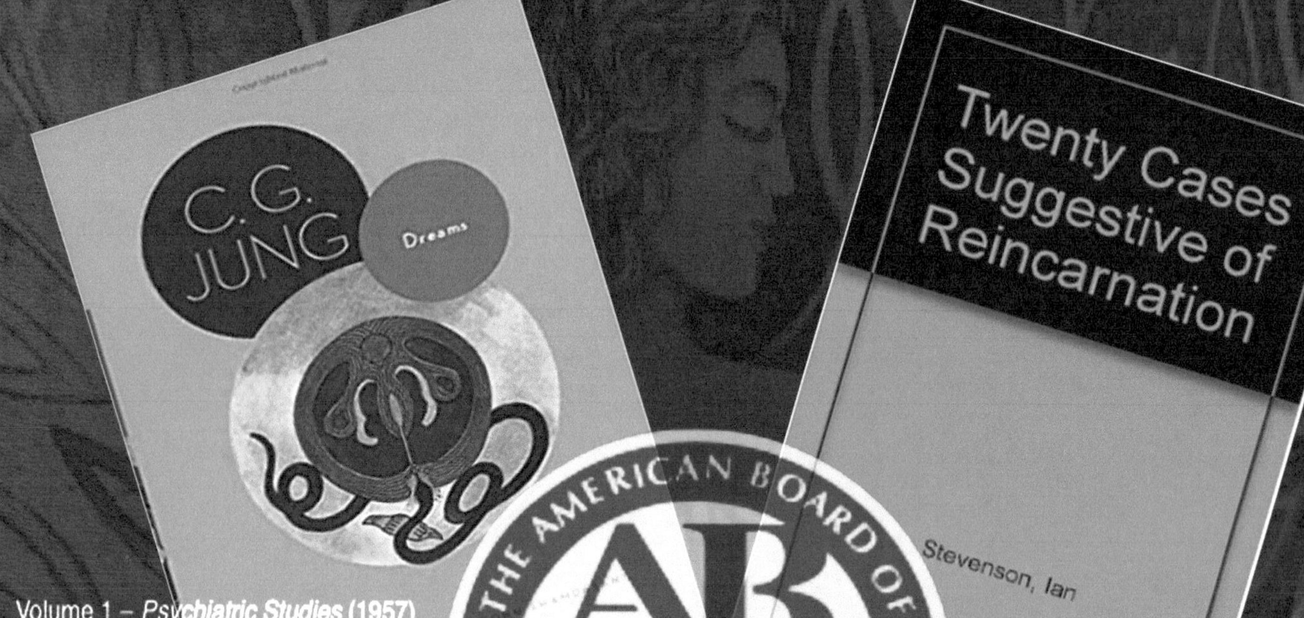

Volume 1 – *Psychiatric Studies* (1957)

Volume 2 – *Experimental Researches* (1973)

Volume 3 – *Psychogenesis of Mental Disease* (1960)

Volume 4 – *Freud & Psychoanalysis* (1961)

Volume 5 – *Symbols of Transformation* (1967; a revision of *Psychology of the Unconscious*, 1912)

Volume 6 – *Psychological Types* (1971)

Volume 7 – *Two Essays on Analytical Psychology* (1967)

Volume 8 – *Structure & Dynamics of the Psyche* (1969)

Volume 9 (Part 1) – *Archetypes and the Collective Unconscious* (1969)

Volume 9 (Part 2) – *Aion: Researches into the Phenomenology of the Self* (1969)

Volume 10 – *Civilization in Transition* (1970)

Volume 11 – *Psychology and Religion: West and East* (1970)

Volume 12 – *Psychology and Alchemy* (1968)

Volume 13 – *Alchemical Studies* (1968)

Volume 14 – *Mysterium Coniunctionis* (1970)

Volume 15 – *Spirit in Man, Art, and Literature* (1966)

Volume 16 – *Practice of Psychotherapy* (1966)

Volume 17 – *Development of Personality* (1954)

Volume 18 – *The Symbolic Life* (1977)

Volume 19 – *General Bibliography* (Revised Edition) (1990)

Volume 20 – *General Index* (1979)

SYNCHRONICITY

Chapter 17

Private Practice - UCSF Faculty - ERA - Jungian Institute

After I had finished my psychiatry residency, I began private practice, seeing a few patients in a colleague's office. I also worked part time at a newly established walk-in, short-term outpatient clinic at San Francisco General Hospital. I received many referrals in my private practice, including from UCSF Langley Porter, and within a year, I opened my own office on Webster Street near Pacific Presbyterian Medical Center. The Medi-Cal program covered private psychiatric sessions for people who could not afford the fees (twenty-five dollars per session) and made entering private practice easy at the time. My office was in a renovated two-story San Francisco Victorian house, which had six offices for therapists. I stayed there until the building was sold, remodeled and restored to a one-family house, from 1968 until 2001.

The movement for women's rights advanced my career in psychiatry as women became more aware of sexism, and institutions were feeling the effects. Consciousness-raising groups, publications, marches, demonstrations such as "bra-burning" and picketing, and conferences proliferated, initially mostly among educated white women and women on college campuses. Freud's theories about the inherent inferiority of women for lacking a penis and the sublimation of this through bearing boy babies came under attack. At Langley Porter, the required curriculum for psychiatric residents included the psychology of women which had been based on Freud and taught by male psychoanalysts. Soon after I graduated from the residency program, I was asked to teach the seminars on the psychology of women. Male experts on women across the country including those at Langley Porter had become wary of teaching Freud. I joined the clinical faculty as an instructor in order to teach these seminars. This was the first step on the academic-clinical ladder, which functions very much like promotions in the US Navy—after a set number of years at each level, officers are either passed over or are promoted depending on their performance. Over the years, I rose through the ranks, becoming first an assistant clinical professor, then an associate clinical professor, and then a clinical professor, which I remained until I aged out a year or so after sixty-five.

My interest in Jung and Jungian theory had grown during my residency. Both Jungian and Freudian institutes required that their candidates be in analysis themselves, and so I had begun mine with a Jungian analyst twice weekly in face-to-face therapy. I'd clocked in whatever the required number of hours were when I applied to the Jungian Institute for admission to the training program. With my liberal arts education, the Freudian focus on just one of many Greek myths (the Oedipus myth) and the effort to apply it to women, which Helena Deutch (*Psychology of Women*, 1945) had done, didn't make sense to me. Besides, the dreams of my patients seemed much richer in potential meaning than a comment on the transference. Then there was the bind that women were put in by this theoretical framework: we were all supposed to have penis envy and, if we protested, we were exhibiting symptoms of a masculinity complex.

When I applied to the Jungian Institute and was asked why I was interested in the training program, I said that I wanted to learn more. I knew that Jungians worked with dreams and myths, valued intuition, and that there was in Jungian theory a place for creativity and spirituality, which I didn't see elsewhere. When I was accepted, I found that I was the only candidate accepted that year (I may have been the only applicant), and I would join the second-year seminar, and the following year, assuming there would be a first year class, I'd join it. Within a few more years, the length of the application grew as did the numbers of applicants. Jung's psychology and writings are often dense reading, but they were a means to understand what young people were experiencing in non-ordinary states of consciousness through music, meditation and hallucinogens. Besides, Jung had a knowledge and respect for Indigenous and Eastern spiritual practices which fascinated many in this generation. Jung's psychology become popular in this new-age culture.

American Psychiatric Association and ERA

While I am hardly a "Forrest Gump" (the character and movie about the intellectually disabled man who was present at important historical events in his time), I have felt a sense of kinship with this character because he turns up at important events, meets famous people, follows his instincts, and makes a difference. So much of what I have done professionally has had to do with historical circumstance. I was there when Langley Porter needed a woman to teach women's psychology.

I was there when John P. Spiegel, MD, the president-elect of the American Psychiatric Association, searched for a woman to be on the Council of National Affairs. He asked around for suggestions and chose me after I had been recommended by Dr. Alexander Simon, the head of Langley Porter, and by Carol Wolman, a young woman psychiatrist on the Task Force of Women. When he called, I didn't know who he was, didn't know how important the Council on National Affairs is within the organization, or why he would want to appoint me to it. Dr. Spiegel was a visionary, a liberal, and was president-elect in 1973, the year that the APA decided that homosexuality was no longer a mental illness. The effects of racism on mental health had been raised by Black psychiatrists, and now sexism was an issue, raised by women psychiatrists. He wanted a woman on this important council, and what mattered was that both feminist women psychiatrists and men active in the APA would be comfortable having me on the council.

With acceptability by both, while not having my identity defined by either—I was in a familiar position of *positive marginality*. I could speak for women and feminism and be taken seriously by the men. I was a member on the Council of National Affairs for four years, then became the chairperson. While the main point was that I was a woman, I also imagine that it helped being a "two-fer" as an Asian and a woman. Thinking this was probably the case, I took care to represent both, and moved that the APA establish a Task Force of Asian-American Psychiatrists, the precursor to the Committee of Asian-American Psychiatrists.

The Equal Rights Amendment (ERA) was the controversial issue in the APA in the 1970s. The ERA was passed by the House of Representatives in 1971 and by the Senate in 1972. The deadline for ratification was 1979, which was extended for three years. By 1977, thirty-five states had ratified the amendment, with thirty–eight needing to be adopted. The APA went on record in support of the ERA in 1974 and 1977. With pressure from the Committee on Women and many leaders of the APA strongly supportive, the Board of Trustees voted to cancel the 1981 Annual Meeting in New Orleans because Louisiana was a non-ratified state. (Organizations that supported the ERA were showing their support and putting pressure on states that had not ratified it by not holding their conference in non-ratified states). Jean Baker Miller, Alexandra Symonds, and I organized PFERA (Psychiatrists for ERA), and with other women psychiatrists on the Committee on Women, Brenda Solomon and Elaine Hilderbrand, created a network of support for the ERA.

Then came the Referendum: a group of members successfully petitioned the Board to hold a referendum stating that APA would "not prohibit the holding of meetings in a state which has not passed the Equal Rights Amendment." This appeared in the January 18, 1980, issue of *Psychiatric News*. Ballots were sent to APA members, and on April 18, 1980 *Psychiatric News* reported that 5,679 members voted not to boycott non-ratifying states, with 4,461 voting to maintain the boycott.

Activism and Individuation

This was just before the May 1980 annual meeting, which was to be held in San Francisco. I was the only PFERA leader in San Francisco and it was a month away. My inner activist—the one that says to me, "silence is consent" —knew that this was a moment of decision. "To do nothing" is a choice; and "to do something" will be a challenge. I took on being the point person for PFERA, with phone conferences with the others. I called Gloria Steinem, whom I had never met, described the situation, and asked her to come to San Francisco to speak. She said yes (!) and did more: she called a press conference when she came, which gave the issue widespread coverage. Once she said yes, the ideas and energy flowed. Inspired by the layout of the *Pacific Sun*, I designed a newspaper-appearing handout that featured Gloria in the center, the headline announcing the ERA issue, with topic-titles that would be covered inside, including petitioning the Board of Trustees.

The Referendum was not binding, and they could vote to continue the boycott. The green ERA-YES buttons were much in evidence, energy was mobilized, and we picketed our own organization to support ERA and withdraw from non-ratified New Orleans. For most of us, this was our first time holding a placard, and chanting slogans like "ERA YES" and "Boycott New Orleans." Most of us were of the Silent Generation and had been too involved in the long hours and years becoming doctors and psychiatrists to take part in demonstrations—much less lead one. Gloria Steinem put us in touch with Del Martin and Phyllis Lyon, who coached us.

At this time, the APA membership was eighty-nine percent men, eleven precent women, and two-thirds of our patients were women. We were making the point that inequality and discrimination has negative psychological effects, which made the ERA a mental health issue. When the Board of Trustees met at the end of the 1979 annual meeting, we showed up, and I was invited to speak. They voted to allocate $30,000 to help ratification efforts and voted to withdraw the 1980 annual meeting from New Orleans. It felt wonderful! And the feeling did not last for long.

The next Board of Trustees meeting was at APA Headquarters in Washington, DC. Reconsidering the previous vote about New Orleans was on the agenda. Between the two meetings, members of the board heard from outraged male members of the APA, and a sexist example prevailed: the board had gone to San Francisco and been seduced, this was the morning after.

The next annual meeting would be in New Orleans, after all. It meant that we who thought we had succeeded, had to decide once more what to do. Would we now lead a boycott of the meeting in New Orleans?

Here I will pause to reflect upon what I had learned. When I made the commitment to organize, beginning with reaching out to Gloria Steinem, who was at this point, a celebrity (not the friend she became), I had never done something so bold and brash (my introvert's view). When I reached her and she not only said yes, but did much more, I felt the truth of Goethe's quote: "Whatever you can do or dream you can, begin it; Boldness has genius, power, and magic in it."

After the Board of Trustees meeting in San Francisco when we were elated, it seemed that we were living up to Margaret Mead's words, "Never doubt that a small group of thoughtful, committed citizens can change the world; indeed, it's the only thing that ever has." While PFERA activism in San

Francisco began with my commitment, there was a "we," not just an "I," doing this. In the morning calls I'd make to Allie and Jean and others on the East Coast, we discussed strategy and ideas, and they lined up support from male elders of the APA, former presidents and others with prestige in our profession. This would become a model for me of how women's circles support the women in them to do what they dream they can do.

I was learning for myself what I now, past eighty, know to be true:

Activism and individuation (to find a meaningful, inner directed, chosen life-path) come together when the choices we make express who we are and who we are becoming. Activism is a thread in my life through which I have grown into being who I am as a person and as a soul.

I had a chance to reflect upon my PFERA activism in a 2017 interview for a story in *Psychiatric News*, a publication of the American Psychiatric Association. The following is excerpted from that interview.

> The ERA episode served a major consciousness-raising role, and that was a good thing. Sometimes you lose, but you still persevere to make a point. We raised equal rights as an issue for every psychiatrist in APA, and they had to decide if they would go to New Orleans. The battle of the ERA was not in vain. It contributed to psychiatry by demonstrating that women were not treated as equal to men and had been kept from achieving their full potential. I think that every woman psychiatrist who got involved in this effort at the national level, and those who spoke about the reasons behind the boycott of New Orleans in her district branch, found her voice—after the years of training and being in hierarchal situations, where maintaining silence on issues related to sexism was a survival skill.

At the meeting of the Board of Trustees in the Washington Headquarters of the APA, the decision to rescind the decision made in San Francisco was made behind closed doors. The San Francisco meeting had been an open meeting. While we waited outside to learn whether the APA would boycott or go to New Orleans, I received a phone call from my literary agent that my book proposal for *Goddesses in Everywoman* had been accepted by a publisher. I was now committed to write this book and be a leader of a boycott.

My efforts on behalf of women patients and the ERA had taught me that while all women psychiatrist members of the APA had gone through similar education and training, they had two distinctly different attitudes toward women and the patriarchy, which were as different as Athena and Artemis. I had learned this from my activism on behalf of the ERA.

In Greek mythology, Artemis was the goddess of the Hunt and Moon. Her realm was the wilderness, in which she often roamed with her female companions. With her silver bow and arrows, she was the archer with unerring aim. She protected young animals and young girls, and was the only Olympian who came to her mother's aid. In contrast, Athena was Zeus' favorite, and the only divinity he trusted with his symbols of power. Her realm was the city. She was the protector of heroes, and the goddess of (strategic) wisdom. The city of Athens bore her name.

The issue of the ERA shook out which archetype was dominant. Women psychiatrists who supported ERA were feminists, archetypally Artemis. Athena women did not have a sense of sisterhood. They admired and were drawn to successful men. They were thinking types who tended toward patriarchal institutions. Their similarity is that they are both Virgin Goddesses (classical mythology designation) whose attributes include goal focus, independence, and autonomy. Archetypes are personality patterns that shape behavior, typology, and values.

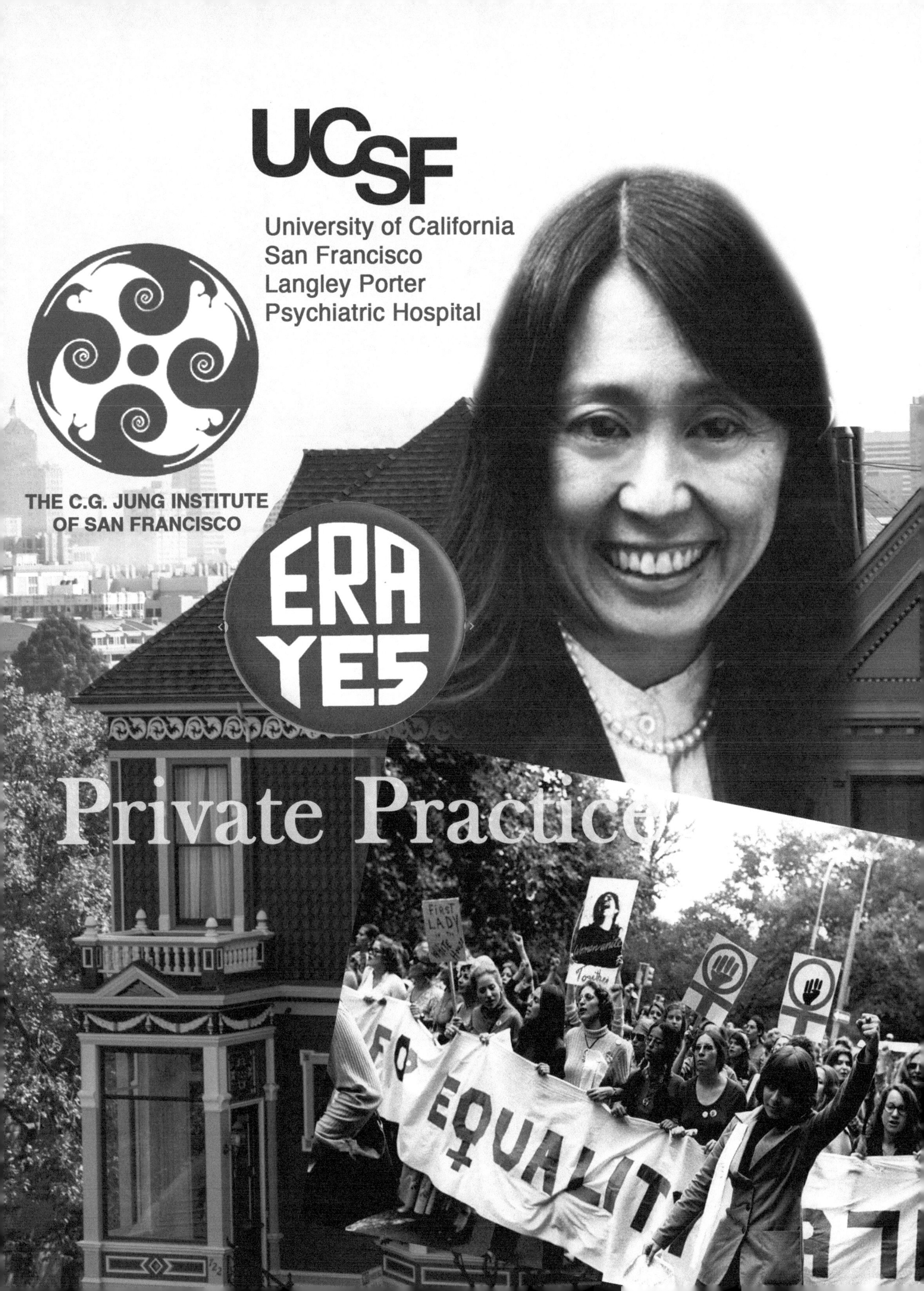
UCSF
University of California
San Francisco
Langley Porter
Psychiatric Hospital
THE C.G. JUNG INSTITUTE
OF SAN FRANCISCO
ERA
YES
Private Practice
FIRST LADY
EQUALIT

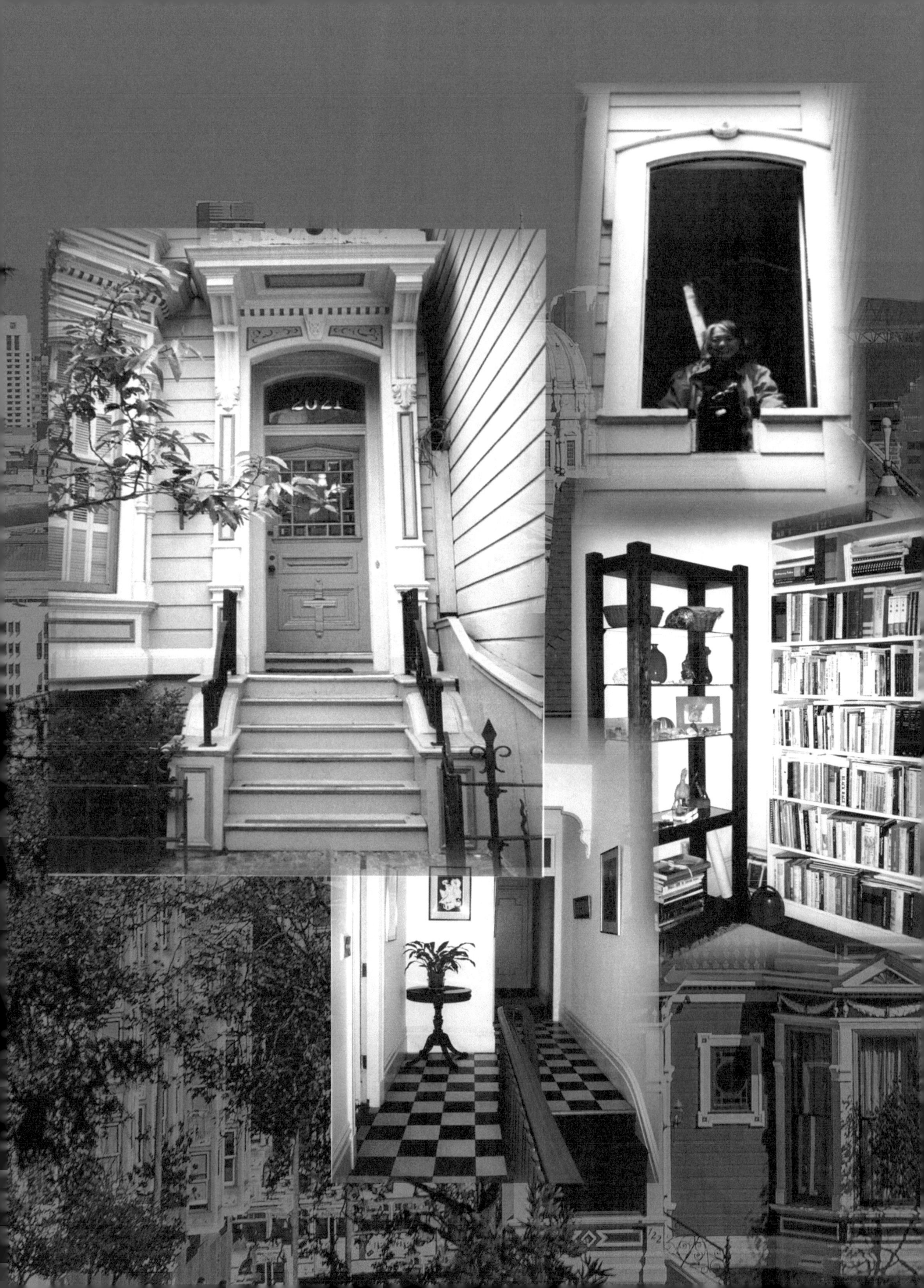
2021

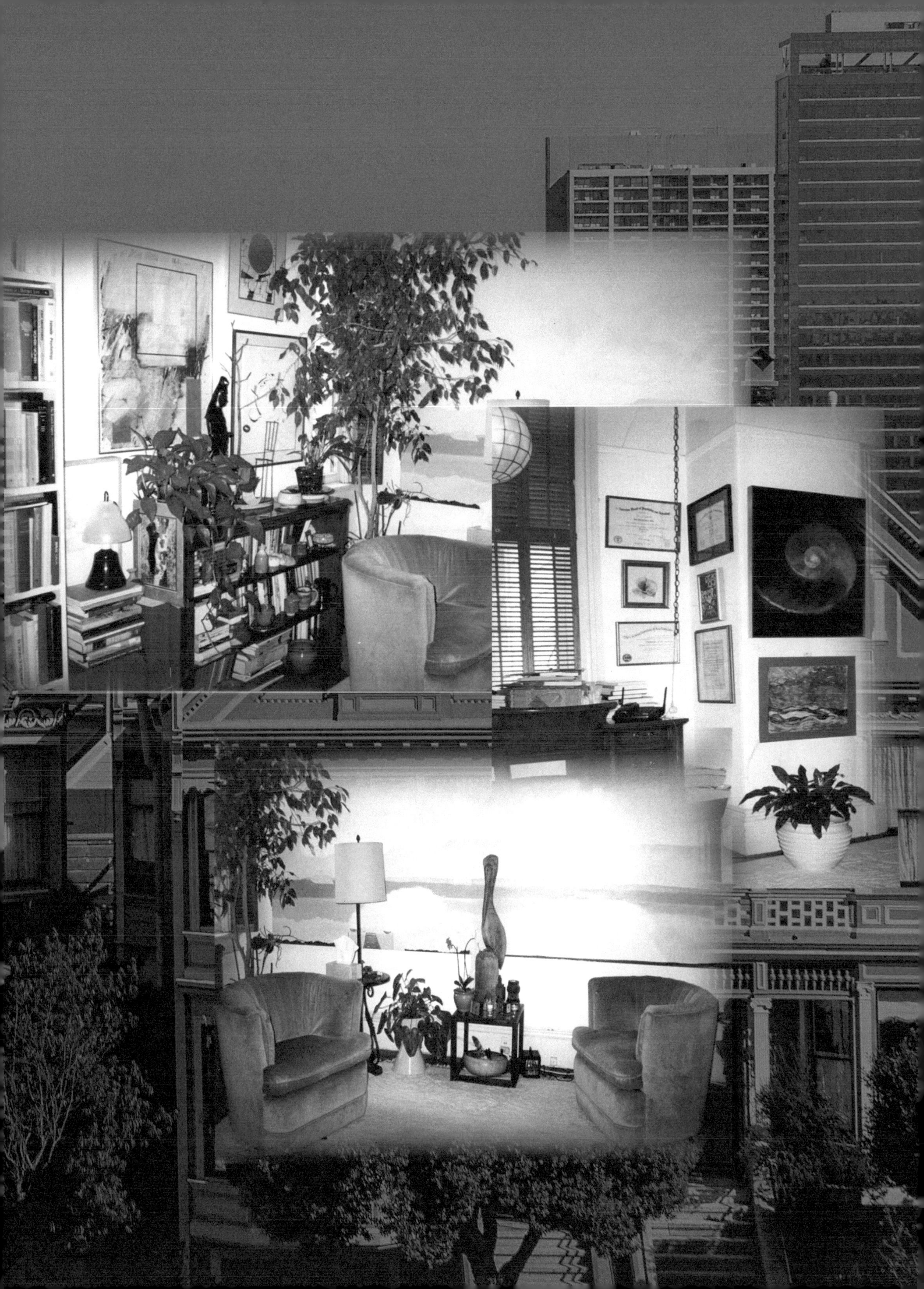

PFERA
Psychiatrists for Equal Rights Amendment

Council of National Affairs
American Psychiatric Association

Comm

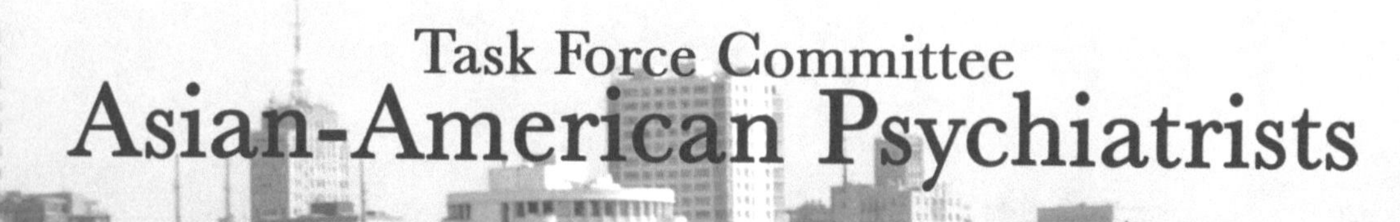

Task Force Committee
Asian-American Psychiatrists

Psychiatric News

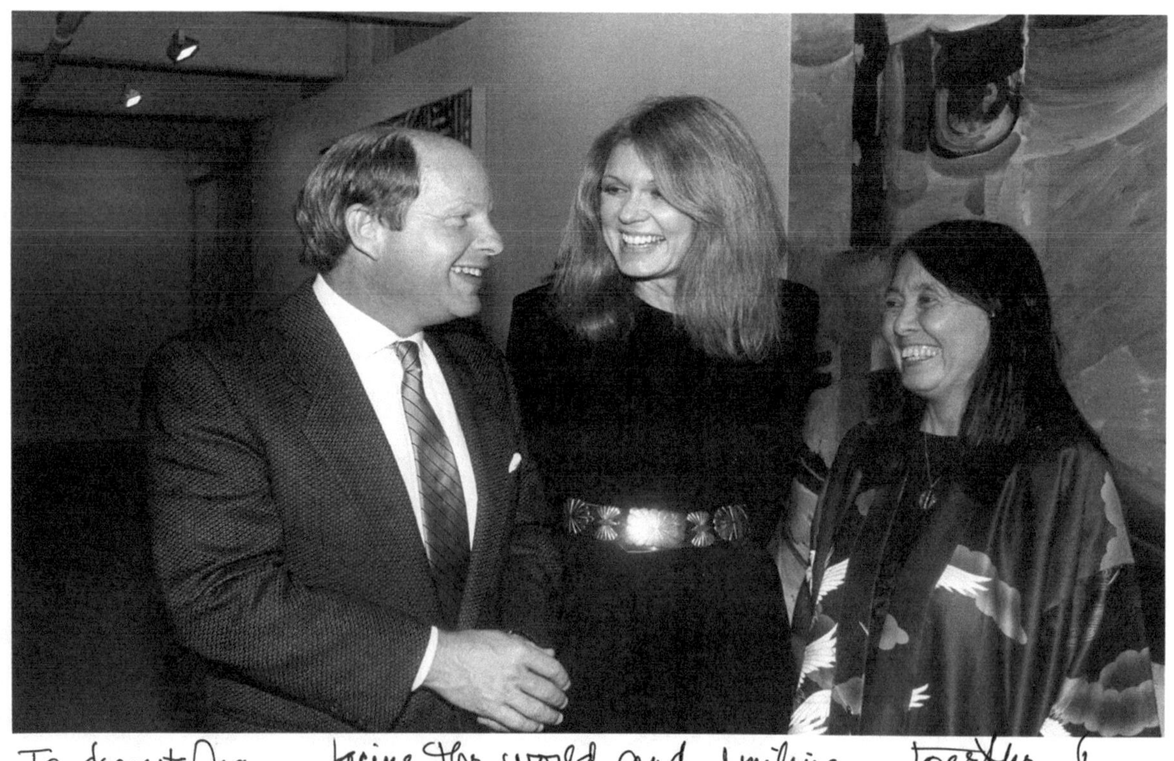

Gloria Steinem

Chapter 18

Becoming a Jungian Analyst

I was a candidate in the training program at the C.G. Jung Institute of San Francisco from 1967-1974. I had applied wanting to know more about Jungian psychology after I'd finished my residency—initially thinking of it in academic terms as a post-graduate program. Wrong metaphor! Within the Institute, the metaphor was often the family. Later while I still was a candidate, Joseph Wheelwright, MD, one of the founders, spoke of needing to change the metaphor from family to tribe. By then, the institute had grown and moved. When I began, the institute was then in a modest two-story wooden Victorian house on Clay Street, between Upper Fillmore (several blocks of small businesses that served Pacific Heights) and what is now the California Pacific Medical Center. We met on Tuesday evenings for two hours of seminars, each taught by a Jungian analyst. I was critical of the teaching, until I got some excellent advice from Charles Klaif, MD, another candidate who had also trained at Langley Porter and was in the seminar class a year ahead that I had joined when I entered the Institute and had been a class of one.

I was used to well-organized and reference filled teaching—the kind that demanded note-taking. This was different. Charles found a seminar valuable if it gave him one new thing to really think about. I soon did also. I was also in my own analysis, a requirement, which had changed my attitude toward my dreams. I had vivid, Technicolor dreams—it had been like going to the movies almost every night. Now I thought about them, it might be that something that was said in a seminar brought more meaning to them. Gradually, I absorbed what I was being taught and what was in the air, and was becoming a Jungian-oriented psychiatrist in my office practice. I had a bookshelf filled with The *Collected Works of C. G. Jung*, all twenty volumes, in their shiny black book jackets. I read the recommended readings from the *Collected Works*, often finding that Jung's writing did not engage my thinking—until it was clearly applicable to something or someone in particular.

Formal schooling with examinations (which medical school epitomizes), or psychiatric training with the emphasis on describing patients, detailing the symptoms, considering causes and arriving at a diagnosis and treatment plan, require turning outward—to have an extraverted focus, to be objective. We needed to take it in what we were taught and had to be able regurgitate it back. Now in Jungian seminars, I was learning to be a discerning introvert, to take in what intrigued me, or clarified something for me, or was knowledge I wanted to learn, and then turn this over in my mind, ideas and images alike. Jung's concepts became like food to digest or marinate—not regurgitate! Or, like cows with their two-stomach digestive system, I'd find myself bringing ideas up and chewing them over later.

Once I became a candidate, I was eligible to go to the North-South Jungian Conferences, hosted in turn each year by either the San Francisco or the Los Angeles Societies of Jungian analysts. There was a theoretical tension between the two training programs. The San Francisco Institute had been founded by psychiatrists, and the Los Angeles Institute analysts had come through the ministry or psychology to Jung. Most of the founders or elders in both institutes had trained in Zurich, and many had been in analysis with Jung. Their analysts wondered if our candidates were analytical or archetypal enough. Ours wondered if theirs were clinical enough. So members from the certifying committees at each institute came together each year as a board to decide whether candidates were ready to become analysts, with our analysts questioning theirs and vice-versa. Members and candidates of each institute met together at an annual North-South Conference with the choice of site and program alternating between Northern or Southern California.

In 1973, I went to the North-South conference, my first since Melody and Andy were born. It was held at La Casa de Maria, a conference center in Santa Barbara that was run by ex-nuns, former Sisters of the Immaculate Heart of Mary (IHM), who had welcomed Pope John XXIII's Vatican II Council's effort to bring the Church into the twentieth century. One of their relatively well-known members was Sister Corita, who created colorful lithographs with quotes or ideas written across them. I had hung one of hers in our house. In 1967, the sisters elected delegates to a special General Chapter meeting held at La Casa de Maria, which met over six weeks, and rewrote their Decrees.

Vatican II (held between 1962 and 1965) took place in Rome over the same years that the second wave of the women's movement had its beginnings and was gaining momentum. The IHM sisters had decided to shed the heavy and hot black "habits" that covered them from head to toe, which had been prescribed for them to wear. They now determined their own prayer schedule and no longer would follow rules laid down in medieval times, and they would choose their service endeavors. Cardinal McIntyre reacted to their new Decrees by firing all of the IHM nuns teaching in the diocese. Efforts at reconciliation failed. The Vatican then sided with the Cardinal, and the nuns were told to return to their former, medieval code or seek dispensation from their vows. About three hundred of the Sisters, more than three-quarters of the order, chose to leave their order and establish a community. They owned the La Casa property which they struggled and succeeded in turning into a Conference and Retreat Center.

In going to the North-South Conference, I was coming back into the Jungian fold. I had been *in limbo* (an inactive candidate), and my time and psyche had been involved with the births of two children and their needs. When I was a candidate, once we were through seminars, we could remain in limbo until we decided to write our Certifying Case and present it and ourselves to the Joint North-South Certifying Board. The case presentation was usually one that we had worked on with our control analysts. It was an example of our long-term analytic work. We chose who would be our control analysts, with the only suggested requirements being that we have a man and a woman, and work with them consecutively on the same case. I had Joseph Wheelwright, MD, and Kay Bradway, PhD, for my control analysts. This was what had been done in Zurich.

Candidates who were ready to present themselves and their work for certification would beforehand have talked readiness over with their personal analyst and met with the certifying committee, who would have heard from our control analysts. The chairperson of the certifying committee in San Francisco would then arrange with his or her counterpart in Los Angeles where and when the two certifying committees (who now would constitute the Joint North-South Certifying Board) would meet. The candidate would make copies of his or her case presentation for all members of the Board who would have read it before meeting with the candidate. After meeting together, the candidate would leave the room to wait outside while the analysts talked and decided. If it had gone well, the candidate would be invited back in and congratulated ("knighted" was Wheelwright's word).

Then came a crisis that shook up the training program. The San Francisco certifying committee was sued by a candidate and the case had gone to court. He was the plaintiff; I think that the defendants were members of the committee, his analyst and the Institute. I knew the candidate before all of this happened and had thought that he was the most Jungian of us all. He had discovered Jung's writings when he was sixteen or so, dove into them and had read the entire collective works by the time he was in college. He was a psychiatrist, an Ivy League athlete, and someone whose deep inner life lay under a socially adapted persona.

His own analyst Joseph Wheelwright had given him reasons to assume he was ready to be certified and yet, when it came time to appear before the certifying committee, I gathered that he and the members of the committee did not agree on his readiness to become an analyst. And he in response ended up suing the certifying committee which did not help him or candidates in general. I intuitively felt that he had such knowledge and affinity with Jung's ideas, that to not be seen as worthy by the certifying committee must have had the emotional charge of a denied birthright. It was not something that he could win in court, organizations such as the Society of Jungian Analysts have the right to set standards and memberships.

As a result of this, the atmosphere toward candidates changed radically. From the changes, it seemed as if all of us were now viewed by analysts as people who could sue them. Limbo ceased to exist; we would be reviewed annually. We were to write a letter to a committee in which we were expected to share "our innermost thoughts and feelings" and meet with them to discuss ourselves and our status in the training program. Other changes affected new applicants; the application form went from one page to over a dozen pages. I had been offended by the tone of the letter and the expectation that I would share my "innermost thoughts and feelings" with committee members, most of whom I didn't know. My reaction was to do something—to organize. I wrote a letter to all of the candidates. It led to having a retreat at Timber Cove on the Mendocino Coast. We met in a large circle and before we started, six of us each threw three coins, to determine which hexagram and therefore what advice we might get from the *I Ching*, the ancient Chinese *Book of Changes*. We got Hexagram 18,Ku: "Work on what has been spoiled."

Introverted intuitive people make up most Jungian organizations, which was the case in San Francisco. Well-meaning people with this typology are often not comfortable having power and authority and often don't use it well, especially when unconscious or in denial. The archetype had been the family, with the analysts seen as role model parents who welcomed us. Now they were being wary of us and were changing the process to examine us more closely. This was a time of mutual misperceptions. I was in the thick of this, as I was the elected chairperson of the new Candidates Organization, with John Beebe, MD as vice-chair. I also needed to decide if I would go for certification.

I remember thinking to myself, "Give me one good reason why I should go through this." I was well-established professionally, had enough patients, and was on my way to Langley Porter where I supervised a talented resident, which is the best kind of teaching. We met in his office. I went in expecting to be brought up to date about patients he was seeing. On this day, however, he wanted to discuss something more personal. He told me he would like to come into therapy with me and he also wanted to know about the Jungian Institute. I considered this a response to what I was muttering to myself: this was a very good reason to go through getting certified! His analysis hours with me would count toward hours required to apply to the training program—but only if I was certified.

My certifying case was an Episcopalian priest who I had seen for several years. It was he who responded to the wooden sculpture of a pelican that is in my office by asking: "Do you know that the pelican is the only feminine symbol of Christ?" I didn't and wondered why. I learned that when there is no food, the female pelican will feed her chicks with her own blood, by wounding herself in the chest with her beak to fed them. The sculpture sits between me and my person, as if on the rim of an invisible alchemical vessel where the work of analysis is done. As a symbol of Christ, it is a Christian symbol of the Self or divinity, or the Tao. "Where two or more are gathered in my name, there shall I be also." It's the symbol of the energy that is invited into a vessel of healing and transformation. Jung's model of analysis was the alchemical or chemical reaction: if the patient is to be affected by the work, so too must the doctor. I am affected by feelings, images, Intuitions, and thoughts that come to me in doing this work which is focused on the patient.

My analysand had some amazing synchronicities, which led me to work with them as if they were "waking dreams," and write about doing this in *The Tao of Psychology*. He also told me a dream that differed from all the others of his that I had heard. I called this a "visitation dream." These kinds of dreams are qualitatively different from usual, familiar dreams. His father appeared to him in this dream, shortly after his death, looking very much alive and healthy. He had something to say to my patient. It took place "nowhere." In the dream, he knew that his father had died, and yet here he was. This dream had the impact of a real experience, which it was. There is a "reality" to visitation dreams that affects the dreamer, and on hearing them, touches the analyst. Once, during the time I was disenchanted with becoming a Jungian analyst, he talked about how the church holds a tension between the essence (revealed wisdom, a numinous experience, a divine insight) and the institution created around it (made up of men with their various agendas, ambitions, and imperfections). I realized it applied to Jungian institutes, which was a valuable perspective to remember.

In 1974, I became a certified Jungian analyst. I went to Los Angeles to go before the North–South Certifying Board and felt I was among colleagues as we talked about the paper that I had sent them. It was not an examination, and they weren't testing me. Rather it was an affirmation, and an outer recognition of an inner shift that I had made from the time I applied to now being an analyst. There was only one other candidate, also from the San Francisco Institute, David Tresan, MD, a psychiatrist who also lived in Mill Valley, a few more turns up a winding road from where I lived. We both had been "knighted" and now were newly-minted Jungian analysts.

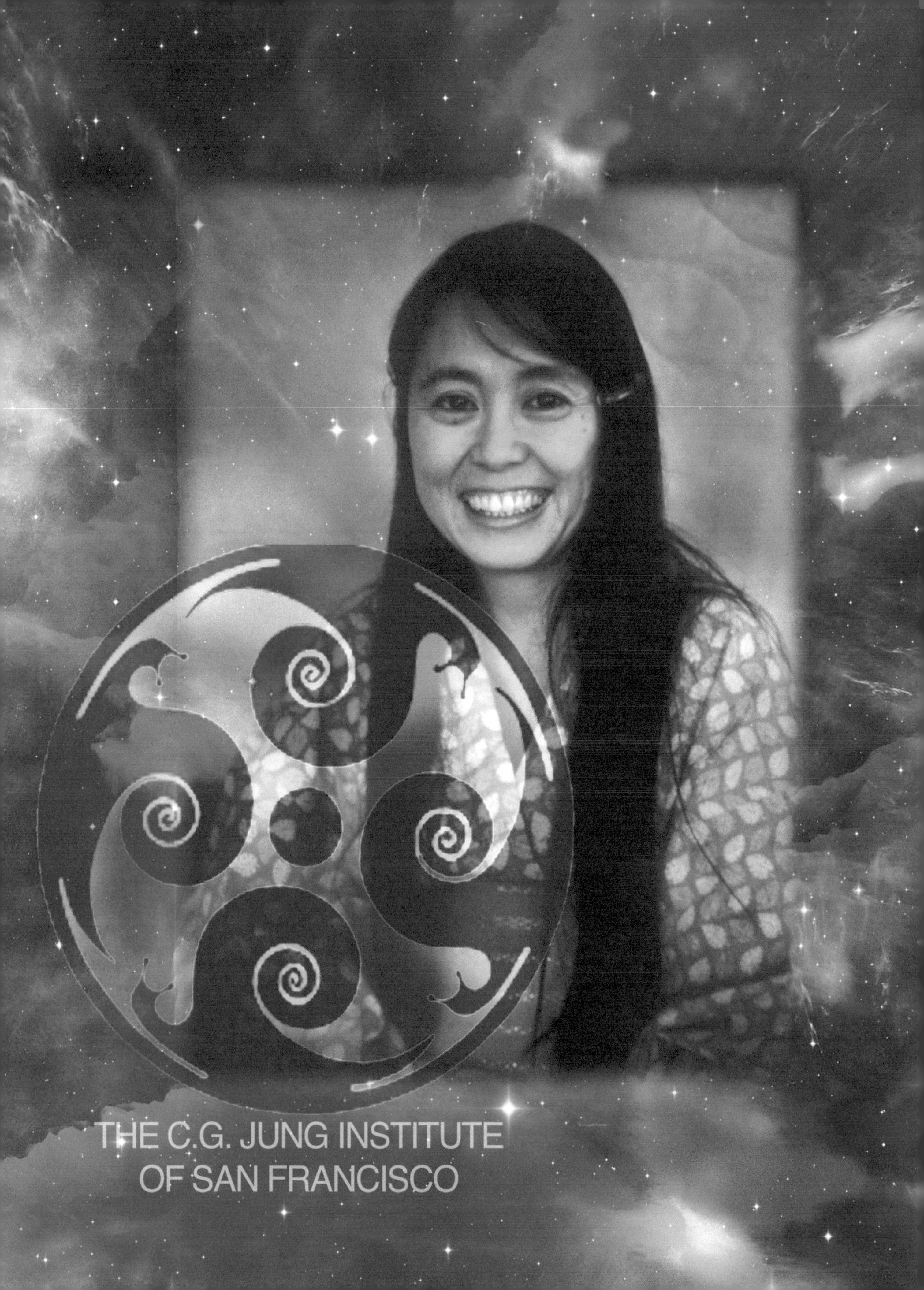
THE C.G. JUNG INSTITUTE
OF SAN FRANCISCO

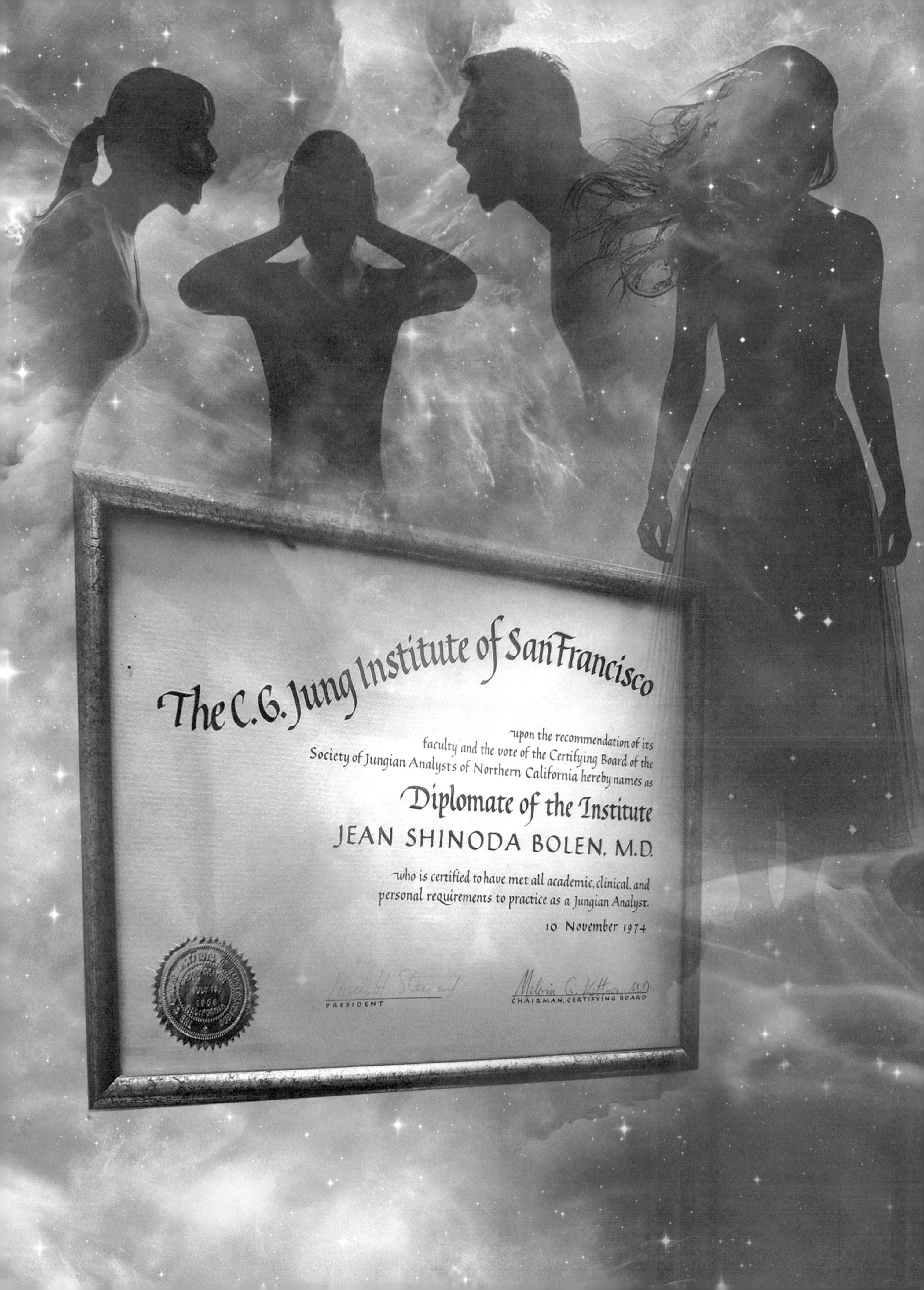

The C.G. Jung Institute of San Francisco

upon the recommendation of its
faculty and the vote of the Certifying Board of the
Society of Jungian Analysts of Northern California hereby names as

Diplomate of the Institute

JEAN SHINODA BOLEN, M.D.

who is certified to have met all academic, clinical, and
personal requirements to practice as a Jungian Analyst.

10 November 1974

PRESIDENT

CHAIRMAN, CERTIFYING BOARD

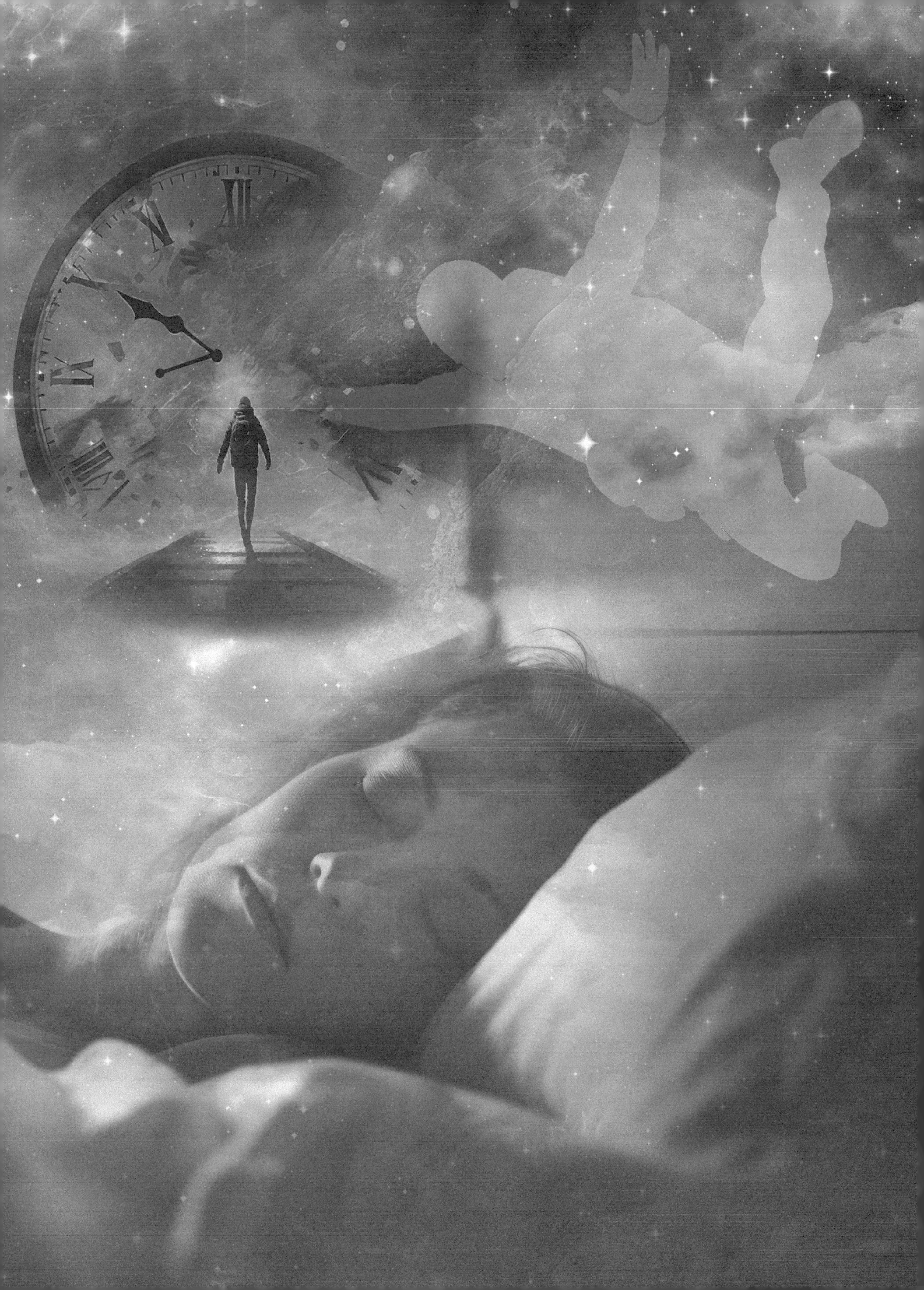

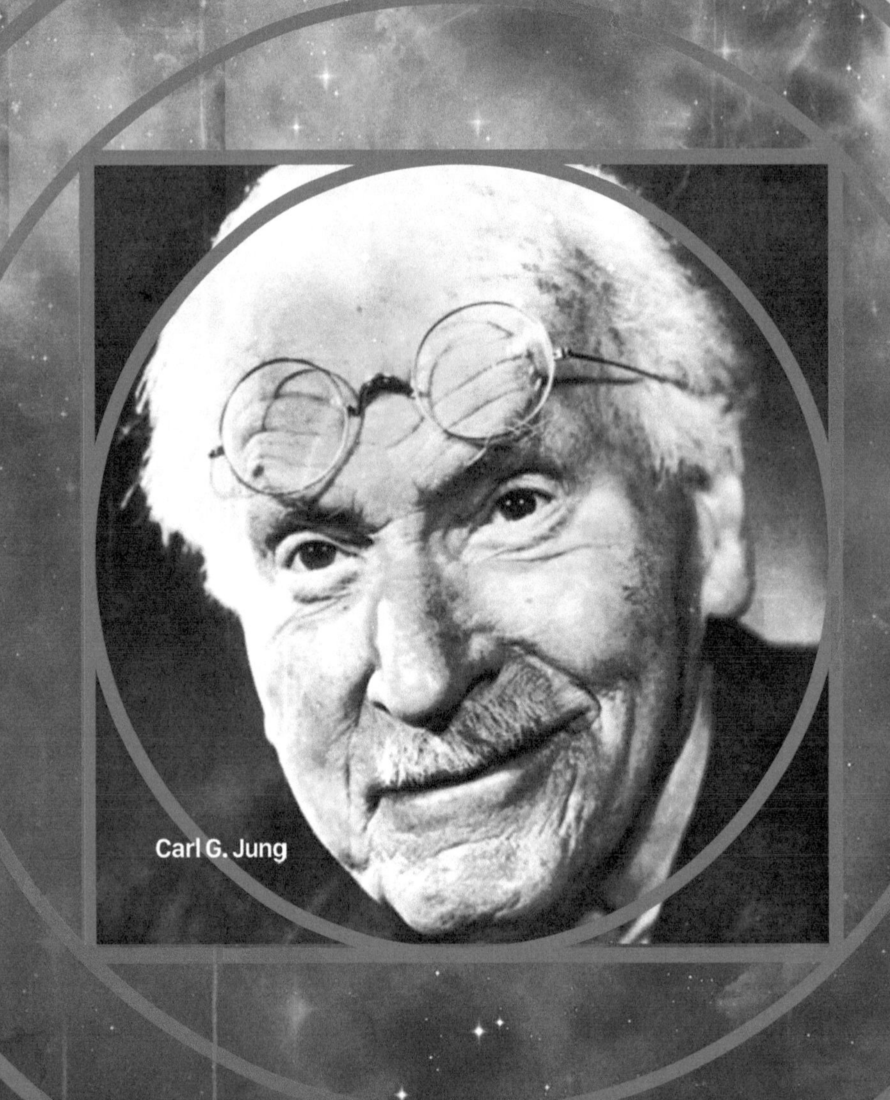

Carl G. Jung

Chapter 19

Becoming a Jungian Whistle-Blower

I became a whistle-blower in the San Francisco Jungian Institute on May 27, 1981, when I wrote an open letter to "The Jungian Family (analysts, candidates, interns, staff, Board of Governors)." I brought into the open what had been known and ignored for years: one of our most prominent analysts had a reputation for sleeping with his women patients. In this initial letter, I had not named him. Most Jungian analysts knew that I was referring to John Weir Perry, MD, as would many professionals outside of the Jungian institute and an unknown number of women who were once former patients of his, some with schizophrenia who had been hospitalized and helped by him, before he then had a sexual relationship with them. Rather than focus on him, the initial reaction mostly from male colleagues was anger at me—to blame the messenger.

The analyst I was confronting publicly had been my own analyst many years before. I was distressed by what I had learned, because I cared about him, valued the years spent in analysis with him, and valued our work together. He had never been unprofessional or physically crossed a personal boundary with me. I was distressed with what I had learned about his unethical and harmful behavior. The knowledge had come to me through a series of troubling conversations with other therapists, within and outside of the Institute.

I would have been a great deal more comfortable *not* being the recipient of information that came my way. But with this information came responsibility to do something, to act from my inner conviction that "silence is consent." This was how felt when I wrote the first letter and then in a more detailed subsequent one on July 13, 1981. I wrote both as open letters because my previous efforts to have the Institute or the ethics committee take action had failed. I had brought this to the chairperson of the ethics committee and had been told that I should bring it up with John Perry, which I had done years before. Initially I believed him when he said it was in the past and then it became clear that it was ongoing.

One criticism to my open letter was that I also included an article from the *New York Times* on "Rights Amendment Issue Divides Psychiatrists," bringing up the related issue which now had national attention. The political element was offensive as it also was implicitly critical of the Institute. While organizations in psychiatry and psychology including psychoanalytic (Freudian) institutes were supporting a national boycott of holding conferences in non-ERA-ratified states, our Executive Committee had voted against doing so, which reflected the majority view at the analysts meeting.

In my open, short letter, I wrote: "We have a reputation for disregarding the damage done to several/many women patients by one well-known Jungian analyst, who has been repeatedly accused of having sexual intercourse with patients and former patients." In contrast, it took only one clearly stated incident of unethical sexual behavior by a former patient to Robert S. Wallerstein, MD, Chair of the UCSF Department of Psychiatry, for Wallerstein to discuss this with Perry after which, he asked for and received John Perry's resignation from the clinical faculty." The woman who reported this was now a resident in psychiatry.

As a result of my open letter, John Perry brought a complaint about me before the Institute's ethics and grievance committee for having written it. On Father's Day, June 21, 1981, he and I would meet with them. While I had not named him in my letter, the community knew who I was referring to, as it was general knowledge that had also been discussed at a regional meeting and at the candidates' organization. I had not said that he had been my analyst in my letter. Or that it saddened me to write, and that I had a deep affection for him and an appreciation of the analytic work I had done with him.

It felt symbolic and therefore synchronistic that this meeting with the ethics committee was to be held on Father's Day. Another remarkable timing: Gloria Steinem and I had lunch together just before I went to this meeting. She was in town for an event and we were able to get together for the first time since she had been in San Francisco to support Psychiatrists for ERA. I think of Gloria as an archetypal big sister of the women's movement. I felt this personally when I asked for her help, and she came.

When I wrote my open letter, it was many years after I had first heard about John Perry having intercourse with a patient. I had heard this from an angry psychiatrist who was outside of the Jungian community. She had been covering another psychiatrist's practice when this patient went into crisis and the story came out. Then the woman psychiatric resident in my seminar at UCSF Langley Porter spoke up and told us that this had happened to her when she was hospitalized and was his patient. It came up again from another source—this time from a psychiatrist in the training program at our institute whose patient had been a former patient of Perry's. I also learned that Perry's unethical behavior had been brought to the Northern California Psychiatric Society's ethics committee which did not report him to the medical board under the condition that he enter analysis, which he apparently did not. At this point, I went to the chairperson of the ethics committee at the Jungian Institute, who told me that this was not an ethics committee matter unless a patient herself formally complained. He said I should talk to John Perry myself.

When I was ready to confront him, which took me a year, the opportunity presented itself. We were both at a Marin regional meeting and during a long break it was possible to have a private one-on-one conversation, which happened outside on the lawn in the sunshine. I told John Perry what I had heard and believed to be true, and that it was as if I had learned something bad about someone who was like a father, which left me feeling ashamed to be his daughter and angry at what he was doing. He listened with what felt like compassion. He wasn't defensive and said that all of this was in the past—that it all took place six-to-eight years ago and just involved three women. I wanted to believe him. I said, "I hope this is true." Since he had been my analyst and did know me, I went on to say, "You know me, and you know that I will have to do something if I hear that what you are telling me is not true." It was like a pledge I was making to myself and to him. His innocent blue eyes and a reassuring smile conveyed that I needn't worry.

More stories came to me after this, trustworthy reports by analysts or candidates who were seeing former patients of John Perry's with whom he had sexual relations and had been damaged psychologically. I talked to the next chairman of the ethics committee and encouraged other colleagues to do so as well. When still nothing happened in response, and bolstered by the response to issues that I had helped raise in the American Psychiatric Association, I wrote my open letter to the Jungian community.

The reaction to my initial open letter was mixed, with the strongest support from Jungians who had been or were treating his casualties. I was criticized for bringing this up or bringing it up the way I did. Discussion at the Board of Governors and Candidates Organization focused on me and the letterhead I had used initially rather than his behavior. (It was on the Institute's letterhead, which I had been using as chairperson of the certifying committee.)

At the following Analysts meeting, which I attended, the subject of my letter was not brought up at all until the very end of the meeting when the president, James Yandell, MD, spoke up and pledged that he wouldn't let this matter slip through the cracks. Silence was the reaction at this meeting, though I did hear from individual analysts who wrote letters to me, mostly supportive, though there was a hostile one. There was a lot of buzz, and I gathered there was talk behind my back that I was glad to not hear. John Perry's reaction was a complaint to the ethics committee, and a request that the two of us meet with them.

I sat in a chair immediately across the table from John Perry. Both of us spoke directly to each other with Kay Bradway, who chaired the ethics committee, creating a *temenos* (a sanctuary in Greek, or safe place which is what the analytic container should be) with four other analysts: Gerry Spare, Paul Kaufman, Tom Kirsch, and Jim Yandell seated around the table with us. It was a solemn and serious meeting. I can remember that the feeling was sadness, not anger on either of our parts. I don't remember specifics of what each of us in turn said—we voiced some of what we had written to each other before this meeting, with copies to the committee members.

John Perry and I had written to each other, he on June 7, I on June 15, 1981. In these letters, our respective feelings and motivations were honestly expressed. He wrote of paying for these mishaps heavily for six-to-eight years, including being barred from teaching at Langley Porter, and stepping away from a mental hospital unit that he inspired, in order that it could continue. (The unit was an innovative, compassionate residential facility for young adults with acute psychosis.) He wrote that "it was like putting my child out for adoption," and about being summoned to various committees, and also to several therapists (who apparently knew or were treating his former patients). He wrote as if he were the victim and that I was making it worse by penning the open letter. "If the humiliation, the grief, the loss, and the reprimands were not enough," he wrote, "you follow upon all these moves and see fit to drive the knife in deeper yet by a very open call to disgrace."

I told him that when I initially spoke to him that he had lied to me saying this was all in the past. John Perry thought of himself as the injured rather than the injurer. I gathered that one of the purposes of the meeting he requested to have with me before the ethics committee was to rein in any further action on my part—and I said so. My hope was that I had done all that I would have to do, and that others in the Institute would grapple with the problem.

On July 10, 1981, a letter went out from the ethics committee to the members and candidates of the Institute, reporting that they had met regarding the issue I had initially raised. "If you have information relevant to this issue," they wrote, "please supply the Committee with relevant, clear-cut information."

On July 13, 1981, I wrote the detailed letter to the analysts and candidates, the second one since the initial open letter to the Jungian community. Near the beginning, I wrote, "Considering the gravity of my statement and the confusion, anger, support, censure and actions taken in the wake of my May 27, 1981 statement, I feel you are entitled to more information. I also feel a need to explain 'where I am coming from,' what my concerns are, the potential direction this could take, and the resolution that I believe is possible. This is a family matter that touches all of us. I believe we are called upon for compassion, wisdom and responsible action."

This letter was an eight-page deep discussion that included events so far, and went beyond the particulars to include process, conceptual and theoretical context, and the alchemical model with which we work as Jungians: transference/counter-transference. It included text from the standards of professional behavior from the American Psychiatric Association, the Board of Medical Quality Control, and the California Medical Association. I concluded, "It's time for us to consider having ethical guidelines."

A special analysts meeting was called on August 13, 1981 to move the matter of John Perry out of the ethics committee into discussion by the general membership. Kay Bradway presented the committee's report with a chronological account of the committee's involvement since 1975. The report covered allegations made about John's sexual involvement with patients and former patients, with information about sources, and excerpts from letters received by the committee from members. My recollection is that the committee heard about fourteen women who had been patients of his with whom he had sexual relations, pledged them to secrecy, and then abandoned them. The report closed with a recommendation to the membership for indefinite suspension of John from the Society of Jungian Analysts.

John Perry attended the next September 10 membership meeting. It was painful for us—including myself— to hear him justify his intentions. He intended "healing" and felt victimized by the reactions of women after he ended relationships with them. I had the impression that if only he had agreed that he had a problem and would go into analysis or be supervised, that it would have been a relief to many who could support what he wanted. He was appealing the indefinite suspension and wanted to be "on probation for a set period of time, but without conditions." The indefinite suspension stayed. Expulsion was beyond what the analysts could consider then.

For many of my colleagues, who had rejecting or absent fathers, John Perry would have healed their father wound and been a role model. Reactions of anger, sadness, and disillusionment led some to deny that what he was doing with women patients could be true, or have a one-sided compassion for his suffering, humiliation, and fears that he couldn't support himself if he lost his medical license (which he eventually did). The experiences that many analysts who once were in therapy with him were, like mine, positive. They had more compassion for him than for the unknown women whose trust and boundaries he had violated, unless they were now treating former patients of his (or perhaps had daughters) and knew the emotional cost of what he had done. I gathered that women patients who had such experiences were reluctant to go into therapy with another male Jungian, would only go to see a woman therapist, or if they did see another male therapist, the work would involve testing boundaries and trust, though once established, could heal what John did and continue analysis.

I was appalled by the enormity of his blindness when he spoke for himself at the analyst meeting. I did wonder if he had been repeatedly enacting the Pygmalion myth, named for a sculptor who had created a statue of a beautiful woman, fell in love with the image he had created, and couldn't feel anything for a real woman.

Women who descend into the collective unconscious and lose touch with reality can regress into infancy and childhood when real life becomes overwhelming. Deeply regressed hospitalized patients often were and still may be kept on locked wards and treated with antipsychotic and antidepressive drugs. The new approach that John Perry inspired and taught helped first time hospitalized regressed women to grow through stages. Possibly, once she becomes an attractive woman, he projects his feminine image or "anima," makes love to her, and then is not attracted to her afterwards. Possibly, he was acting out a positive fantasy—though there is nothing known, and this is only speculation.

To a temporarily overwhelmed, regressed, hospitalized woman patient under his care, he became like a father who saw and helped his little girl grow up to become a woman, and then violated her body and her trust when he became attracted to her sexually. The father who raised her, the man she may have seen as strong and protective became exploitive, but it may take time for her to know this. Initially, there is the specialness of his attention, perhaps the power of supplanting her mother, and the sexual initiation which the father may delude himself as the tender lover transforming her fully into being a woman.

This was to be kept secret, like John Perry's patients promised him. A daughter whose father has committed incest with her will usually have psychological and relationship difficulties, be left with anger, shame and guilt, which gets further complicated in some families when her mother seems to know what is going on. Harm that is done within families can usually be traced through several generations, as can the effect of the attitudes and realities of the historical time.

The effect of patriarchy results in male superiority and dominance over women. "Sexism" came into consciousness in the late 1960s and 1970s. This was followed by the psychology of addictions which defined dysfunctional relationships as between a narcissist and a codependent, or an addict and an enabler. While becoming a Jungian analyst had become my primary training after residency, and the model of the psyche with which I worked, I also was learning from social movements that were outside the Jungian sphere.

I was a member of the Jungian family who went out in the world and brought back what I learned—in my usual and familiar position of *positive marginality*. So, when the Institute family kept not addressing the "elephant in the living room" (a metaphor from the addiction model), like a dysfunctional family, I could see what was going on in a larger context of patriarchy and unconscious sexism, when others did not or would not. It was also a shadow of Carl Gustav Jung. When I entered the institute as a candidate, Jung's relationship with Toni Wolff who had been his patient, his mistress, his colleague, and a contributor to analytical psychology was like a family secret. He had a similar relationship with Sabrina Spielrein, who, like Toni Wolff, also became a colleague. I became a whistleblower because I learned information I couldn't ignore, which came through uncannily synchronistic events.

My only glimmer of John Perry's shadow came in a dream while I was in analysis with him, long before I knew about this dark side of his psyche. My analysis with him led to relating to my dreams and learning about myself through them, as well as all the other ways an analysis helps. In this particular dream I was looking at a uncomplimentary, vivid painting of John Perry. In it, he looked very dissipated. He said it could be a compensatory image for my idealizing him, which I knew I wasn't doing. Sometimes an important dream image can remain in the mind, as this one did. In the years after I finished my analysis with him, I began hearing about his sexual encounters with women patients. At the time when I had the dream, it was puzzling, later its meaning became clear. I called it a "Portrait of Dorian Gray" dream, after Oscar Wilde's novel about a handsome man, whose moral corruption and downfall was visible in the changes in his portrait but not in his actual appearance. John Perry initially seemed to be a good man, which is how I saw him, but as time passed, he caused harm as he disillusioned and emotionally wounded others who trusted and looked up to him. The Northern California Psychiatric Society learned of his ethical transgressions, which would have led to reporting him and the loss of his medical license, except that Dr. Wheelwright accompanied him which apparently assured them that John Perry needed and would go into analysis. He apparently did not.

The New York Times

Rights Amendment Issue Divides Psychiatrists

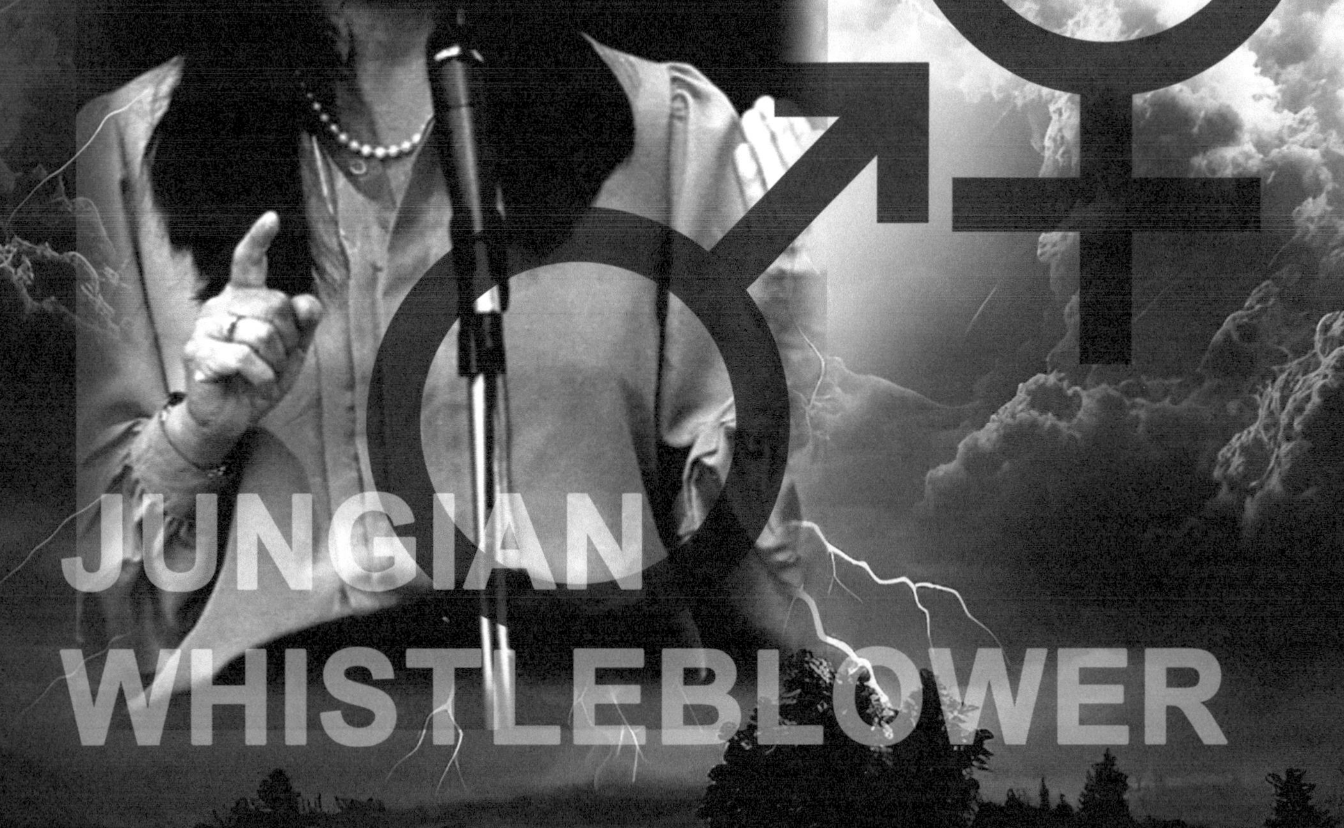

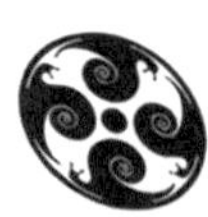

THE C.G. JUNG INSTITUTE
OF SAN FRANCISCO

OPEN LETTER

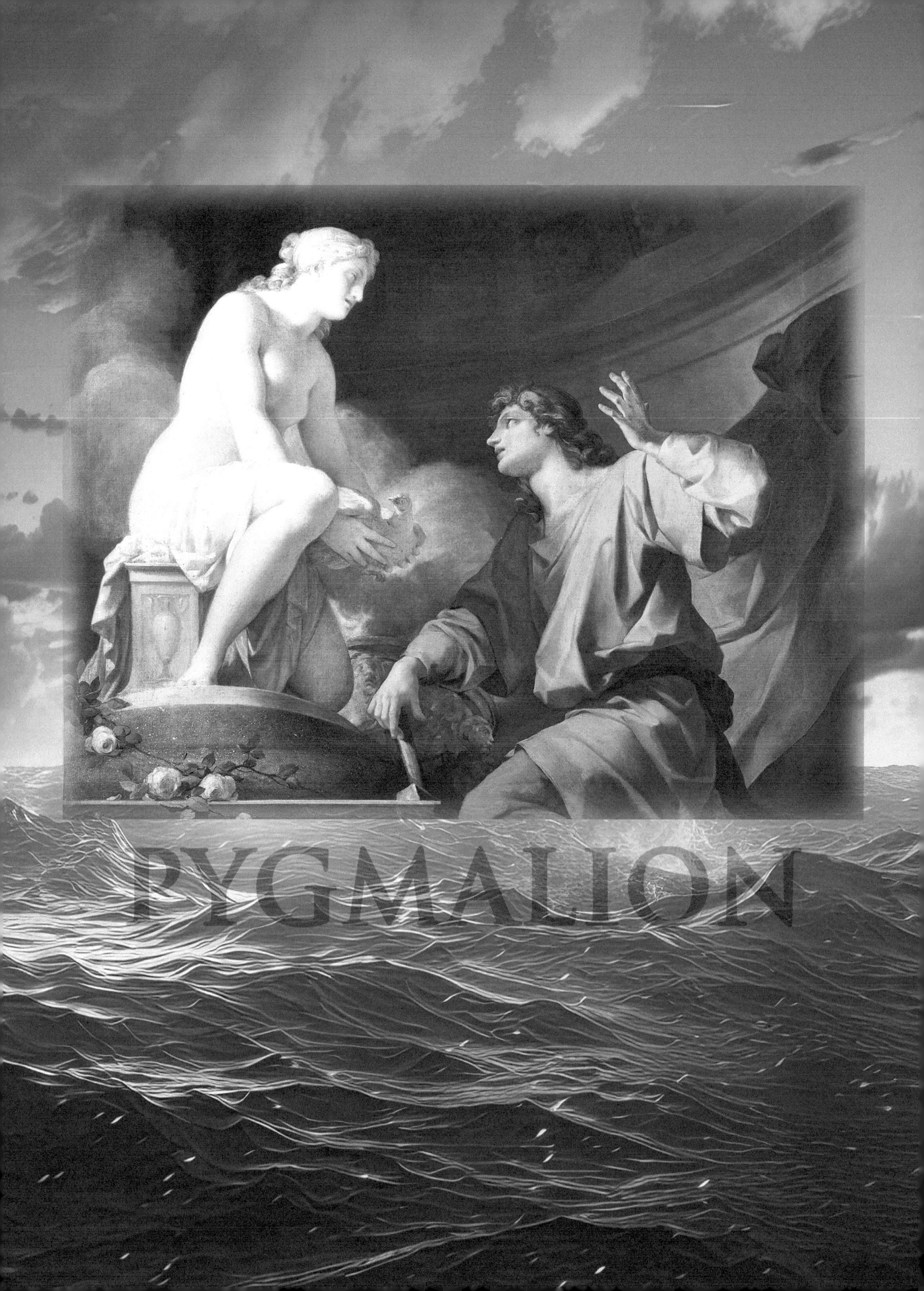
PYGMALION

ETHICS

Section 4

Women's Spirituality, Activist, Solo, Mother & Son

Chapter 20

Pulling Together – Growing Apart

Our daughter Melody Jean Bolen was born in 1970, our son Andy (Andre Joseph Bolen) in 1972. The Sausalito apartment with a stunning view was no place for active little ones. There was no yard, and the living room opened onto a deck that was a couple of stories above the ground. It was time to move. We leased a one-story house with a fenced in, big grassy backyard in Tiburon, eight miles northeast of Sausalito. Tiburon was a bedroom community across the bay from San Francisco where both Jim and I had our respective offices. It would now be a longer commute. Many who lived there chose not to drive and instead took the ferry to work in the city.

I had taken time off with each birth and could determine my own working hours. Our childcare support was stable and exceptionally good: "Ivy" (Mrs. Mary Ivy Dekker) and "Ty" (Gertrude Norris) were two long-time residents with grown children. What began as supplementary income turned into meaningful relationships for them and for my children and me. I had to feel fine about leaving my children in someone else's care when I went to work. My most important initial meetings were with potential babysitters, not patients! I chose by instinct, intuition, and information women freely gave me, and by observing them with my kids. Over a relatively short time, these two became part of my children's lives and our lives for years.

At the time and in retrospect, our marriage was a good one. It was an egalitarian marriage in regards to household responsibilities. Both of us shopped for groceries and cooked, and we pitched in to do whatever needed doing, and we didn't keep score. Both of us were thoughtful and considerate people. We were like horses who were in harness together, going in the same direction, pulling a heavy load. We did this very well. Some of the elements of this are common to couples with young children. I'm thinking of films taken in malls of couples without children and couples with small children. Couples without children looked at each other a lot. Couples with children hardly made eye contact with each other, even while talking were looking at store windows or the kids.

With work and children, gender differences in communication, extraversion and introversion, and a lack of available time and energy, conversations that could deepen emotional intimacy between husband and wife are difficult to have. There are, after all, only twenty-four hours in a day, and what has to be done takes up most of the time. When is there time or privacy for a deeper conversation with a tired spouse?

I can look back with compassion at the situation, which is common. Both of us had been single through our twenties, were used to being independent, and when we became parents we sacrificed for the family important archetypes which Jung had named *puer eternus* and *puella eterna* (Latin for "the eternal boy" and "the eternal girl,: or inner child/inner dreamer-adolescent). We had a shared capacity for fun and adventure, symbolized by Jim's French beret and white two-seater Mercedes convertible. It was not long after we were married that he sold it and got a used four-door sedan. While neither of us were Peter Pan or Wendy in Never-Never Land, once we stopped sharing delight and fun and instead took on the roles of responsible grownups, an inner connection between his *puer* and my *puella* was lost. In Jungian psychology, these are Latin words (boy/girl) that are linked to *eternal,* often indicating a lack of maturity in an adult. In responsible adults, some, but not all, still have a capacity for delight and can experience these moments in the midst of ongoing responsibilities. Both Jim and I had chosen people with ability and responsibility to help us do what we had taken on. In this stressful period of our lives, I was still in the training program at the Jungian Institute and also in private practice doing psychotherapy in depth.

Later I learned that it was not just Jim and me who responded differently in this stressful period but was characteristic of gender. When a department at UCLA came under stress, the researchers noted how the women and men responded differently; the men followed the "flight or fight" reaction. In the academic and corporate world, the threat isn't a saber-toothed tiger, it's that a project won't be funded, or that a layoff may happen. The threat of unemployment or business failure can result in loss of role, prestige, sense of competency, self-esteem—even manhood. "Flight" then is the tendency to withdraw, to not want to talk, to go into the office and shut the door, or go home, sit in front of the TV and keep everyone away. "Fight" is the irritability, road-rage, lashing out, and projecting "loser!" on others. This was an adrenaline response that is enhanced by testosterone.

The researchers at UCLA saw that women responded differently. They wanted to talk about this threat, they gathered together, and cleaned up the workplace. At home, they tended children and gardens, and neatened up the house. As they did what the researchers named the "tend and befriend" response, stress levels went down, and oxytocin (the maternal bonding hormone) went up. The oxytocin response is enhanced by estrogen.

There is another difference between men and women that comes up in couple conversations, and it is a generality that doesn't universally apply. Women usually want to talk through a problem, which includes the circumstances and their feelings. Men want to fix the problem, which leads to telling her what she should do, or him doing something about it. When a problem is shared and feelings about what happened are voiced and heard with love and understanding, a bond of connective tissue grows between them.

Sometimes, psychological type differences are a source of tension in a couple. When they are discussing a family or a business decision, the extraverted response is usually faster, especially if it is an extraverted-intuitive response. An introvert's process requires that the issue be taken in and not responded to immediately. Feeling and thinking are our assessing functions, usually decisions are best made by considering both, and even better if both intuition and sensation (getting specific information) are considered. Sometimes passive-aggressive and slower introverted responses overlap. The introverted partner's need for more time is legitimate, but unvoiced resentments can also be passively expressed, through the power to withhold decisions held by the introvert. Extraverted feeling-intuitive types usually feel certain about people and decisions, while thinking types can look at all angles of the situation. These gender and typology generalities applied to us as a married couple with children, as they probably do in many families.

In addition, there was for me, and for those of us who do depth psychotherapy, an occupational hazard. We become used to quality conversations and we are affected by the work we do. Our people reveal what is in their hearts and souls. We hear raw feelings, see tears, are privileged to hear big archetypal dreams, and we may be trusted with a secret, a shame, or a hope. Our words and responses can heal childhood wounds and support growth—and some of our sessions are as significant to us as they are to those who come to us. The relationship work we do as analysts (to paraphrase Jung) is like an alchemical reaction. For one person to be transformed by it, the other must be also.

We who do this work go off to work like everyone else, and come home after. In between, we may be accompanying a person into the underworld of irrational fear, hear about a wonderful synchronicity, glow in shared pride at an accomplishment, or hear a dream as affective as a work of art, or grieve with someone that touches the place in me that has known loss. I may help people who need support to keep on keeping on, and at the end of the day I may be wrung out. I may have made a life-or-death decision in a session with someone for whom suicide is a possibility. None of these are everyday conversational topics.

I am reminded of Robert Paul Smith's illustrated children's book, titled as a conversation between mother and son: *Where Did You Go? Out. What Did You Do? Nothing.* The boy had all sorts of experiences, explored, was surprised, and it was quite a day! The title is similar to conversations between spouses: "How was your day?" "Fine."

When I returned home after my last patient, there was dinner and childcare, household to-dos, and my natural role as a supportive wife who can relate to the subjects and to the business challenges of *Psychic Magazine*. The magazine was a creative success, but the business side was a struggle, and seeking financial support had gotten entwined with our social life.

As we pulled together, we were growing apart. It looked as if we were partners in a successful two-career marriage, and for a long time, I thought we were. But as time went on there was less and less between us because deep conversations and the soul connections made through them were not happening. I was increasingly busy and lonely. Up until I married, my friendships were important and had lasted over years. Circumstances had changed that. With children, time for friendships diminishes, and my former close friends were now in New York City, New Haven, or Los Angeles. Then we got into roles or ruts in the marriage, and maintained the form, which we did well, while talk between us became superficial, mostly logistical details.

Maybe it would have been different if I had a different occupation—but for me, this work was a calling. It was soul work. Work for me was gratifying on many levels. The metaphor was the analytic container or alchemical flask, keeping confidences, respecting what was told to me, and it left me with little I wanted to say about work when I got home.

When I was upset after the death of a patient under questionable circumstances, and needed to share what I was feeling, there wasn't anyone but Jim to talk to about it. When I tried to, we missed an opportunity. It wasn't something he could fix, or feel as I did, and I couldn't say, or even know clearly, that what I needed was a quality of listening that would give me comfort. *Maybe.* Like many unresolved complex situations, the effect of what might have been remains unknown. It also was a death that sent rings of emotional reaction out from it like a stone thrown into a pond: I met with her young son, and one of her close friends was in my practice. My task was to support them in their grief and confusion.

We moved from Tiburon to Mill Valley toward the end of the 1970s. We bought and remodeled a house in the Old Mill school district. This project, and other activities on both of our parts, kept us occupied and pulling together. There were, however, major new interests that we separately were engaged in that would further us growing apart. In 1979, *Psychic Magazine* became *New Realities.* The first issue introduced *The Course in Miracles,* which would be the major focus of the renamed magazine. In 1979, I attended the first Women's Spirituality Conference at Asilomar and *The Tao of Psychology* was published.

The first Women's Spirituality Conference was the beginning of a deepening soulful opening for me to the divine feminine. At about the same time that this was happening in me, Jim received a copy of the manuscript for *The Course in Miracles* from Judith Skutch. When he held it in his hands, he had a numinous response. The *Course* was channeled through Helen Schucman, a research psychologist at Columbia University, who heard a voice say, "This is a Course in Miracles, please take notes."

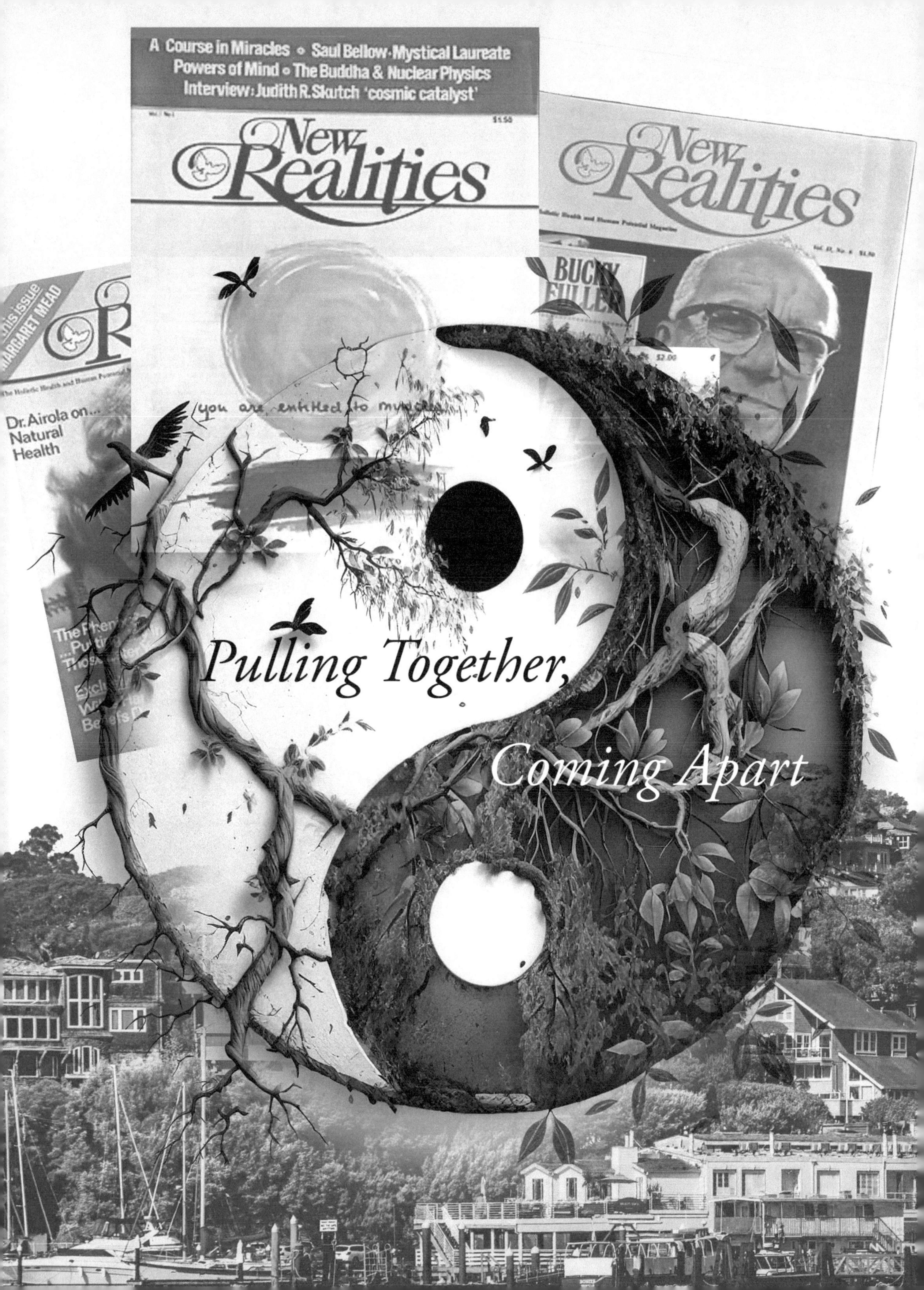
A Course in Miracles • Saul Bellow-Mystical Laureate
Powers of Mind • The Buddha & Nuclear Physics
Interview: Judith R. Skutch 'cosmic catalyst'
$1.50
New Realities
you are entitled to miracles
New Realities
BUCKY
$2.00
this issue
MARGARET MEAD
Dr. Airola on...
Natural
Health
Pulling Together,
Coming Apart

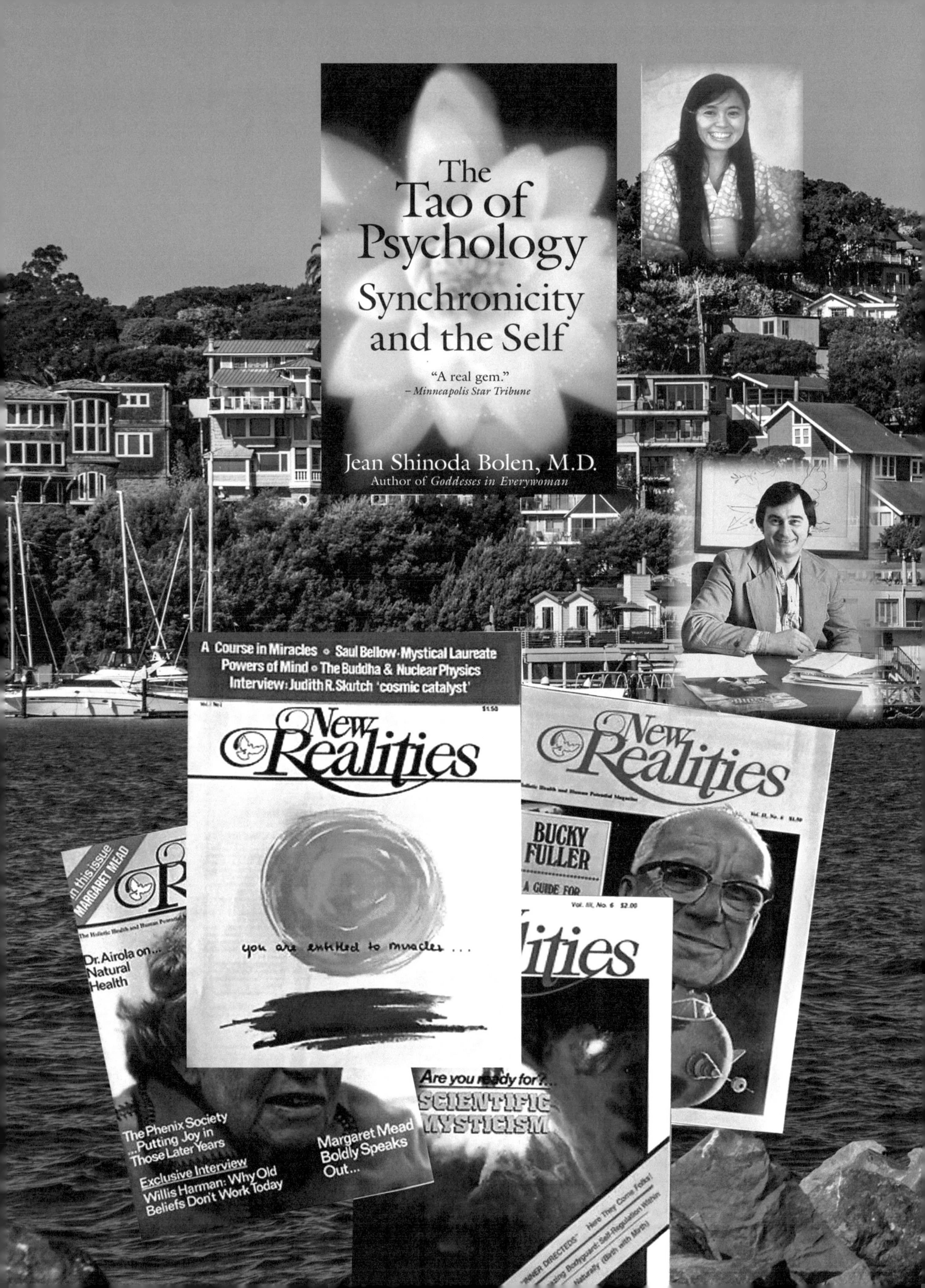
The Tao of Psychology
Synchronicity and the Self
“A real gem.”
– Minneapolis Star Tribune
Jean Shinoda Bolen, M.D.
Author of Goddesses in Everywoman
A Course in Miracles • Saul Bellow-Mystical Laureate
Powers of Mind • The Buddha & Nuclear Physics
Interview: Judith R. Skutch 'cosmic catalyst'
$1.50
New Realities
you are entitled to miracles ...
New Realities
BUCKY FULLER
A GUIDE FOR
In this issue
MARGARET MEAD
Dr. Airola on... Natural Health
The Phenix Society ...Putting Joy in Those Later Years
Exclusive Interview
Willis Harman: Why Old Beliefs Don't Work Today
Margaret Mead Boldly Speaks Out...
Vol. III, No. 6 $2.00
Are you ready for?...
SCIENTIFIC MYSTICISM
Here They Come Folks!

Fight or Flight vs Tend and Befriend

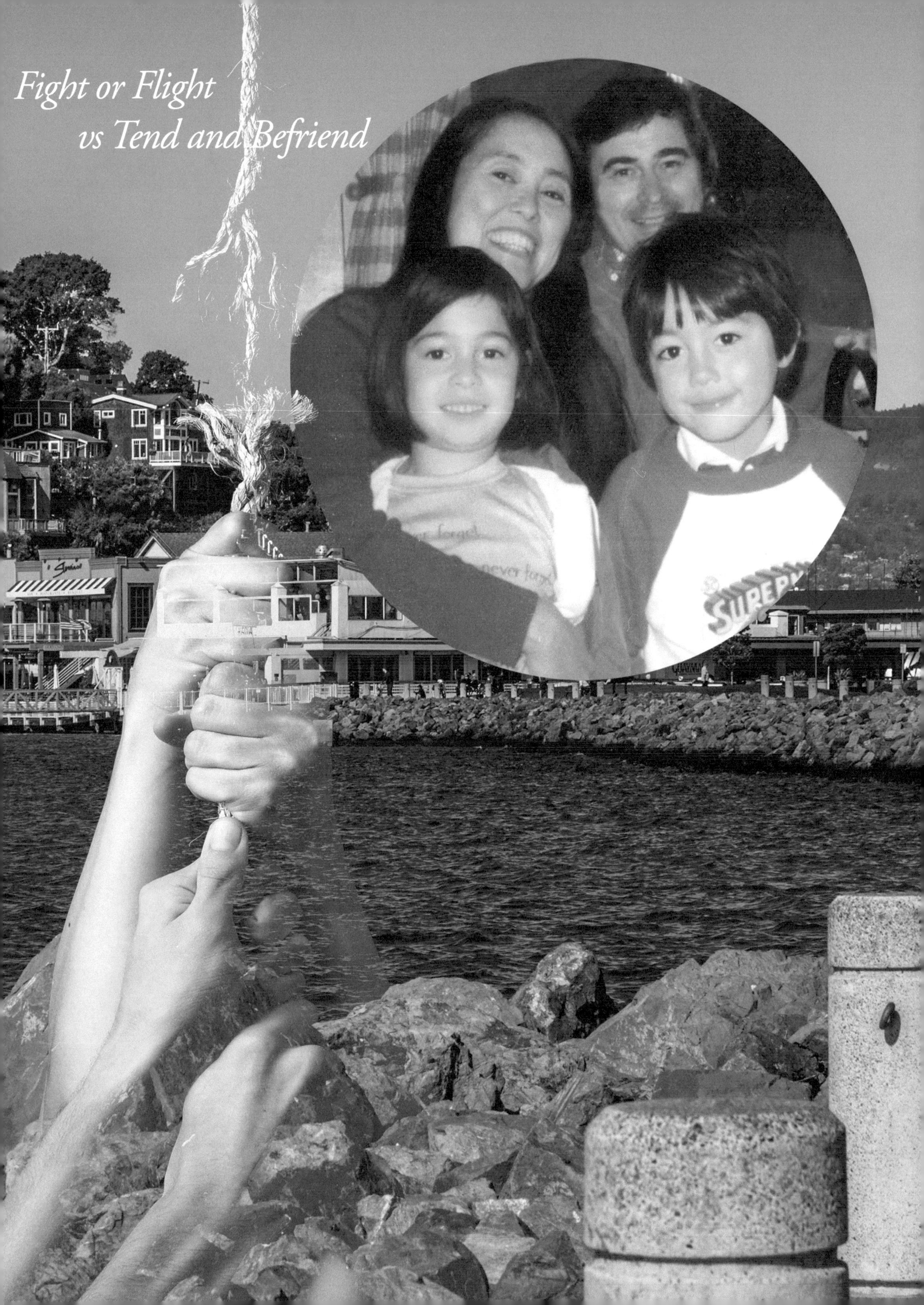

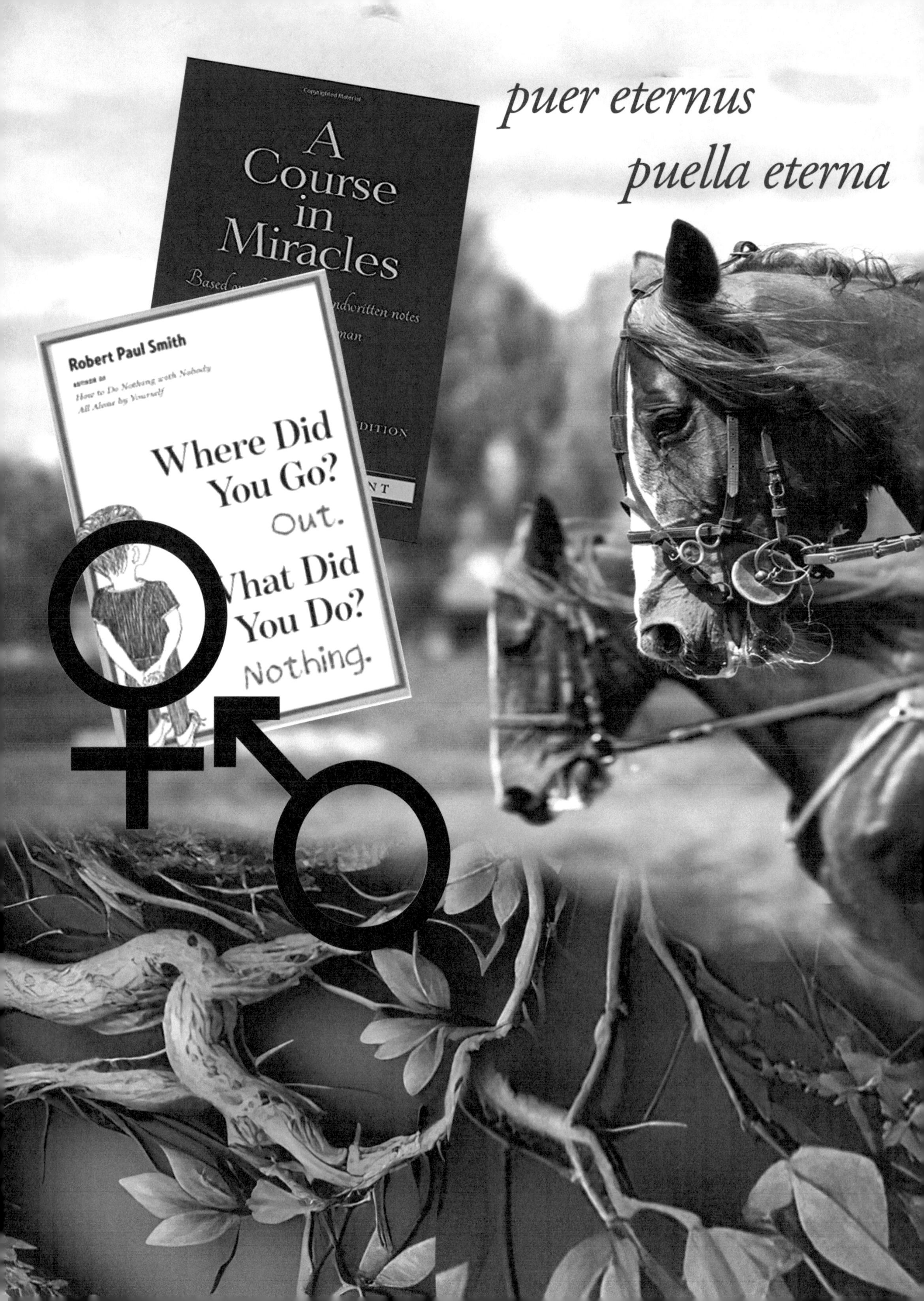

puer eternus
puella eterna
A Course in Miracles
Robert Paul Smith
How to Do Nothing with Nobody
All Alone by Yourself
Where Did You Go?
Out.
You Do?
Nothing.

Chapter 21
Women's Spirituality - Goddess

My first experience of women's spirituality was as a participant in an invitational pre-conference at Asilomar, near Monterey, California, held before the annual Association for Humanistic Psychology Conference in the summer of 1979. Each woman who came had been invited in a chain letter fashion: the inviter extended the invitation to others, as it had been to her, by a woman who thought of her as a woman in whom spirituality was important.

This gathering was brought together by two psychologists, Karin Carrington and Nancy Scotton. It was called "Women's Spirituality: A Dream of a Common Language," a title inspired by a work by poet Adrienne Rich. We met in circles. There was ritual, music, personal sharing rather than a person in authority speaking, laughter, and spontaneity. It was a new model for me to find that each of us was the only authority on how we felt and were affected by whatever was spiritual for us. Some called divinity "Goddess." As a Protestant, the Bible was the textbook, the pastors and theologians, the experts. I hadn't realized that religion and spirituality are not only separate but often in conflict until I read the words of women who were discovering the Goddess, had experiences of my own, and found words myself.

Over time, after this experience, I grew to realize the power of being in a circle of women who told their truth, each of whom spoke from their own experience. A circle of women, or a women's circle with a spiritual or sacred center, changes the women in it. Each is a mirror to see a facet of herself and each can model something arising in another. It was a model for change that I would use in workshops, write about, and bring to the United Nations two decades later. On the way, two other conferences had an influence on me and on the Women's Spirituality movement.

Later that year, I was on book tour with *The Tao of Psychology*, giving talks and signing books at different venues. One was in Atlanta in a Unitarian church with an African-American woman minister. She suggested we pray before I spoke to those gathered in the church. I closed my eyes and unexpectedly heard her say, "Dear Mother-Father God." It touched me by the rightness I felt when we prayed. Synchronistic moments have a quality of magic and grace about them. They bring an awareness to us that an invisible world or the universe somehow, inexplicitly, takes an interest in us. "Mother God" was a phrase that entered my psyche then; it was a body-soul opening to Goddess Spirituality, which is sometimes used interchangeably with Women's Spirituality. "Mother God" resonated in me and moved me. It felt right that God be both male and female, that divinity be Mother as well as Father.

It reminded me of an experience that I had in which I felt held in the arms of a Mother Goddess. This had occurred in my office after the death of a patient who I thought had been murdered. My analysand-patient picked up on grief I thought was not showing. She asked if I was okay. I was touched by her concern, because I had felt so alone with my sadness, with no solace elsewhere. When my eyes filled with tears, she got out of her chair, came over to mine, put her arms around me, and I felt in that instant that both of us were held in an energy field of loving maternal comfort. This was a powerful and significant experience. Afterwards, I began thinking about the difference between my sense of God and this. The God I knew as a Christian was the trinity of Father-Son-Holy Spirit, and sometimes Heavenly Father. The personal sense of a transcendent God had set me on the path to become a doctor and then a psychiatrist. This was also a numinous moment that filled me with awe, but it was different—a woman comforted me and the Goddess held us both.

I thought back to the middle-of-the-night feedings when I got up to nurse my daughter Melody in the quiet of the apartment we had then—sitting in the rocking chair, with her at my breast, and me with enough milk for her. I remembered the feeling of this being a holy moment. It was transpersonal, archetypal—we were in an energy field of great mother and divine child.

There was excitement and a rippling of organizing creativity that followed the Asilomar meeting. Some were directly connected, but as it is with movements, ideas seemed to rise into the consciousness of individuals as if unseen seeds had been widely scattered. The major manifestation in the Bay Area was the first Women's Spirituality Conference that was open to all who wanted to attend. It was held at Fort Cronkite in 1981 or 1982, a decommissioned former military base in the Golden Gate Regional National Park, south of the Golden Gate Bridge. I was one of several hundred women who came. It was organized with help from John F. Kennedy University. Women were invited to offer a class, a ritual, a creative experience, and to actively participate in this conference. The result was a rich and diverse choice of activities, a menu of offerings. Many attendees were women whose names would become known in the next decades.

The first evening, there was a huge bonfire on the beach, with chanting, dancing, and rituals. Talks and classes in a variety of subjects were given. Angeles Arrien gave a talk based on several tarot cards that was an extraordinary tour de force on archetypes. (I suggested that she be invited to speak at the San Francisco Jungian Institute and wasn't able to cause it to happen.) The value of this women's spirituality conference and ones that followed was that individual women were connecting with and expressing the deep feminine in creative ways, and had role models.

I came to the conference with a college friend, Ann Morris, an artist and a philosophy major at Pomona who had an interest and knowledge of Jung. She later went on to create Sculpture Woods on Lummi Island, one of the San Juan Islands in Puget Sound. This is a permanent installation of sixteen life-sized or larger bronze mythic figures. They are exhibited in nature among the trees where they become part of the landscape, where the metaphoric connection between them and nature actually come together.

My contribution was a talk about Artemis, goddess of the hunt and moon, and archetype of the sister and feminist. I was working on the manuscript for *Goddesses in Everywoman* and speaking about the different goddess archetypes that women who responded to the conference invitation could have. The talk was scheduled at night. We gathered together to walk on the road from where we were to the chapel at Fort Cronkite. There was some moonlight and the stars overhead. I led the way. In the small chapel, where many religious services had been held, I stood and talked about Artemis. The power of an archetype when it is described and named comes from the "Aha!" of recognition in the listener, who is drawing images and patterns up from the collective unconscious. When we walked together in silence and sisterhood with the world around us—mostly hills without houses and lights—under the nighttime sky, we were in Artemis' realm. I was as affected as my listeners.

In 1984, *Goddesses in Everywoman* was published after a minor saga of wresting it from the initial publisher, who wanted extensive changes, to have it accepted and published as I wrote it by Harper San Francisco. It was introduced at a weekend workshop sponsored by Women's Quest, a Berkeley-based and goddess-centered organization that grew out of the Women's Spirituality Conference. Women's Quest was inspired and led by Anthea Francine, who had come to Berkeley to study at the Graduate Theological Union. She had come from England via Zurich where she studied Jung. She was a soul friend who had kept personal dream journals and saw the value of women meeting in circles centered in beauty and in the feminine. Her height, presence, voice, and dress when she led events made her a personification of an archetypal priestess.

I introduced each goddess, told her mythology, and spoke of the meaning of the archetype. Then women from Women's Quest enacted the particular goddess in costume, through dance or mime, art, and music. The workshop was held in a large room in a church which had been transformed into a feminine space. This was a model for subsequent *Goddesses in Everywoman* events held elsewhere and led by others. Women read the book, identified with particular goddess-archetypes, and in their small circles told their own stories about having lived out aspects. Some who realized that they needed to cultivate a missing goddess, and enacted her with others for whom that goddess was primary. The music chosen for each of the goddesses helped to evoke them—sensual music for Aphrodite, for example. I recall how the orchestral music for "Chariots of Fire" (a film that was very popular then, about an Olympian runner) was used to power up Athena.

Goddesses in Everywoman: A New Psychology of Women became an immediate San Francisco Chronicle bestseller, and it stayed on the list for weeks. A year later, it was published in paperback by HarperCollins in New York, and promoted as a bestseller. I was sent out on a book tour to major cities in the United States. I would be met at the airport by a media escort, who had a full schedule for me: there would be a bookstore talk and book signing, interviews scheduled with print media people, radio and daytime TV appearances. Then, every big city had its own afternoon talk show with a man and woman as co-hosts. Authors guesting on the show would cross paths coming and going in the studio's "green room," or waiting room, until it was our turn.

My book was a psychology of women based on the major Greek goddesses (Hera, Demeter, Persephone, Artemis, Athena, Hestia, and Aphrodite). Gloria Steinem wrote the foreword, which was personally meaningful. It gave me a "big sister has my back" feeling. She wrote: "I would like to invite you into this book, especially if you are one of those readers who might be, as I was, resistant to its theme. After all, how can mythological goddesses from a patriarchal past help us to analyze our current realities or reach an egalitarian future? Just as we are most likely to buy books recommended by trusted friends, my inspiration to read this manuscript came from knowing its author." There followed a description of how we met because of Psychiatrists for ERA, comments about seeing me in action, and now seeing or calling on the goddess-archetypes in herself. Word-of-mouth recommendations, its use in mythology and psychology college courses, and over time, translations and foreign editions have kept this as my most well-known book. The thirtieth anniversary edition with the subtitle "Powerful Archetypes in Women's Lives" was published in 2014.

In 1984, Sherry Ruth Anderson had a powerful and detailed dream that she described in *The Feminine Face of God: The Unfolding of the Sacred in Women,* written with Patricia Hopkins. They first met in the summer of 1985 at a Women's Quest gathering. They made a commitment to research and write a book about women's personal spiritual lives. To do this, they set out "to hear directly from women about the unfolding of the sacred in their lives in their own words, in the language of their own hearts." It was a four-year project that was published in 1991. I wrote the foreword, which began: "*The Feminine Face of God* is as significant as Betty Friedan's *The Feminine Mystique* and Carol Gilligans' *In a Different Voice* were in articulating a growing edge of conscious awareness in women. . . it does for women's spirituality what these two books did for women's roles and women's ethics. . . This is a book that invites women to define for themselves what is sacred, to find an indwelling source of spiritual sustenance in themselves, in communion with others, and with the divine as they know It/Him/Her."

In 1985, the first Women's Alliance Solstice Camp, started by Charlotte Kelly, was held for two weeks outside of Nevada City, California in the Sierras. Over the next decade, these camps were a growth-medium for the early seeds of Women's Spirituality to flourish, find support, and grow. They were the beginning of women's summer solstice camps that are now held in many other places. I learned and made friends, became conscious of a bigger world of ideas, learned by doing, risked looking foolish (to myself), and stopped being self-conscious as I participated in dance, drumming, and keening.

In many parts of the expressive world, women wail or keen in sorrow and mourning. Joanna Macy taught us how to keen, and then she slowly read a long list of now extinct animals, fish, and birds that once shared this earth with us as we expressed our sorrow. Barbara Marx Hubbard introduced the idea of resonating circles and the influence through resonance of each circle. Brooke Medicine Eagle brought Indigenous wisdom and ritual for us to do. We each belonged to a small circle with an altar in the center and met in much larger ones as the occasion determined. The effect on us was not immediate but part of a process that would lead to a deeper and more personal expression of ourselves, to the development of academic Women's Spirituality programs, to ecological activism, and appreciation of Indigenous wisdom. Books were written and read, ideas rippled out, music was sung, and women reinvented themselves and their spirituality. Small initial changes led many women to change their lives as well as deepen their spirituality. Words from a goddess song, "Everything She touches, changes," are true.

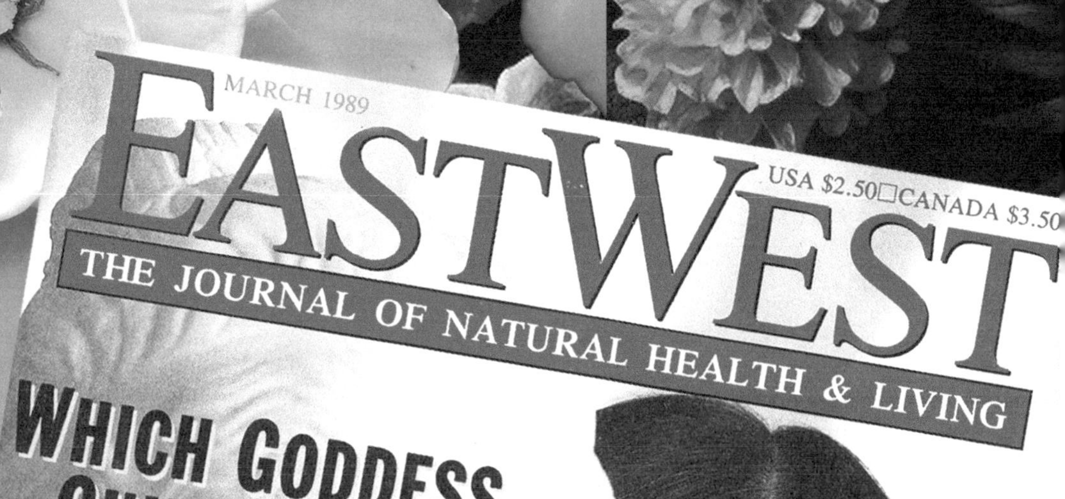
MARCH 1989
EASTWEST
USA $2.50□CANADA $3.50
THE JOURNAL OF NATURAL HEALTH & LIVING
WHICH GODDESS GUIDES YOU?
An Interview with Jean Shinoda Bolen, M.D.
Norman Cousins' Healing Equation
Spotlight on Full-Spectrum Lighting
Animal Research Under Fire

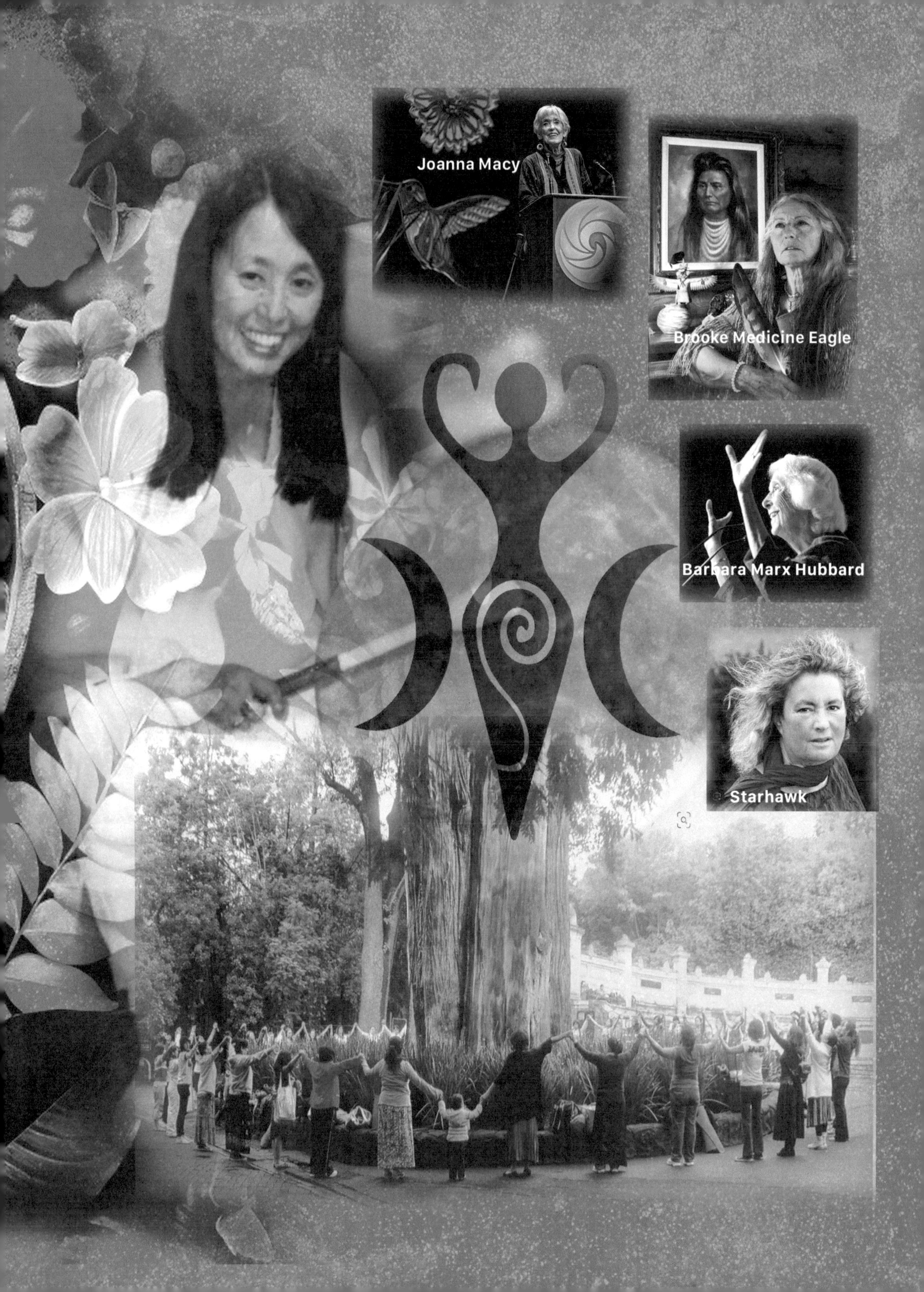
Joanna Macy
Brooke Medicine Eagle
Barbara Marx Hubbard
Starhawk

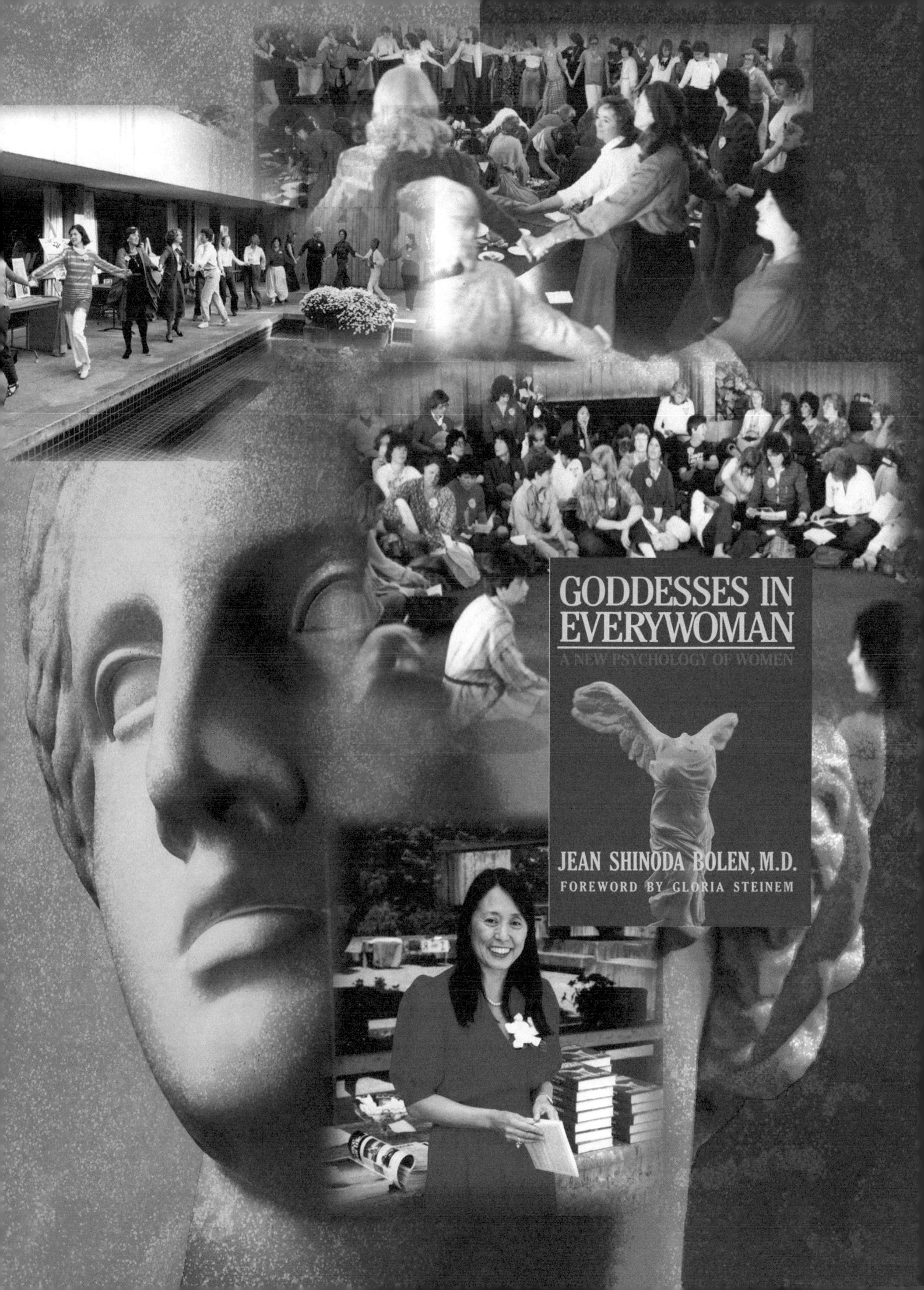

GODDESSES IN EVERYWOMAN

A NEW PSYCHOLOGY OF WOMEN

JEAN SHINODA BOLEN, M.D.

FOREWORD BY GLORIA STEINEM

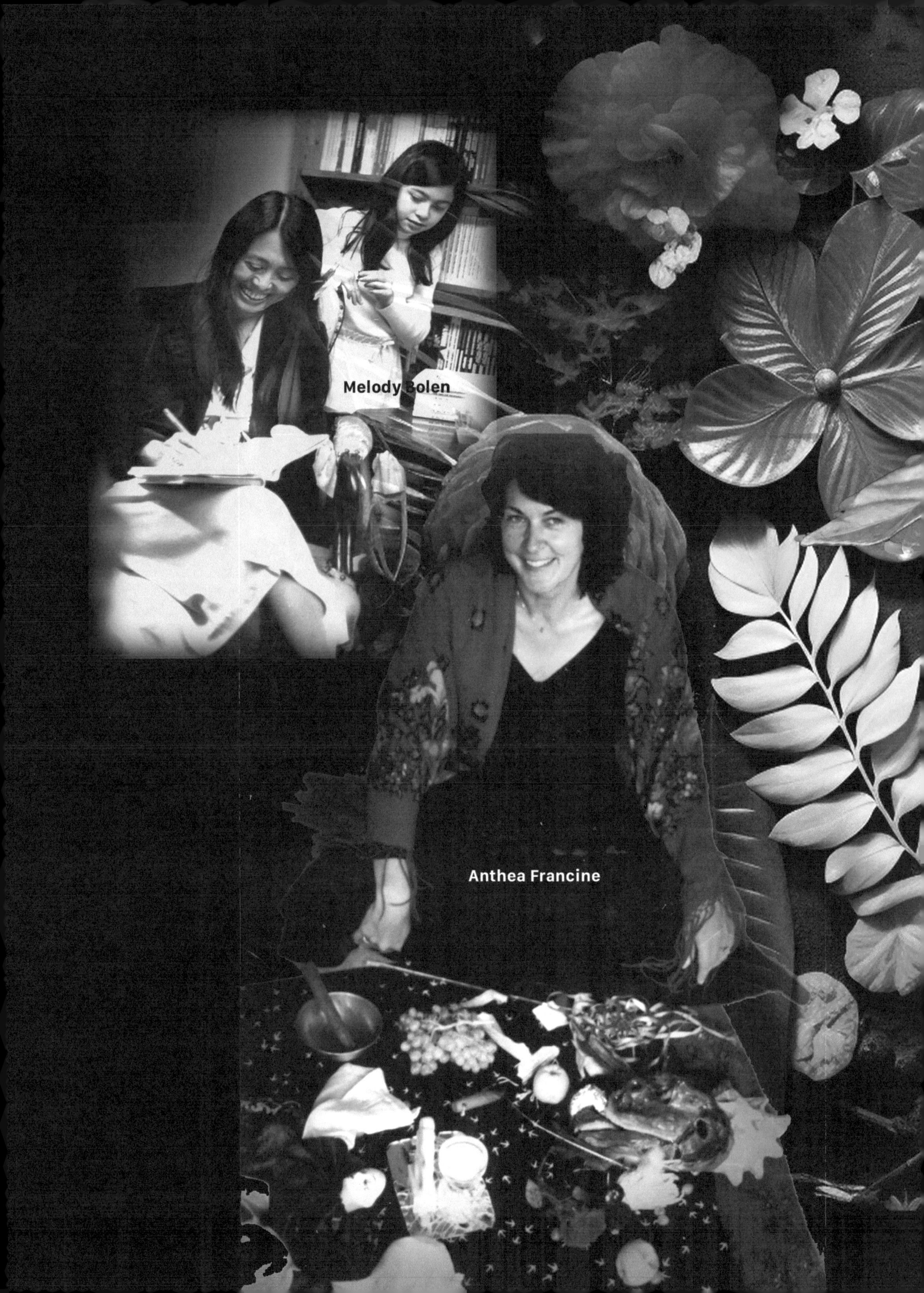

Melody Bolen

Anthea Francine

Chapter 22

Solo Journey - Hestia

In the middle of the 1980s, I left my husband and home, which led to divorce several years later. California has a "no fault" divorce for "irreconcilable differences," which could be said to be true for every marriage that ends in divorce. While our life as a couple ended, our roles as parents continued, and the family archetype would be reconstituted as the enduring connection between us. After the separation and before the divorce, we individually and together saw therapists. Neither of us remarried. Lots of marriages stay together, almost no-matter-what, and many do with the help of therapists (including those who have done so with my help).

Irrational as it seemed even to me, and as good a marriage as it was, when I left, there was no turning back. My physically leaving seemed impulsive and in the moment, as it happened after we had a heated argument—a rarity. My experience in the marriage was of being alone and lonely, while together. The marriage phase of my life was over, and I had not anticipated or planned for it. In the immediate interim, I stayed at a motel, then with friends, then for a month or so in a furnished corporate rental apartment near my office where my kids could stay. In our house in Mill Valley, they had their own rooms at one end of the house, with parents in a master suite at the other end. In contrast, the rental was cozy. This nomadic period ended when I moved back to Mill Valley and into a Shelter Ridge condominium.

While they were crowded and cozily with me in my San Francisco rental, Rainbow, our Bernese Mountain dog, fell ill. She had been with us the whole time that we lived in the family house in Mill Valley. With the children in school and working parents, she spent a lot of time by herself in an enclosed area behind the house. Bernese Mountain dogs had been bred as working dogs—they are beautiful, large dogs. Rainbow was mostly an outside dog. Now I was gone, and Melody and Andy were away when they spent overnights with me, as they were the evening we learned she was ailing. The children returned while she was still alive, and she died shortly after. The next day I joined them and their father when we buried her next to the house. Hers was a real and symbolic death. I thought at the time that she was a sacrifice, and by on taking on whatever she did, she may have spared us some illness. Her health would have been affected by the change in the household, by the absences, by emotional neglect, by absorbing feelings of depression, loss and anger that were in the house.

Shortly after the separation, I came back to get personal items on the way to a documentary filming in a house in Mill Valley. The film's theme was based on an epic museum installation: Judy Chicago's *The Dinner Party*, which was a monumental work of art that functioned as a symbolic history of women in western civilization. Laid on a triangular banquet table, measuring 48 feet on each side, were places set for thirty-nine "guests of honor." Each had a larger-than-life painted porcelain plate with an individual image based on the butterfly to symbolize the vulva, ceramic flatware, and a chalice. Placements were on textiles and runners with images drawn from each woman's story in needlework. The work was premiered at the San Francisco Museum of Modern Art in 1979, where it drew major audiences, and would go on to be exhibited in sixteen venues in six countries. It is now on permanent exhibit at the Elizabeth A. Sackler Center for Feminist Art at the Brooklyn Museum, New York.

Starhawk—writer, activist, neopagan and ecofeminist—had invited a dozen or so of us to bring symbolic placemats and objects to put on them, and then to discuss women's spirituality among ourselves while it was filmed for a documentary. It became part of *Goddess Remembered* (1989), the first film in the Canadian Film Board's trilogy directed by Donna Reed. The documentary is based upon goddess cultures that date back 35,000 years (according to Maria Gimbutas and Merlin Stone) and its connection to the women's spirituality movement in the late twentieth century. I was with Merlin Stone, Carol Christ, Luisah Teish, Kim Chernin, Starhawk, and Susan Griffin, among others.

I also did my first firewalk shortly after leaving my marriage. A short workshop was being offered that I signed up for and went to by myself. Could I do what I believed in? Could I walk bare-footed on hot coals and not get burned? I saw this as a challenge to myself—if I truly believe something, will I put my body on the line? I was, in a more metaphoric way, doing this by leaving my husband. I listened to the talk, listened to testimonials, had knowledge of this being done in India, and believed in mind over matter. Science and common sense says that if coals are hot enough to ignite a stick of wood or paper, putting bare feet on those same coals will cause burns. When it was my turn, I walked on the coals that glowed under my feet. There were two spots on the bottom of one foot where something hot had "stuck" to my skin. This imperfect firewalk made me ask to do it again—which I did, this time without the uncertainty that had taken courage to do it the first time. The coals were hot, but not to my feet.

Another new experience that I sought out myself was getting my first astrological reading. I heard about an astrologer in New York from a trusted source, and made an appointment to see Dr. Julie Bresciani for a "cold" reading, so I told her nothing about myself ahead of the reading. This was in probably in 1985, when I was on the Ms. Foundation board which regularly met in New York City. I learned that when I left my former life, it coincided with a major event in my chart: "Uranus had hit your Grand Cross." While this made sense only astrologically, I welcomed the information because as I learned of its significance, it made sense internally and nothing else had explained or justified what I was choosing to do (or not to do). I couldn't go back.

The planet Uranus is called the awakener or liberator or the call for authenticity when it "hits." When it hits a grand cross, it affects the four areas or houses that can be in conflict with each other. In my chart, they represent family, personality, career, and marriage. Over the years, since this first reading, I have come to understand that the grand cross is a difficult configuration of opposites within the personality, which can make life very difficult. Putting the problem into my own metaphor, I could be "crucified on this cross" by the conflicting energies pulling me in opposite directions, or I could become psychologically big enough to hold these tensions of opposite within me consciously.

What I did grasp immediately and appreciate was that the basic three planets that defined my personality accurately accounted for who I perceived myself to be. The rising sign has to do with the face or persona with which we meet the outer world. Mine is Leo: the lion and fire sign, the extravert which explains my social skills and friendliness as a child that got me through the many schools and situations which the forced evacuation caused, and the warmth and ease with which I speak to groups. My sun sign or essential nature is Cancer: the crab in her shell, the sign of the introvert, and a water sign that I came to understand only after I could spend time alone. It takes energy to be in my Leo persona, and that energy is limited. Solitude refuels me. My moon or relationship to the unconscious is in Scorpio: the scorpion, a water sign, and the most complex of the twelve astrological signs.

I was told that many people with moon in Scorpio take people into the underworld and abandon them there, but because my sun sign is in Cancer, which is known as the maternal sign, I go into the underworld to bring people back. This would explain what I discovered when I became a psychiatric resident and was assigned my first inpatients on a locked ward: I was comfortable in their world. I was unafraid of psychosis, and had an affinity for images that arose from the unconscious in dreams and creativity. I could see the potential in the person and help that potential become realized. Later with the further guidance of Jung's writings and Jungian analysts, I've come to know my way around this watery realm where personal and collective unconscious forces and images flow together. A much later added insight of potential qualities was the position of Neptune on my chart that meant "muse and medium."

After I left and moved to Shelter Ridge, Melody and Andy were in high school. They spent half of the time living with me, and half the time living with their father. When they were not with me, I lived by myself for the first time in my life. I had lived with my parents, with roommates in dorms or housemates, and then with my husband. I loved living alone. It was my first experience of solitude and the serenity that I could experience being by myself. I moved into an empty condo which was carpeted but not furnished. The emptiness created a sense of spaciousness which I liked. Other than taking my books and art, I had not taken anything from the family house.

I was creating and living in a "Hestia" space. Hestia is the Greek goddess of the Hearth. It was her presence that made a house a home, and a building a temple. She was the third Virgin goddess, who, like Athena and Artemis, retained her virginity in a patriarchal cosmology and mythology in which all women could be possessed or raped or married as decided by gods or men who desired them. As archetypes in women, they represent that part in a woman that can stay one-in-herself when married or even after being raped.

Hestia is the least known Greek goddess; she was not personified in sculptures or paintings, and did not take part in the intrigues, conflicts, or romances in mythology. Yet, she was considered the most honored and revered, and given offerings in homes and temples. She was considered to be in the fire itself at the center of a round hearth. Hestia's fire provided light and heat for home and temple, fire that also cooked food. Metaphorically, Hestia was a provider of illumination, warmth, and nourishment. Her geometrical image is that of the mandala, a Sanskrit word for circle within a square or rectangle, which is the shape of Tibetan Buddhist sacred paintings. It is also the word and image that Jung used for the archetype of the Self, or the archetype of meaning. She is the eldest sister in the Olympian pantheon of gods and goddesses.

In women's retreats, it's instinctive to meet in circles. In workshops or retreats that I do, there is a lit candle at the center, often placed on a beautiful or symbolic cloth. In lighting the candle, we are inviting Hestia's presence in the candle's flame, just as it was her presence in the fire at the center of a round hearth that made home and temple sacred places. I have spoken of Hestia and then led a guided meditation using some of these phrases: "Your body is a temple with a glowing fire in your heart center. Imagine light and warmth emanating out from there to all the cells in your body. Your body is sacred. You are at peace and can go deeper into that place in yourself which is quiet—to the still point, where Hestia is."

There is a tension in the psyches of women between the archetypes that have to do with independence and lack of need for another person to complete them, and those archetypes that need another person to fulfill their meaning as wife, mother, or lover: Hera the archetype of the Wife, Demeter the archetype of the mother, and Aphrodite the archetype of the lover. All of the archetypes are potentials in us, what matters deeply to us depends upon the strength of archetypes in us which seems to be innate, like other inherited attributes or talents.

I've thought about Gloria Steinem's response to why she was not married—the assumption being that a woman as attractive as she would be among the chosen. She would say, "I don't mate well in captivity." It was good for a laugh and ended that line of questioning.

I've also thought about Kay, a close friend in high school and in college, and the depth of her grief over her boyfriend's betrayal. We were in high school at the Forest Home Christian camp when I heard her sobbing, inconsolable. They did eventually marry. Her marriage has endured over fifty years and remains the deepest source of her meaning, even though, like me, she was a beneficiary of the women's movement, and was advanced at work to become a full partner in a law firm before she retired. While Kay, Gloria, and I have developed and been affected by more than one archetype, Artemis is clearly the dominant archetype in Gloria Steinem and in me, while Hera the Goddess of Marriage and archetype of the wife must be the strongest and most meaningful archetype in my friend.

Imagine a horizontal scale, with the independent archetypes at one end, and the relationship archetypes on the other, and a sliding marker that you can place anywhere between the two poles. Where do you put your marker? Does the question "stay or go?" even arise? "Go!" came through loud and clear for me.

This course-change might not have happened if I were not a Jungian analyst for whom individuation, depth, and meaning were deeply held values, or if I could not be financially independent, or if I felt and responded to social or religious pressure, or if I had felt guilty of a sin, or if my archetypes were different, or if this were a different historical time and not the San Francisco Bay Area, or if our paths had not diverged over spiritual differences. I had been affected by feminism and consciousness-raising about patriarchy, by the goddess and women's spirituality. *The Course in Miracles* had transformed Jim's thinking and as a result, *Psychic Magazine* became *New Realities*, with *The Course in Miracles* the subject of the first issue and a core belief for him and content for the magazine. Sadly, we could not share and appreciate what had become spiritually sustaining for each of us. We could not talk as soul friends. The deep connections I was feeling at a soul level threatened the marriage, and his angry, judgmental reactions to me took it over the edge.

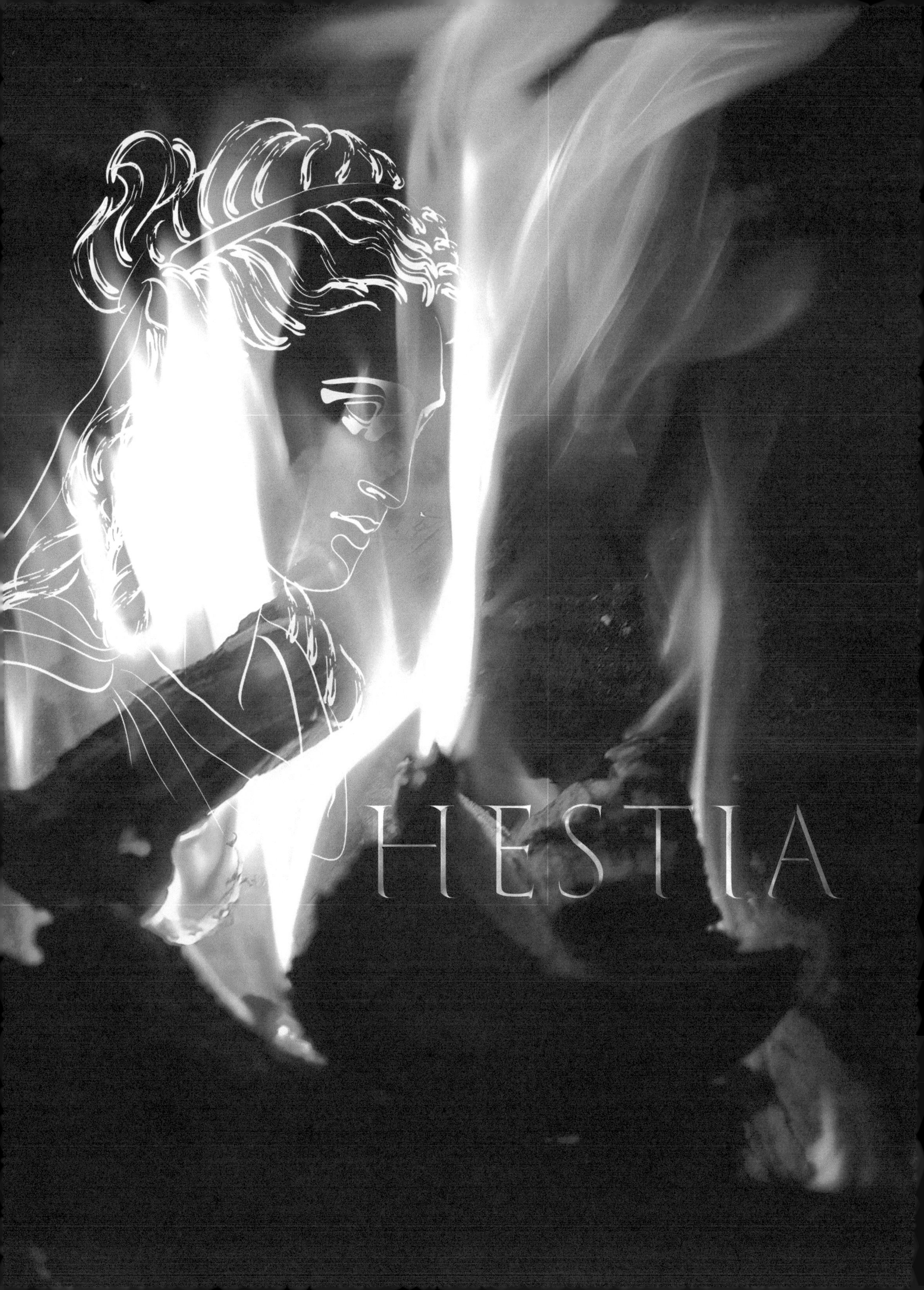

HESTIA

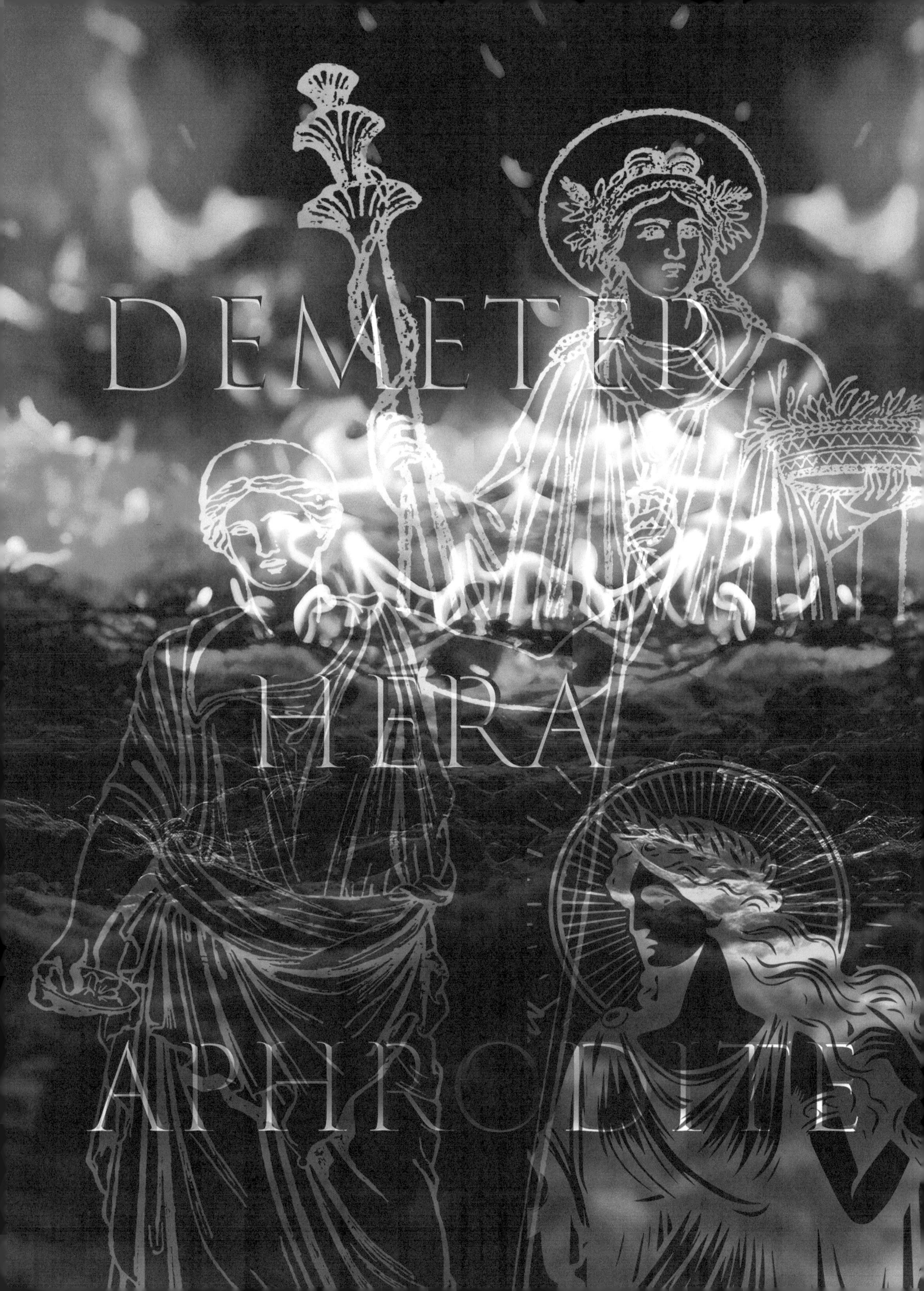
DEMETER
HERA
APHRODITE

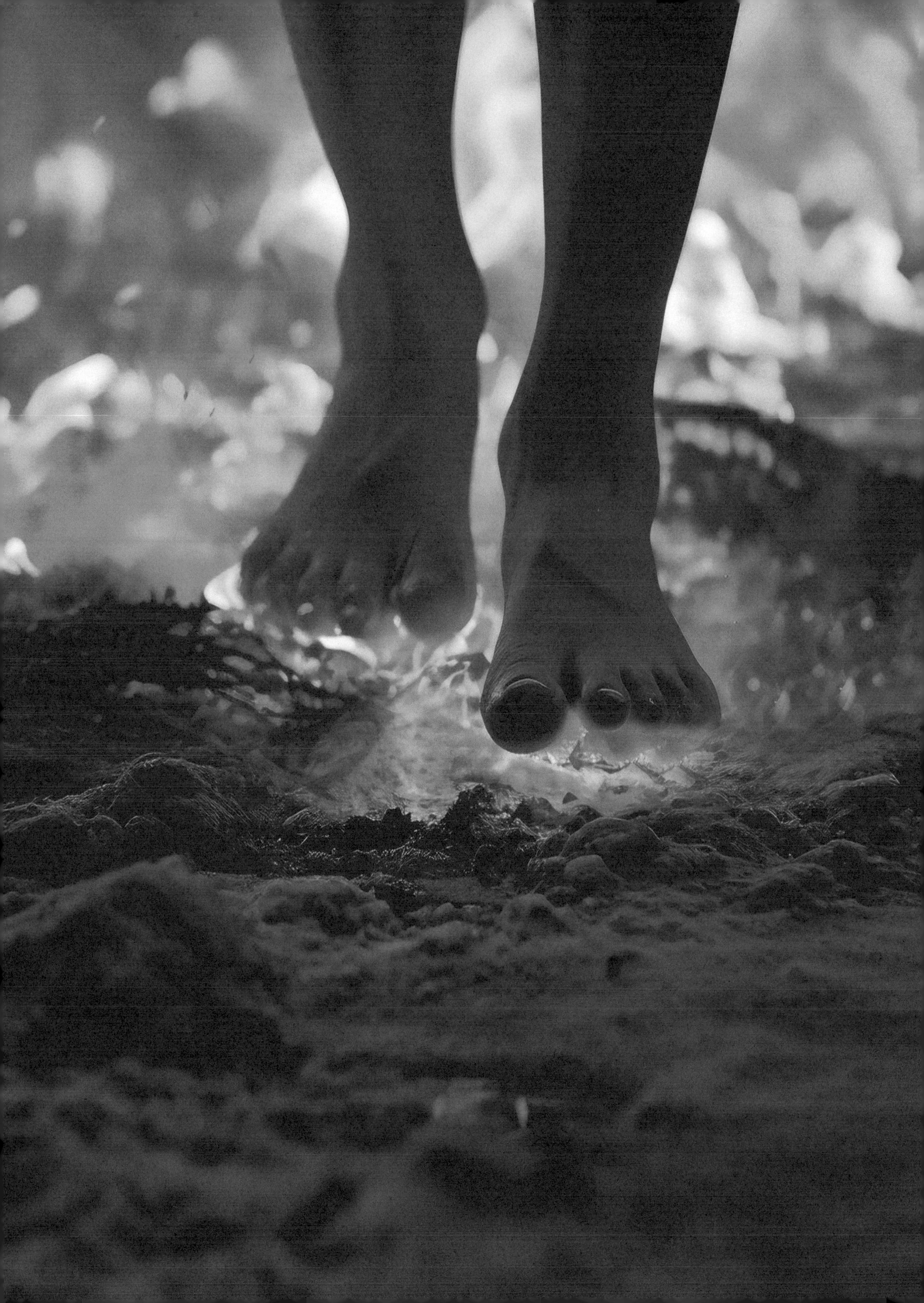

Jean Bolen

ARTEMIS

Chapter 23

Doctor-Mother and Son

Andy's "birth bump" had been removed in September 1981 when he was nine. The birth bump's proper name was neurofibroma, a non-malignant tumor. The pathologist who reported his findings at the time suggested that it could be part of generalized neurofibromatosis, in which tumors multiply on nerve fibers anywhere and everywhere. However, as far as was known, this was the only neurofibroma he had. At fourteen, after his growth spurt in puberty, he shared a concern he had kept to himself: the muscles in his right shoulder had become less developed and weak. His shoulder and upper arm muscles were normal before; he had been able to swing from one bar or rung to the next on gym equipment. This was a very serious sign that something neurological was wrong. It made my heart heavy. Since I was also a doctor, it added another layer of knowledge, dread, and responsibility.

After I had my own experience of pregnancy, labor, and delivery, I felt a deep respect and profound connection with women who had given birth. It was a physical experience that had dropped me into the archetypal depth of being a mother, specifically, "the mother" of Melody and Andy. My well-being and theirs became linked. I would forever be vulnerable. I would learn that there is truth in the saying that "we are only as happy as our least happy child." While this is how I learned that to be a mother is be vulnerable, I have also learned that this can be true through adoption, as taught to me through a women's circle, with Pauline Tesler and Grace Dammann, who became mothers through adoption. I know it doesn't require giving physical birth for the archetypal depth of bonding between mother and child to form.

My friend Terry Tempest Williams was fifty when she and her husband Brooke adopted her twenty-four year old Rwandan translator, and she dropped into the mother-archetype. In her book *When Women Were Birds,* she wrote:

> I am not Louis's mother, but I have become a mother, which is an unspoken agreement to be forever vulnerable. Unbidden, my eyes slide to the clock day and night and I wonder where he is, if he is safe, on the road or at home, if he has had enough to eat, if he is healthy, if he needs anything from me. It doesn't matter the age of our relations, conventional or unorthodox, we suffer and learn by heart.

On becoming the mother of an African son, Terry's heart became concerned for her adopted son, as do Black mothers who know about racism firsthand. Young Black men can be in danger, just by going out and about.

The vulnerable-heart of mothers may become attuned when her child of any age is in danger. When Dr. Louisa B. Rhine collected stories of ESP, the commonest example of ESP communication was between mothers and sons who were away at war, when their lives were in danger, or as they died. I'm also recalling early Russian research into ESP. Scientists wired a mother rabbit to a device in a laboratory, while her litter of young were taken into a submarine that was deep underwater. When her babies were killed—one at a time—the exact time was recorded. Meanwhile hundreds of miles away in the laboratory the device that measured subtle changes in skin electrical conductivity reacted, at the exact moment.

Demeter and Persephone are mother and daughter in the ancient Greek myth on which the Eleusinian Mysteries were based. They are also archetypal patterns in the personalities of contemporary women. I describe Demeter as a Vulnerable Goddess archetype in *Goddesses in Everywoman*. When this is an active archetype in a woman, being a mother is a deep source of meaning. It is the primary one in women who yearn to be mothers and are fulfilled when they do and feel a deep loss when they cannot. Being a birth mother physiologically does not automatically call forth the archetype, which can be sad for both woman and child; something is missing. As in the myth, when Demeter is an archetype, a mother's well-being and the fate of her child are deeply linked. Demeter suffered when she could not prevent her daughter Persephone's abduction into the underworld.

When the danger is a disease, as it was for my son Andy, a doctor is the usual bearer of the news, which takes parents as well as patient into the underworld. In the myth, Persephone was gathering flowers in the meadow. Her only decision was which beautiful flower to pick next. The sun was shining, and all was as usual. Demeter was going about her goddess business, her ordinary life, when suddenly Persephone is abducted into the underworld.

In my personal variation of this, it is my son who brings me the news. He tells me what he has been keeping to himself until he was ready to face whatever comes next. Privacy, competency, and trust are mutual givens between me and my fourteen-year old son—he has come to me with expectations that I will respond as I do, without drama. I see how much less developed the muscles are in his right shoulder, and check on the weakness of muscles. It's clearly a serious matter. While muscle weakness is the problem, I know that it has a neurological cause. I mentally trace shoulder nerves to the brachial plexus to cervical nerves to spinal cord. I am able to think like a doctor objectively, and I have an optimistic nature, the two qualities that keep my mother-worry angst for him out of this moment. I am aware of this aspect of myself. It's as if a silent Demeter is behind my left shoulder.

The neurofibroma pathology report from when he was nine was a forewarning. The good thing about being a doctor is that I knew or could find out who the best doctors could be for Andy. His neurologist was Maire McAuliffe, MD, who functioned as his primary physician. She was smart and had common sense. She was also a doctor-mother, and she and Andy had a mutual liking for each other. Her humor and his counted as a plus. She had been one of my instructors at UCSF and was respected and liked by surgeons that she often worked with.

In December 1986, the doctors ran an MRI to diagnose the cause of Andy's shoulder weakness, and the findings were ominous. There was a dumbbell-shaped neurofibroma in the spinal canal in his neck. It was inside and outside of the dura (the tough protective covering of the spinal cord with openings where bundles of nerves connected the spinal cord with everything outside of it), narrowing where it went through. Andy would now have follow-up MRIs to track this. As a doctor, I saw his MRIs and often went with him and could be in the room with him. Later, after the results had been read by the radiologist, we would go to see Dr. McAuliffe, who would examine him and they could talk. I'd wait in the waiting room while Andy would see her by himself, and I would hear the summary with them both present at the end.

Andy was able to live with not knowing until something definite was known. It was natural for him to live in the present moment, not compare himself with others, and not fear what lay ahead, a quality that I hadn't appreciated before (when he didn't look ahead to when a school project was due, or an exam was coming up, and would be engrossed in something else). I framed one of those sayings that are printed on cards and tacked it up in his room: "Remember, It Wasn't Raining When Noah Built His Ark." Now, I was thankful for this.

A conversation when he was about five reminds me of how he dealt with having neurofibromatosis. Melody and Andy were in the car with me, and she was voicing her concerns about starting at a new school in the fall. She was worried about what it would be like—the new school, the other kids, the new teacher. He listened for a while, and then said, with finality: "When we move, we move." Message: we find out then, no point in "what if's." This illustrates their difference in perception styles: intuition is looking ahead; sensation is in the present.

We were watching and waiting, with regular follow-ups on MRI and neurological examinations. This was a course of non-treatment. Andy's tumors were not cancer, but when one is located in the spinal canal, it would become very dangerous if it kept growing. Which it did. On a follow-up MRI, the dumbbell-shaped neurofibroma had grown. It was now compressing the spinal cord and pushing it to the side against the bone. Compression could cause paralysis from the neck down, below the level of the tumor. Its location made surgery very complicated, and could also cause paralysis if something went wrong.

By now, Andy was eighteen, fully informed about everything to do with his neurofibromatosis and in on all decisions. In April 1990, the decision was made to have surgery, to be done by Charles Wilson, MD, the head of neurosurgery at UCSF. The surgeon and the hospital were the best choice for this major surgery. To reach the tumor, the lamina—bones that protect the spinal cord—are removed. Then the delicate work is done to take out the tumor with the least amount of damage to the cord and nerves.

During the surgery, his father and I waited and learned hours after it had begun that the operation had gone well. In the post-op period while Andy was hospitalized, one of us stayed with him day and night. We were working as a team, as parents in tandem. We were by now divorced, but where our children were concerned, tension between us was set aside. Andy's best friend, Jeff Ravetto, visited him, as did Melody, who was now at Pitzer College. Soon afterwards, Andy came home to rest and restore body and psyche from the ordeal and relief that all went well in surgery.

By June Andy graduated from Tamalpais High School, class of 1990, which was a joyful occasion. Some of the best photographs of him were taken at graduation, beaming. He had a gift for music. He had perfect pitch and had taken up the electric guitar and played with a group at Tam High. He had a wonderful experience on his own taking the summer session for high school students at the Berklee College of Music in Boston. I think he was disappointed that Boston didn't seem familiar—after his "I used to be a Boston judge" comment to me had become a family story. No memories from a previous life! He followed his sister Melody to Pitzer College, the newest of the Associated Colleges of Claremont, where he took part in a student music program.

Andy had many other surgeries to take out neurofibromas in the soft tissues of his neck and forehead, and then ones in his scalp, hand, wrist, and leg. In March 1992, there was a merciless new finding on MRI. There were tumors growing on both auditory nerves. These were recognized as "bilateral acoustic neuromas," which defined the specific condition that Andy had as neurofibromatosis type two, or NF2. It meant that he would lose his hearing—the gift that brought him joy. Now in addition to the MRIs, he would be tested regularly for hearing loss. He came back to live in Mill Valley, took courses at the College of Marin, and continued his interest in music. He had an interest in new technology. Even knowing it was a matter of time before he became deaf, which was the prognosis for NF2, he enrolled in a program to learn audio engineering—mixing. Andy was focused on what he wanted to learn while he still could.

As his mother, I learned that Andy was his own person way back in pre-school. I took him to be enrolled in an excellent school where Melody had gone and had thrived. I brought Andy there and saw that he was more interested in where overhead pipes went than what the teacher was saying. This made me look at alternatives to find what would be best for him. It called on me to be a "Sky Mother." In contrast to "Earth Mother" who physically and emotionally can care for her child in the present moment and is nurturing, a "Sky Mother" senses or sees what may be missing or needed by her child, assesses the situation, and seeks what would help. The alternative for Andy that I found was a Montessori preschool which adapts to what the child wants to learn. This was a better choice, as were other changes in schools as he went along. As he grew older, he was fascinated with computers and the internet. In true introverted style, he had a couple of good friends, and was not one to go with the crowd.

I used to say that Andy listens to his own drummer, and as I was writing this. I looked up the whole phrase from Thoreau's *Walden*:

> If a man does not keep pace with his companions, perhaps it is because he hears a different drummer. Let him step to the music which he hears, however measured or far away.

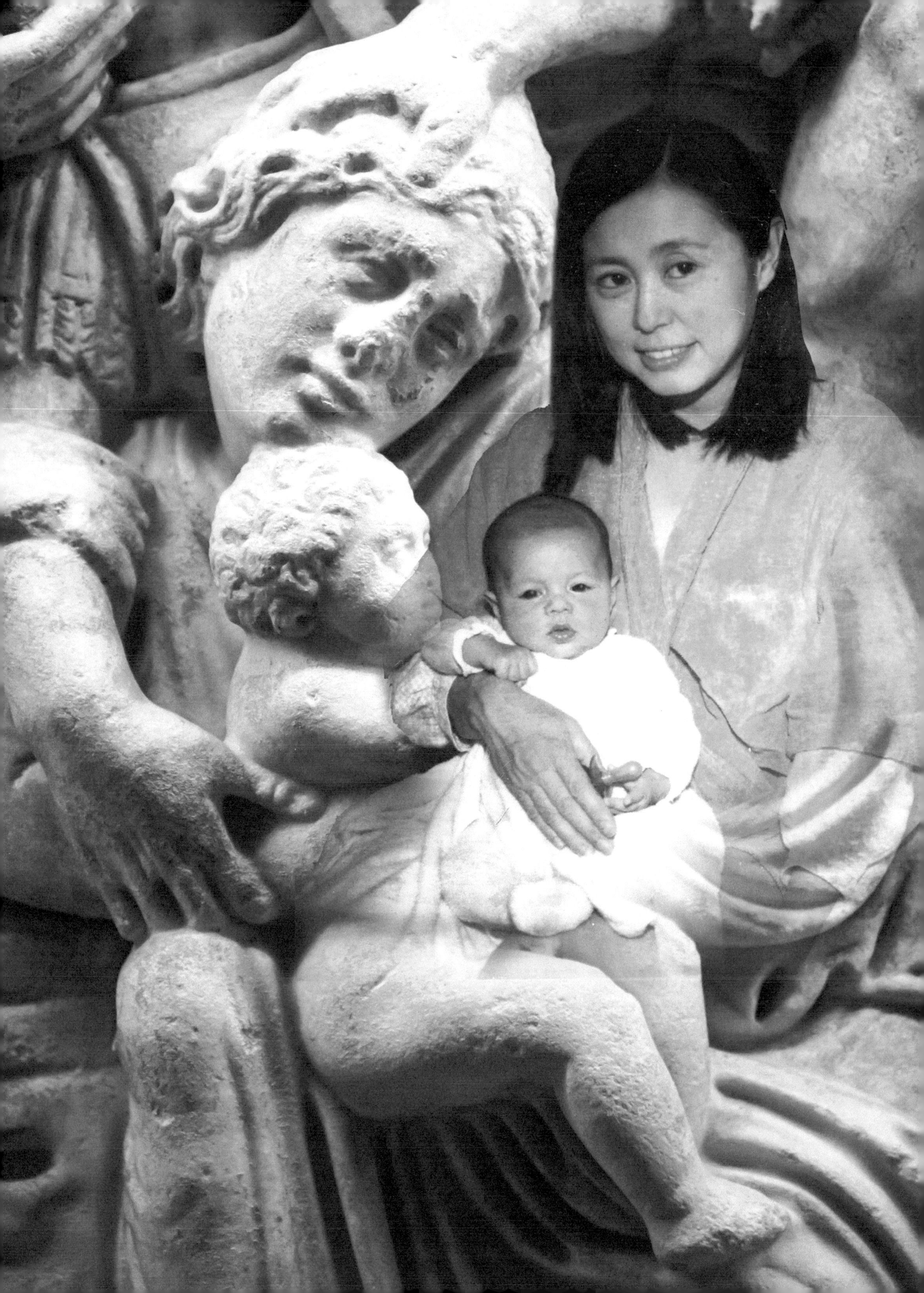

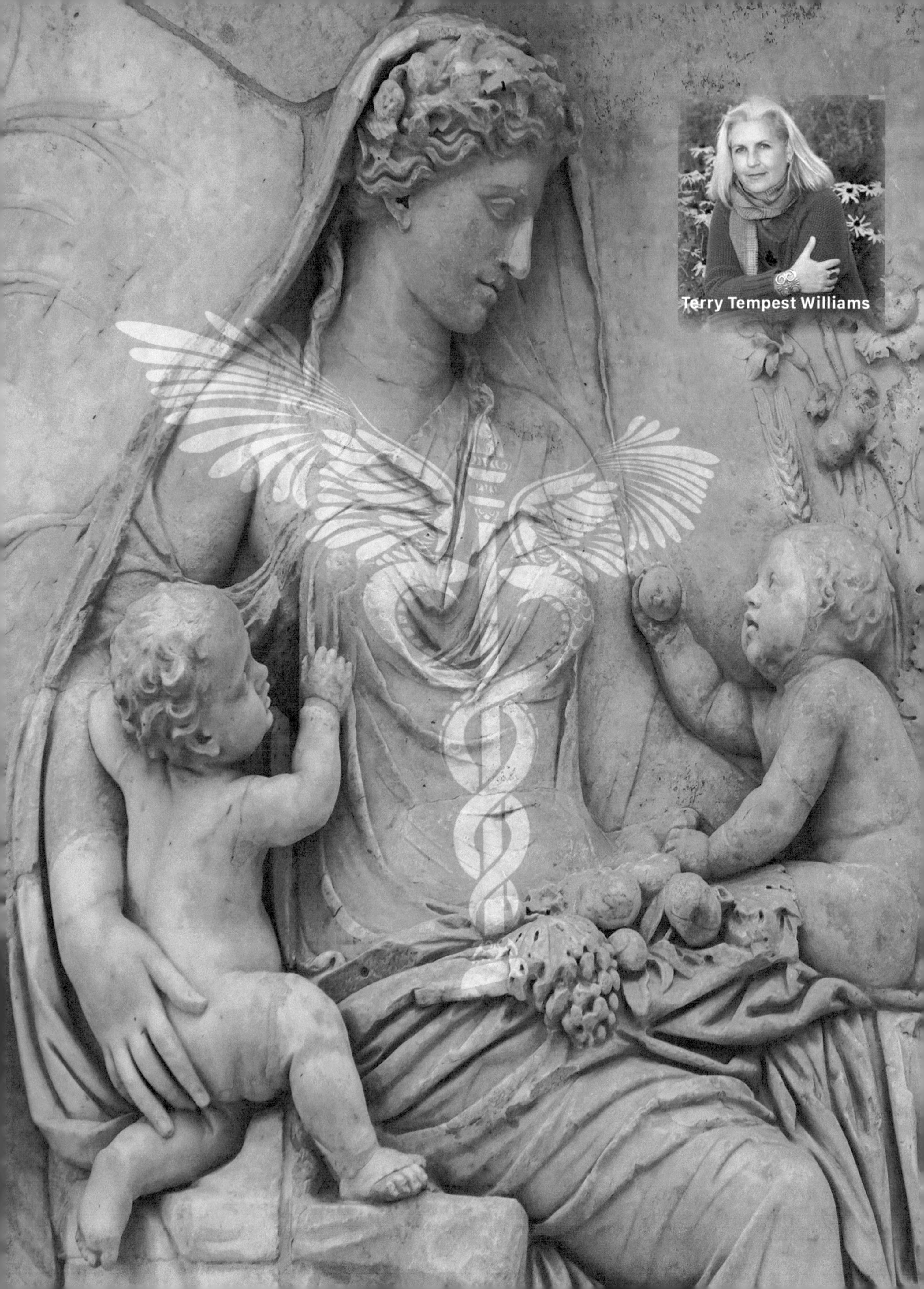
Terry Tempest Williams

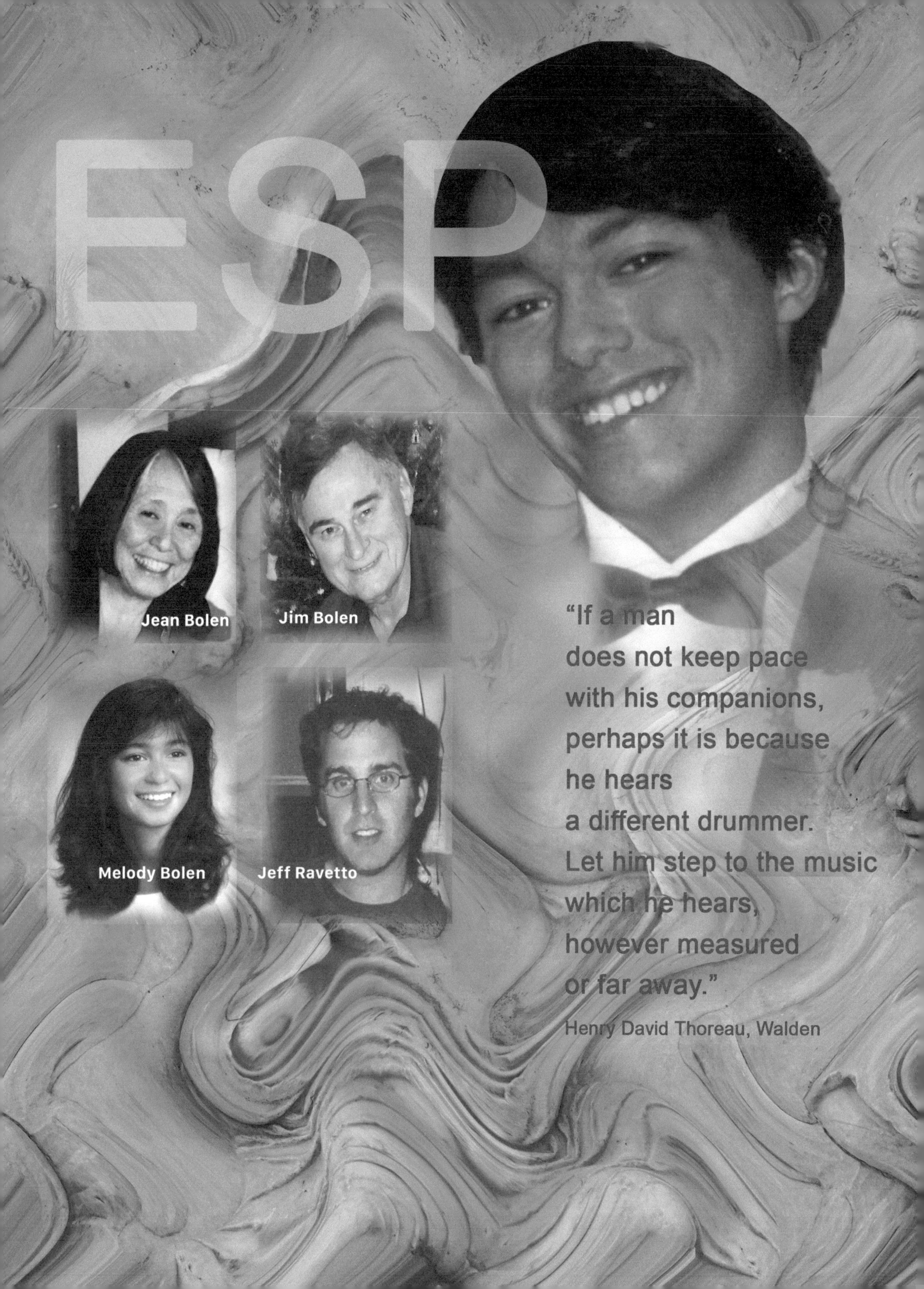
ESP
Jean Bolen
Jim Bolen
Melody Bolen
Jeff Ravetto
"If a man
does not keep pace
with his companions,
perhaps it is because
he hears
a different drummer.
Let him step to the music
which he hears,
however measured
or far away."
Henry David Thoreau, Walden

PERSEPHONE & DEMETER

Section 5

Pilgrimage, Travel, Mysticism

Chapter 24
Pilgrimage – Heart Center/Chakra

"I opened the bulky envelope that had come in the day's mail and found an invitation that would change my life. A total stranger was inviting me on a pilgrimage." This is how I began Chapter One of my book *Crossing to Avalon: A Woman's Midlife Pilgrimage* (the subtitle is now *A Woman's Quest for the Sacred Feminine*). The invitation was from Elinore Detiger, a woman I had then never met or heard of, who became a major influence in my life—because I said *yes.* I can also say in retrospect that this was an amazing example of the aphorism, "When one door closes, another door opens." The invitation came shortly after I had settled into the Shelter Ridge condominium.

It had come when I was in a muddled, painful, and perplexing time of my life. I was forty-nine years old and was trying to get my bearings. In the previous year, I had separated from my husband after nineteen years of marriage, and was in a period of uncertainty, disillusion and transition. I had left the conventional path of marriage. Only now, thirty years later, do I know how true Robert Frost's words were true for me.

> Two roads diverged in a wood, and I—
> I took the one less traveled by,
> And that has made all the difference.

Mrs. Detiger suggested I visit Chartres Cathedral in France, Glastonbury in England, and Iona, an island off the coast of Scotland. It included having a private audience with the Dalai Lama in the Netherlands.

I responded, "Somehow this trip feels like a continuation of an unfolding midlife path, an initiatory rite perhaps, and certainly an introduction to something I only have vague intimations about."

I went on to say: "I am venturing beyond 'my known world,' heeding a call to live my life more authentically even as it puts me in conflict and uncertainty."

Joseph Campbell's *The Hero's Journey* begins with the call to adventure that will take the protagonist beyond his known world. I had never been to Europe or on a pilgrimage before. I had to write *Crossing to Avalon* in the first person in order to tell the story; it is the precursor to this memoir-based book. Going on an adventure was easy compared to the vulnerability of sharing my own story (I have similar feelings about this book as well.) *Crossing to Avalon* was the book I wrote after *Gods in Everyman: Archetypes that Shape Men's Lives,* but not the next one to be published. I wasn't ready. In the meantime, I had been inspired by Richard Wagner's four opera *Ring* Cycle (*Der Ring des Nibelungen*) to write *Ring of Power*: *The Abandoned Child, the Authoritarian Father, and the Disempowered Feminine; a Jungian Understanding of Wagner's Ring Cycle.*

This call to adventure came after Elinore Detiger had held a copy of *Goddesses in Everywoman* and received the psychic impression that this is what she should do. The invitation came with a check to cover time away from my office, and a beautiful handmade gold pendant in the shape of a *vesica piscis*, which I would later learn is the design on the wellhead-lid of the Chalice Well at Glastonbury, the well in which the Grail was once supposedly hidden.

Mrs. Detiger invited me to come to Europe on pilgrimage. The first sacred site was not a place but a person. I was to meet the fourteenth Dalai Lama, Tenzin Gyatso, considered to be an incarnation of Avalokitesvara, the Bodhisattva of Compassion. Since that first meeting in a private audience with others, I would, in the years following, be in small meetings or in an onstage dialogue with him a half a dozen times. Something real, an authentic essence of him invites a similar response in those who meet him. He is unguarded, unselfconscious, curious, and receptive, which invites the same. I believe that the openness of his heart has an effect on those in his presence, which it did on me.

In Jungian psychological terminology, he *constellates* or brings out a reciprocal response in others who are receptive. I had been surprised, the first time I met him, by the chortling happy sounds he made while listening or pausing, and how he answered questions in English, infrequently checking with his translator to repeat the question to him in Tibetan. In later situations where he was giving an important teaching, I heard him speak carefully in Tibetan to be translated line by line into English. His heart and mind, an inner divine child, and a wise person are clearly present and vitally alive in him. I now intuit how by being in his presence, being open, curious and receptive myself, I'd be affected by the field of subtle energy or (invisible to me) aura that surrounds him. In Eastern traditions and beliefs about the chakras in the body (which are not medically recognized), the chakra associated with a bodhisattva of compassion is the heart. It is considered to be in the center of the chest, and center of the chakras; there are three above and three below. These centers, the subtle energies each has, combine in ways into our personal subtle fields. Which is to say we do "give off vibes" or have an aura and unconsciously respond to those of others.

After meeting with the Dalai Lama, what happened next opened me to my own heart chakra. I flew to France and went from Paris to Chartres Cathedral with a driver, and without the guide who was supposed to accompany me in the Cathedral. Thus, I had my own experiences without anyone else in the space with me. Whatever "regretfully and unexpectedly" had come up for the guide—their absence was a gift! I enjoyed seeing the Cathedral as a tourist who had taken courses in art history and in medieval history in college. Then I saw a sign that there would be a tour of the crypt that lies under the cathedral, and I went on it. The guide only spoke in French, which made me call on my imagination and be open to impressions. There followed a return to the Cathedral that was now filled with organ music. Now I walked into the cathedral without assumptions and found that I had an inner compass in the center of my chest that could sense where the energies were the strongest.

This was a subjective interior-in-my-body experience, an introverted sensation (Jungian psychological typology) or body-psyche perception (Marion Woodman's phrase). It was like having a tuning fork or a dowsing willow in my body—in the center of my chest—which I later learned to think of as my heart chakra. I began paying attention to sensations and noticing how I and others place one hand over the heart chakra as a gesture of being emotionally moved, or might even put both hands, one over the other over it, as we bow our head in an act of reverence or deep respect.

When I returned home, now aware of this place in my body, I noticed that the tuning fork vibration was just one sensation. I found there were others. I had been aware of "feeling for" or "feeling along with" when I listened and was moved by what I was hearing. This is intuitive-feeling typology. People pour their hearts out or tear up in the safety of the analytic vessel. I had not noticed until I returned from this pilgrimage that my body-psyche now also responded—with a heart-chakra ache. It would be decades later that I sensed the existence of a deeper layer of compassion, and learned that the heart chakra in Sanskrit implies that beneath our personal knowledge or experiences of suffering and pain, there lies boundless love and compassion.

The thought that boundless love and compassion could lie beneath my conscious mind was an accessible idea. After all, I have been living and working with the reality of archetypes lying beneath the personal unconscious for years now. The collective unconscious (or the *human morphic field* in theoretical biology) makes intuitive sense to me. It is accessible to all of us—our dreams tap into it, bringing up images, symbols, and emotions that we often are not aware of when we are awake. Just thinking of boundless love and compassion brought the ocean to mind, and then images of the water that lies beneath land came—the aquifers, the water-tables, the sources of sweet drinkable water that we and all life needs to live and grow. Just as people need love and compassion; it is essential.

What if we all have access to this boundless love and compassion that lies beneath and all we have to do is remember its existence to tap into it? So, we get ticked off by thoughtlessness, respond with anger to provocation, become fearful thinking about the future, and so on. This is when our offended or fearful ego needs to stop running us. This is the time to remember the existence of boundless love and compassion, to put hand over heart center, to go quiet, and let your heart center fill up with compassion for yourself and for those that had constellated your negativity.

This may seem like a digression—I include it here because I got a lesson that illustrated this to me. I came home late from my office with groceries and laptop, hadn't eaten for seven or eight hours, and my parking space was taken! I was irritable, annoyed, muttering. Then I remembered that I could tap into the layer of boundless love and compassion that lies beneath the ego's irritation and entitlement, and my anger dissolved. It wasn't a big thing, I just needed to remember to connect with this deeper layer.

As the pilgrimage continued on to England and Scotland, I continued to pay attention to what I was sensing in the center of my chest as I walked into and around ancient and current sacred sites. I would come to trust it as much as I would a device (if there were such a thing), especially in the next decade when I led pilgrimages myself. In this part of the pilgrimage, we were a foursome. My companions were Elinore Detiger, Freya Reeves, and Soozie Holbeche. We had gone to Glastonbury, to the Chalice Well, the Tor, and then we wandered around the ruins of Glastonbury Abbey. There once had been a Celtic monastery on those grounds, then the first Christian community in the British Isles, and before it became a ruin, it was the site of the richest and most important church and Benedictine monastery in England. A marker notes where the bones claimed to be those of King Arthur and Guinevere were once interred.

The ruins are in the midst of acres of soft green grass. We entered the grounds early, led there by Ann Jevons, who guided us to a rectangular area outlined by a thin chain with posts about six inches high that marked the place where the High Altar once stood. She said that this was the power point of the abbey, the place where two ley lines crossed (telluric energy currents, which Chinese geomancers call *lung-mei* or *paths of the dragon*). I took off my shoes and stood bare-footed on where the High Altar had been when England had bowed to Rome, before King Henry VIII had broken with the Pope and destroyed the abbey, before the Church of England had come into existence, which in the United States is the Episcopal Church. Grace Episcopal Cathedral in San Francisco was my home church, where I was married, where my children were baptized, where I would speak from the pulpit on Mother's Day, where I would sleep in the Cathedral overnight as part of the Women's Dream Quest, and where I would participate in the conversations that were the beginnings of the Quest at Grace Cathedral.

Standing barefoot on the grass where the High Altar had been, I entered an altered state of consciousness as I prayed. It felt as if energy from above, transcendent divinity (my Christian sense of God as Father, Son, Holy Spirit) came down and met divine energy coming up from the earth below (the Goddess, Great Mother, Sacred Feminine), with both energies meeting in the center of my chest, in my heart center. Mother-Father God came together in me. It was an "Episco-Pagan" moment. In the chakra system, the heart chakra is situated in the center of the body and can be thought of as balancing the world of matter (lower three chakras) with the world of the spirit (upper three chakras).

I sense that we who are bringing our spiritual insights forward, in whatever way we do this, are in an endeavor together. I think that we are like the jewels in Indra's Net (Hindu mythology). We are linked by strands of meaning, whether we meet each other personally or are linked through someone or something that matters to us—a person, an ideal, an experience of awe, or words or music that touch us and resonate in us. The strands of the net or web that connects us might then respond like the strings of a harp (when a harp string is plucked and sounds, that same string in another harp some distance away, vibrates). This is what I mean by *resonate.* Our heartstrings/harp strings vibrate when we are attuned and responsive. When I thought of each of us as jewels on Indra's net, I thought of crystals. I remembered that crystals were used to transmit in the first radios. I heard from people who work with crystals that they pick up emotional energy from people and sometimes need to be purified in ocean water.

The wider meaning of Indra's Net extends to the entire cosmos and is used as a metaphor for the interconnectedness of all things. Stephen Mitchell, in his book *The Enlightened Mind,* wrote:

> The Net of Indra is a profound and subtle metaphor for the structure of reality. Imagine a vast net; at each crossing point there is a jewel; each jewel is perfectly clear and reflects all the other jewels in the net, the way two mirrors placed opposite each other will reflect an image ad infinitum. The jewel in this metaphor stands for an individual being, or an individual consciousness, or a cell or an atom. Every jewel is intimately connected with all other jewels in the universe, and a change in one jewel means a change, however slight, in every other jewel.

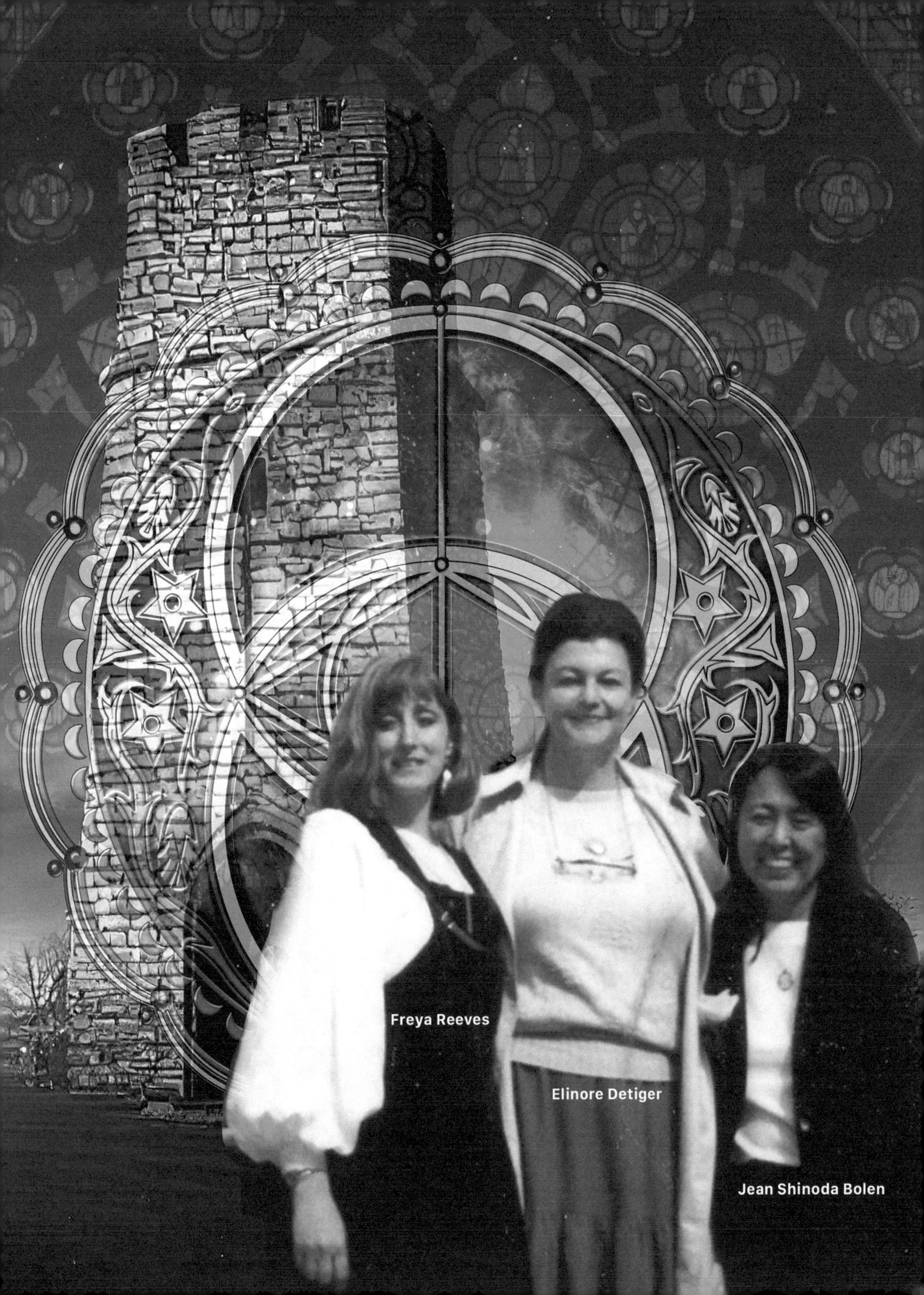

Freya Reeves

Elinore Detiger

Jean Shinoda Bolen

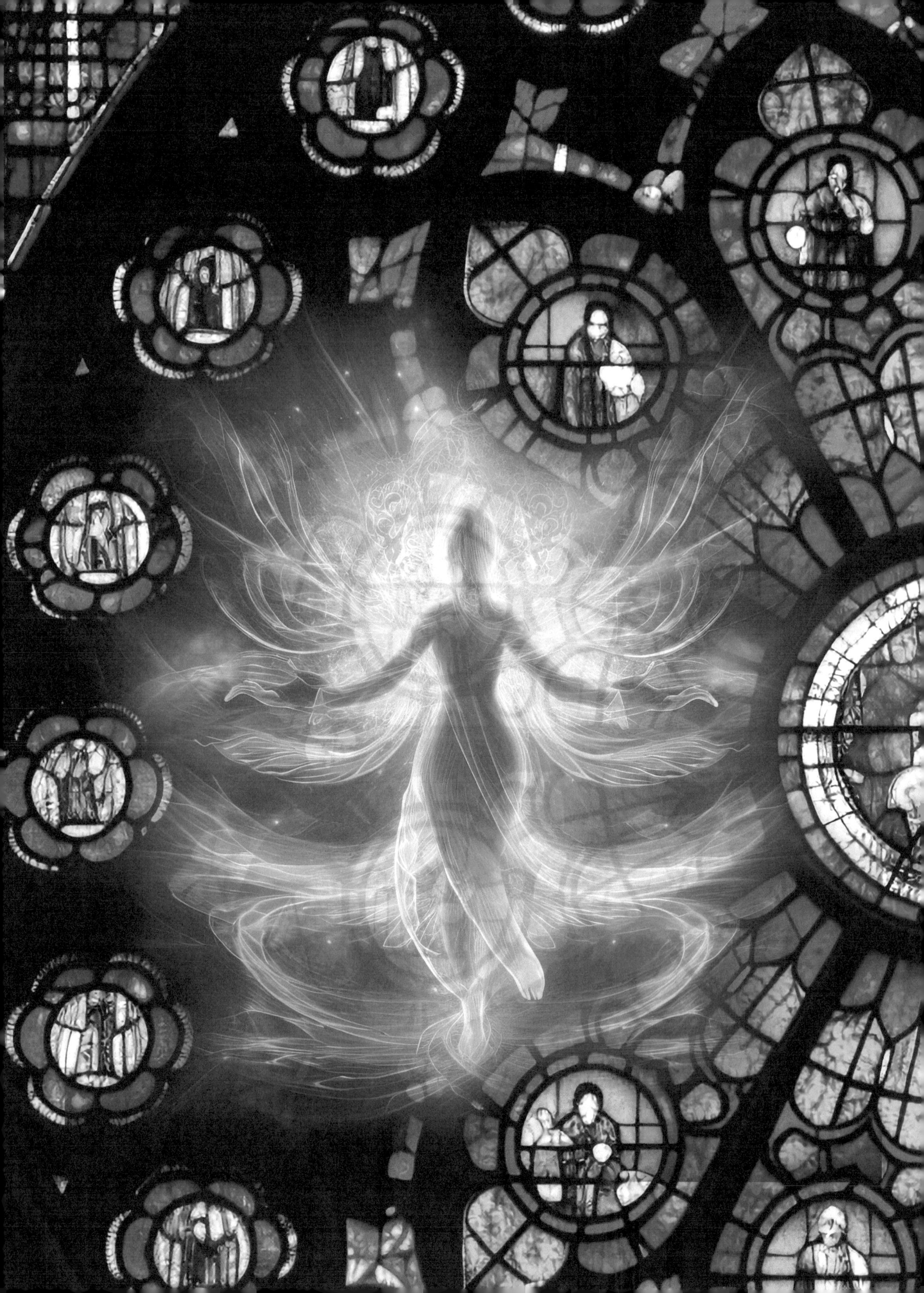

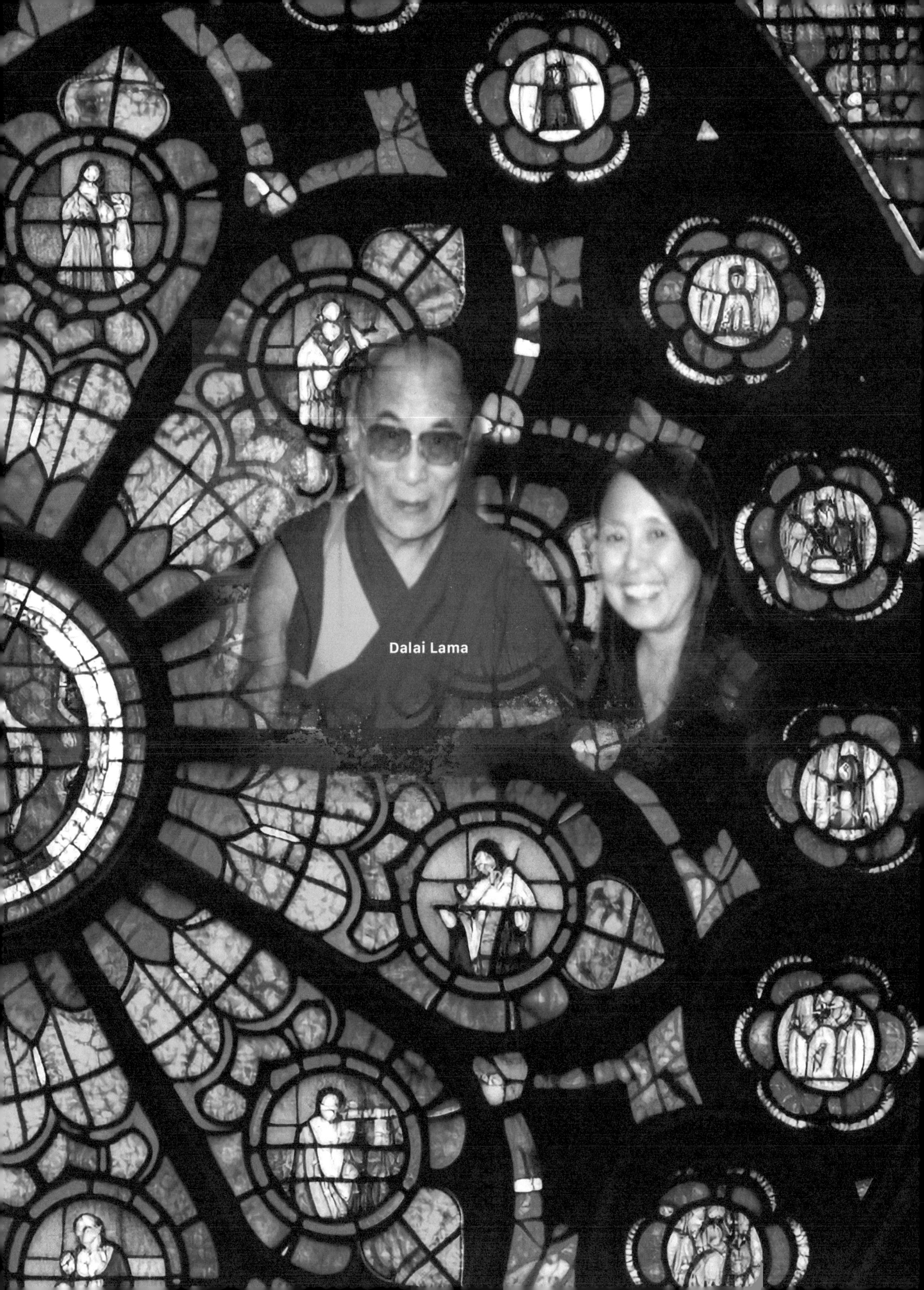
Dalai Lama

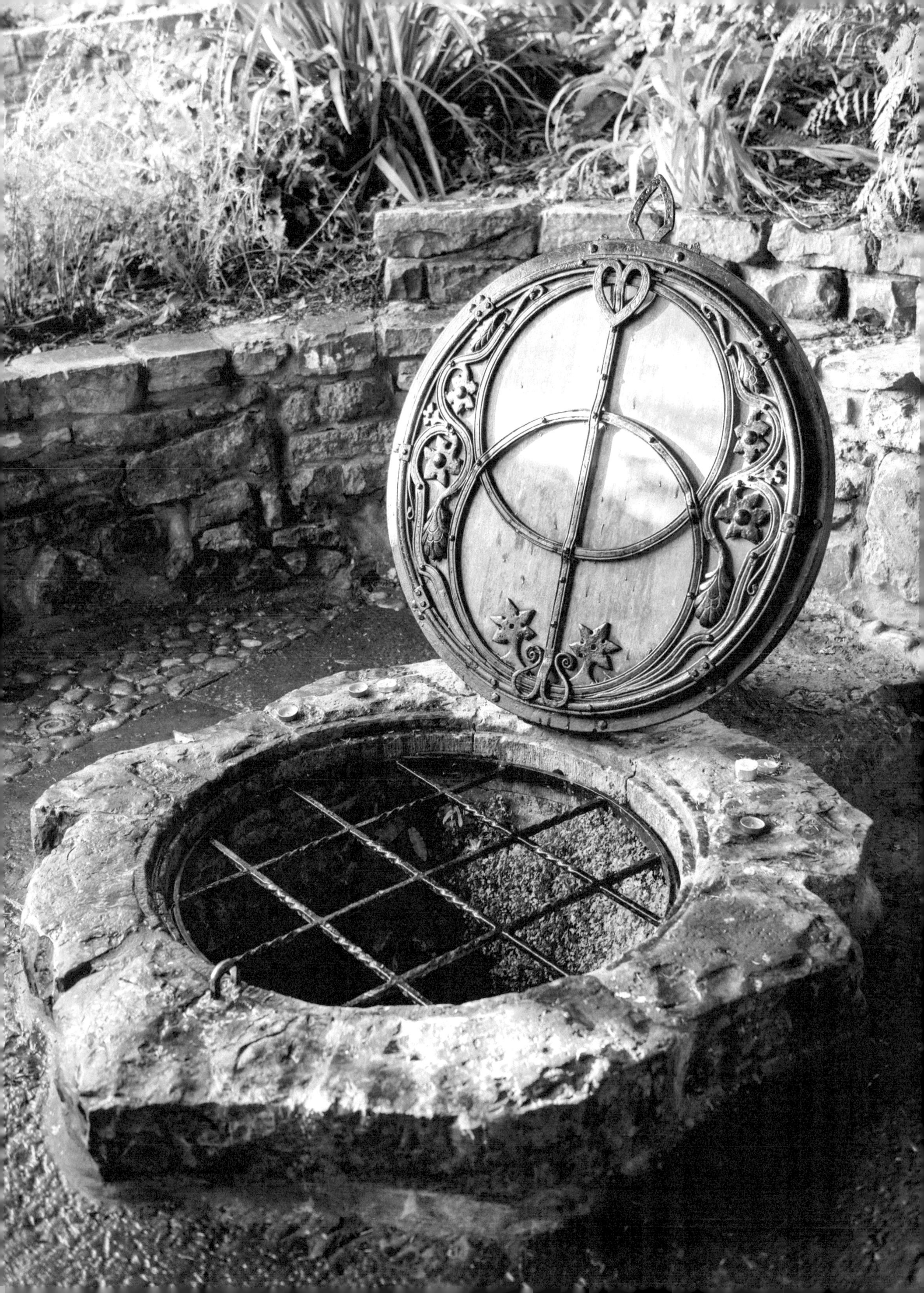

Chapter 25

Feathered Pipe - Greece - Peru

The first women's retreat workshop I ever led was at Feathered Pipe Ranch outside of Helena, Montana. And, it was also the first time that I set eyes on the place. I had agreed to do this sight unseen, at the invitation/pitch from India Supera, who came to Marin from Montana to ask me to do this. We got off to an awkward start—meeting me as a bestselling author, psychiatrist, and UCSF clinical professor made her nervous, and she poured the salad dressing into her coffee by mistake. We laugh about how this was the beginning of almost forty years of friendship, joint work, and adventures together. She is a practical visionary, dyslexic, former hippie, Sai Baba devotee, and the founder and executive director (a position she retired from and then returned to) of the Feathered Pipe Foundation.

The first workshop in August 1989 was called "Women's Wisdom: Celebrating the Sacred Dimension of the Feminine." I would be co-leading it with Jan Lovett-Keen. This was the beginning of doing women's retreats and pilgrimages with India Supera and the Feathered Pipe Foundation. Jan and I had gotten to know one another through women's spirituality conferences in Northern California in the early and mid-1980s. We were such opposites that we could not be more complementary. Jan was a classically trained flautist, who could play any instrument that could be blown through or drummed upon. She could improvise music to go with anything, while I seemed able to turn anything into a metaphor.

Jan was also a massage therapist who had helped me to unlock my ankles. This also freed up my inner physically adventurous child—the one who emerged in Grand Junction, Colorado, jumping over ditches and climbing trees—and soon would be climbing up steep slopes in Peru, ruins in Greece, or riding a camel near the Pyramids in Egypt. I'd sought her help after I had been to Tassajara Hot Springs, the Zen Mountain Center Retreat in the Ventana Wilderness of California. There I found that I no longer had the flexibility to cross a stream by stepping from rock to rock that were there for that purpose.

We figured out the cause was that I was short and ladylike. I sat with my ankles crossed when my feet didn't reach the floor in chairs that were too big for me. She improvised how she did massage like she did music. I got a combination of Esalen-Swedish for tension and touch, and jiggling my ankles and other joints to bring back the flexibility that I had lost. I had been carrying tension in my body as an aftermath of separating from my husband, and it had made me literally and figuratively uptight. What she did worked. Since chair sizes and my height would remain the same, a preventative solution was to always have something serve as a footstool. We laughed at how different we were, this big-boned Earth Mother and me—and yet women in our workshops often called her Jean and me Jan. We were as unlikely a pair as the separated-at-birth twins were in the comedy-buddy film *Twins* played by Arnold Schwarzenegger and Danny DeVito.

We had begun co-leading women's workshops in the living room of the Big House (now called the Murphy House) at Esalen and had done so for two summers. Now we were going to Montana to do the same. We arrived the day before our workshop was to begin to check out Feathered Pipe Ranch.

We would be doing our workshop in a big high-ceilinged room, with a huge fireplace and windows through which we could see a large lawn which sloped down to a lake.

At twilight, India led us up the road to a high point to see the total lunar eclipse. It turned out to be an eerie sight and experience; as the eclipse began, dogs that had been yapping went silent, and as the shadow of the earth went over the moon, the moon turned blood red. I had no idea whether this was an auspicious beginning at the time. It was awesome. It was a dramatic expression of the feminine, like the moon and mother nature.

As I was writing this book, I came across the brochure for this first Feathered Pipe women's retreat and realized how it described the subsequent workshops that we would do at the Feathered Pipe Ranch in the next two decades, up until Jan developed early Alzheimer's dementia and could no longer co-lead workshops with me. We did, however, do one more poignant and yet wonderful event; she joined me in the Big House at Esalen in the workshop that I called "Our Last Hurrah." With the help of her daughter Jessamyn Griffin and my assistant Betty Karr, who shepherded Jan through the airport security and looked after her on the airplane, we were reunited for one last women's retreat circle. Music, it seemed, was the last to go—Jan might not know the words anymore, but all she needed was the beginning tune to take it from there. Jan sat next to me with her flute and participated with her presence and with her music; we had come full circle and were back at the place we had started from.

This is what the brochure for our first Feathered Pipe workshop said:

> When we tap the intuitive sources of wisdom and spirituality that are within us all, life takes on a deeper meaning, and we are nourished by what we feel and know and dream. . . . Jean will lead us through myth, guided meditations and inner journeying to seek the trusting child with a sense of wonder; the grown woman who is a choice-maker; and the wise woman aware of the sacred dimension of ordinary life. Jan will invite the child in us to play, and make us aware of what our bodies know, perceive and can tell us. We'll find that music touches the sacred within us, reminding us of the profound connection between women's nature and Mother Nature, between music and body knowledge.

I have learned to savor experiences, to take in moments of beauty and grace, to feel events in my heart as well as register them in my mind. Sitting with Jan—most of whose fine mind was no longer there, yet *she* was still there—I had a moment of insight about how absurd it is that western thought since Descartes had accepted "I think, therefore I am." The essence of the person and personality, soul or spirit, remains after mind is gone. I doubt if Jan remembered our history of doing workshops and leading pilgrimages, but once she sat next to me in her co-leader position in the circle, she was in her place, comfortable, trusting, and when called upon instinctively could do it. Music would be the last to go for her, probably not because of some brain anatomy alone, but for the soul with which she had been drawn to music all her life.

A month after the lunar eclipse and our first workshop at the Feathered Pipe Ranch, Jan, India and I set out for Greece, taking a group of women who were brave to join us on what turned out to be an adventure as well as a trip. India Supera's ability to improvise was, in her way, as adaptable to circumstances as mine was to make meaning and metaphor out of it, and Jan's was to make music and do massage. The trip called upon all that we could do. It was called "Into the Arms of the Goddess: A Women's Journey to Greece, " and occurred September 15-30, 1989.

It was intended to be a pilgrimage to temples and natural sacred sites throughout Greece, the Greek islands, and Turkey. Our home for the entire trip would be our own private wooden sailing vessel, which we discovered was not meant to carry the number of women we had onboard. We renamed this journey "Into the Armpits of the Goddess," when everything that could go wrong, did—especially the weather. Small boat in rough seas is not a good combination. In the midst of a storm, I made my way down the deck, clutching the rope hand-over-hand to find Jan in the stern, ministering to our seasick travelers. She was holding a wastebasket to catch what they couldn't keep down. When I marveled at what she was doing, her response was, "I don't know what yuck is!"

"I wonder what is going to happen next?" became my mantra on this journey, with which I ended *Crones Don't Whine: Concentrated Wisdom for Juicy Women,* in anticipation that the time would come when I would cross over to whatever will be "on the other side." It is what I said when I woke up in port on a different island than I had been told we would be when I went to bed. It was the unknown outcome when we all met in a circle and every voice was heard—women were either fine with the adventure, in which case they took off to walk around to explore where we were, or unhappy and wanting to consider the alternatives. This included leaving the trip and going to a hotel in Athens, which India would arrange for, and rejoining us at the airport when the trip was over. The complainers left. All hands now on deck would be adventuresome souls, open to wondering what would happen next.

What happened was a weather change, gray skies turned blue, the sun came out, the rough sea turned into a serene mirror— where we anchored, dove into and swam. I learned from Jeanette Hermann, the astrologer who was with us, that Mercury had turned from retrograde to straight on the day the unhappy campers left, after which everything changed, and would stay this way for the rest of the journey. I had never heard of "Mercury retrograde" before. I learned that when Mercury (or Hermes the Messenger God, Guide and Trickster in Greek mythology) was retrograde to expect miscommunications and travel difficulties. This had been a dramatic example. Since then, I learned it worthwhile to pay attention to when Mercury goes retrograde—before the fact, rather than after the fact.

Whether the journey is to Greece or is a metaphor for our lives, to whine about events or people not living up to expectations assumes entitlement, focuses on blame, and misses out on what otherwise would have happened if we changed our inner weather. This trip turned out to be the most memorable of them all—as difficult as it was at the beginning, and how joyful it became. The most awesomely beautiful sight was seeing the sunset over the caldera (remains of the volcano) from the top of Santorini, where we left our boat. From there we took a ferry to Athens where we ended the journey.

More Feathered Pipe workshops and travel-pilgrimages followed, out of which, many friendships and circles began. Artemis was the prevailing archetype in women who signed up to go with us and other women. This is the archetype that responds to exploration, spirituality in nature, and sisterhood. I led trips to sacred sites that Elinore Detiger had introduced me to, saying she was following her psychic assignment. She took me to sacred places and brought me to meet people in Greece, England, Scotland, Ireland, and India. These trips expanded my consciousness, touched and (I believe) affected my soul, ethereal body, and aura field. After Elinore's introductory tours, I returned to all of these places, leading women's pilgrimages and adventures.

There were two places in the world that India Supera brought me to, places familiar to her that she had taken many others to before. She knew people there as well as the places. The first was to Peru. The two of us went there together to scope out the situation before we invited others to join us on a Feathered Pipe journey. She knew guides and others who could tell her if it was safe and what the conditions were.

The second place that she had led many trips to and also knew many people was Egypt. It was another place that I had not been to before and, having never been there before, I was hesitant to be the lead person who would draw people to come. We came up with a solution. It would be an invitation-only group, those who had been on trips with us before, and travelled well—no whiners among them! They would know from the beginning that I'd never been to Egypt and that this was an exploratory-expedition for me. We went into the chamber of the Great Pyramid at Gaza, sailed down the Nile and met the ancient goddess, including Sekhmet in the form of a standing statue with the head of a lioness and the body of a woman (who, with the Hindu goddess Kali, I described as Goddesses of Transformative Wrath, who symbolize the "enough is enough" archetype in *Goddesses in Older Women*). I came away from this trip knowing that I didn't want to lead a women's trip to Egypt. Egyptian men did not respect American women. They moved too close, got into personal space, and treated us as they would never have treated a woman they considered worthy of respect.

The last Feathered Pipe trip with India and Jan was to Peru. We took twenty or so women to Machu Picchu and from there to the high desert to see a total solar eclipse in the clear sky of Arequipa on November 3, 1994. There were very few others there, and the luxury hotel where American tourists once stayed was empty. Our group waited to see the eclipse while we were around the hotel pool with our eclipse glasses, sitting in lounge chairs or on chaise lounges.

The hotel was empty because the Maoist guerilla insurgents known as the Shining Path were active in the area and perceived as dangerous. India had talked with her friends in Peru and gotten porters through them, who turned out to be Shining Path soldiers. We were then under their protection—something I didn't find out until much later. They also were great porters.

The full solar eclipse that we could see from the high desert toward the end of South America was as clear a picture as anyone could have gotten anywhere. Like the blood-red full lunar eclipse we had witnessed the night before our first Feathered Pipe workshop, the dogs that had been barking went silent and there was a hush—or was it a collective in-breath of awe? At the moment of totality, day turned into night, the only sight in the sky was the coronal flares that surrounded the dark full circle. It appeared that the sun had "gone out." It looked like a black hole surrounded by flares and was visually dramatic. A full solar eclipse occurs only when a new moon passes in a direct line between the Earth and the sun, which makes this relatively rare.

Many times during workshops or travels, we dropped out of ordinary linear time. Whether we were meeting in a circle or on a bus or at a sacred site, we were in a sacred circle. After I acquired a Tibetan bell, I learned to rim the edge of the bell with a wooden dowel, building up the sound and vibration until it was "singing." The vibration was felt in the body and it became an almost instant way to bring everyone into a circle, whether seated in one or not. In my mind and heart, the sound and vibration of the bell linked every circle I had ever called together through time and space, and linked everyone in the moment to each other. It also is a link to Dharmsala, India, where the Tibetans in exile and the Dalai Lama live and where the bell, and the dorje that comes with it, was made. The two are paired ritual objects in their tradition. The dorje represents the masculine spirit, the hand bell is feminine—its handle echoes the image that is doubled in the dorje. I removed the clapper inside the bell. If I hold the bell upside-down, it becomes a chalice, which I use to invoke synchronicity by filling it with small slips of numbered paper. Each woman in the large circle draws a slip of paper that designates which small circle she will be in.

Tibetan bells come in different sizes. I chose mine, which is a large one, to vibrate with my heart chakra. I don't ask that people close their eyes as the sound of the bell grows and is felt as a vibration, but most everyone naturally does so. It centers people in their body-psyche. It does the same for me by becoming a focus without words. When I stop rimming the bell edge, the sound and vibration continues as both wind down into silence. There is a natural pause, and then as the convener of the circle or the speaker, I begin—not with prepared words, but with what comes to me to say.

During most summers in the 1990s, I went to Montana to do a women's retreat at Feathered Pipe, or co-led a pilgrimage with Jan Lovett-Keen and India Supera sponsored by the Feathered Pipe Foundation. The pilgrimages did not conflict with the workshops at the ranch because of the long winters that far north, and many of the ancient sacred sites were best visited in spring or autumn because summers could be uncomfortably hot. During this time in which Jan and I regularly led women's retreats at Feathered Pipe, we took everyone to the back country at Black Tail Ranch. We'd lead them down into what probably is the oldest inhabited cave system in North America, specifically into what is called the Shaman's Cave. The descent into the cave took time and caution. It was cold regardless of what the weather was outside and no light from outside reached it. There was what appeared to be a raised stone altar. The cave floor was irregular, and it had a natural chimney or vent at the end that went up and up. This was a natural "sound system." Anyone standing under it (or was hidden on the ledge) who spoke or sang had his or her voice amplified. Jan and I went in first and positioned ourselves at the end of the cave near the natural vent. Women came in one at a time—the narrow path down and into the cave curved into somewhat of a spiral as it descended. They could hear Jan's drumbeat, and later when everyone was seated the flashlights were turned off. One candle on the altar was the only source of light with which we could see the walls of the cave and something of each woman.

The cave experience came after we had been together at the ranch and knew something of everyone's stories. Here was a place and resource that amplified whatever was said and would be held by the others who knew them and were witnesses. I would speak about the metaphor we were enacting, how certain caves were sacred places in the past— wombs of the earth/goddess as well as the underworld in ancient Greece. There is no sense of time passing while in this cave. Everyone was invited to come to where Jan and I were seated and then be led to stand under the chimney—to speak, to pray, to sing, to do what each was moved to do. There was surprise and, for some, delight at how their voice carried. All, however, seemed awed and took seriously how they would use their time. I was especially moved when several over the years spoke directly to someone who had died.

When it was time to leave it was usually because of the loss of body heat; women left when they were ready to go, leaving Jan and me and sometimes one or two others. The spiral path up led to the place where there was a wooden ladder that we had gone down. We stood for a moment in this hollowed out space where sky and the beginning of the cave system could both be seen. As each woman climbed the ladder and emerged out at the top, women who had come out before would shout: "It's a girl!" It was a spontaneous, participant-created natural part of what was a ritual descent and return. After our first couple of journeys to the "Shaman's Cave," the Black Tail ranch put in a light system to light the path which could be turned on and off at the top or in the cave. This made it safer as we grew older.

For a time, I stopped doing workshops at the ranch, then several years later, India asked me to come back because of the financial situation. As soon as I arrived, saw the ranch house, the lake, the lawn, and all that was familiar, the beauty of place and memory came alive. I thought how much I loved this place and loved the work I do here. Instead of the cave experience and the metaphors that go with it, we've run a river in small inflatable boats, the same river that was in the film "A River Runs Through It" with Brad Pitt. Without Jan, I've co-led Feathered Pipe workshops with Brooke Medicine Eagle, Barbara McAfee, and Monika Wikman, and always with India.

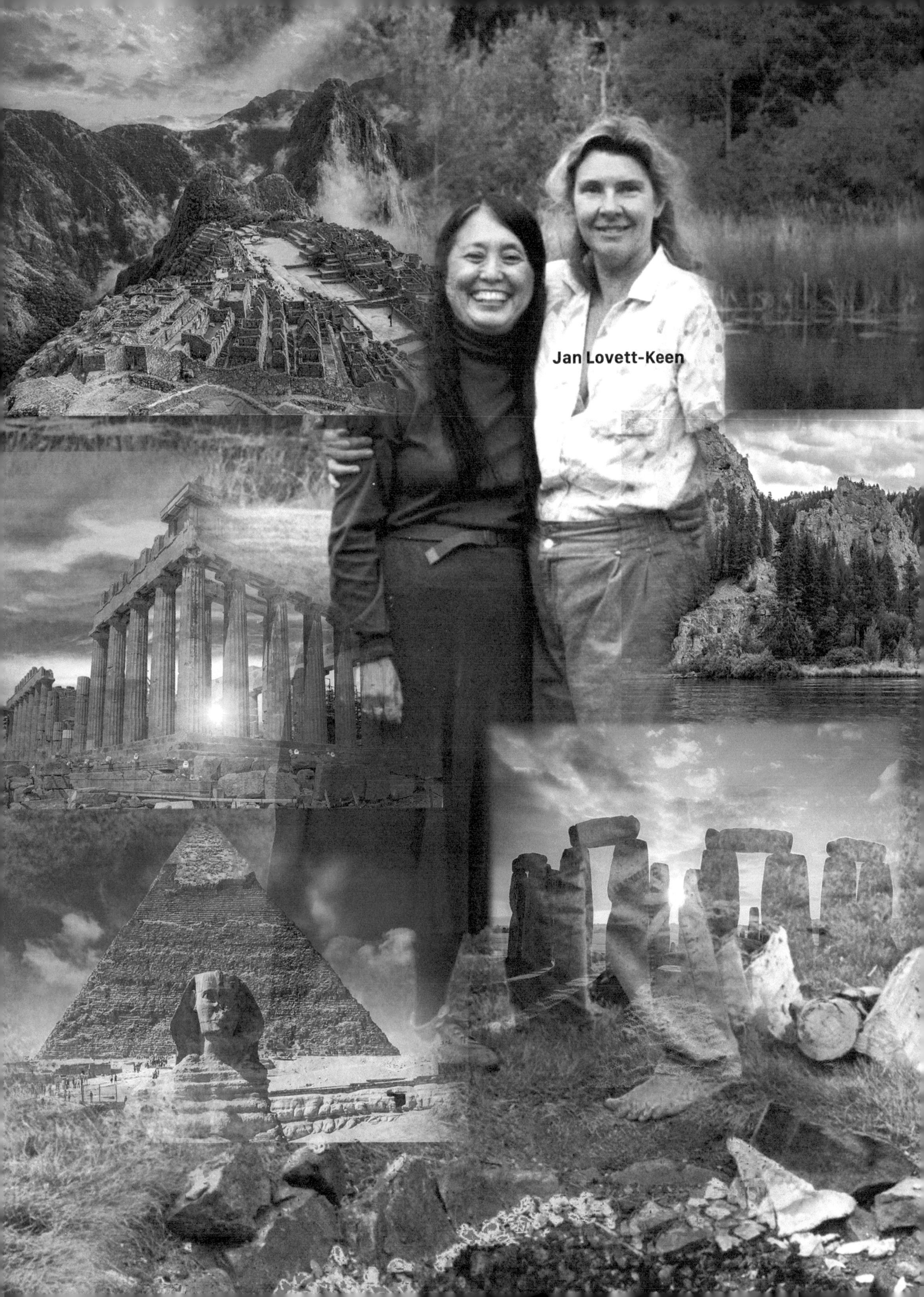
Jan Lovett-Keen

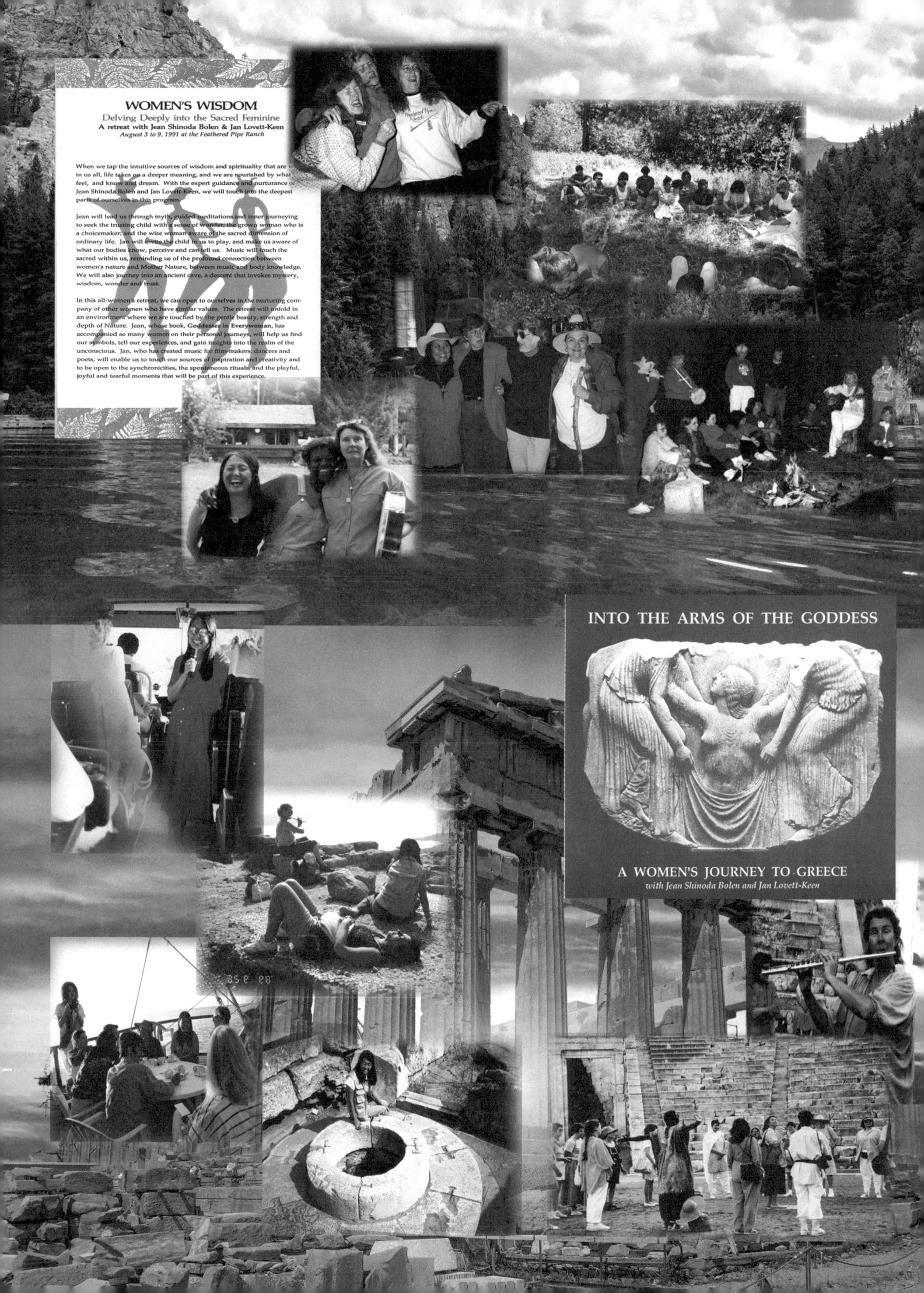

WOMEN'S WISDOM

Delving Deeply into the Sacred Feminine

A retreat with Jean Shinoda Bolen & Jan Lovett-Keen

August 3 to 9, 1991 at the Feathered Pipe Ranch

When we tap the intuitive sources of wisdom and spirituality that are in us all, life takes on a deeper meaning, and we are nourished by what feel, and know and dream. With the expert guidance and nurturance of Jean Shinoda Bolen and Jan Lovett-Keen, we will touch into the deepest parts of ourselves in this program.

Jean will lead us through myth, guided meditations and inner journeying to seek the trusting child with a sense of wonder; the grown woman who is a choicemaker; and the wise woman aware of the sacred dimension of ordinary life. Jan will invite the child in us to play, and make us aware of what our bodies know, perceive and can tell us. Music will touch the sacred within us, reminding us of the profound connection between women's nature and Mother Nature, between music and body knowledge. We will also journey into an ancient cave, a descent that invokes mystery, wisdom, wonder and trust.

In this all-women's retreat, we can open to ourselves in the nurturing company of other women who have similar values. The retreat will unfold in an environment where we are touched by the gentle beauty, strength and depth of Nature. Jean, whose book, **Goddesses in Everywoman**, has accompanied so many women on their personal journeys, will help us find our symbols, tell our experiences, and gain insights into the realm of the unconscious. Jan, who has created music for film-makers, dancers and poets, will enable us to touch our sources of inspiration and creativity and to be open to the synchronicities, the spontaneous rituals, and the playful, joyful and tearful moments that will be part of this experience.

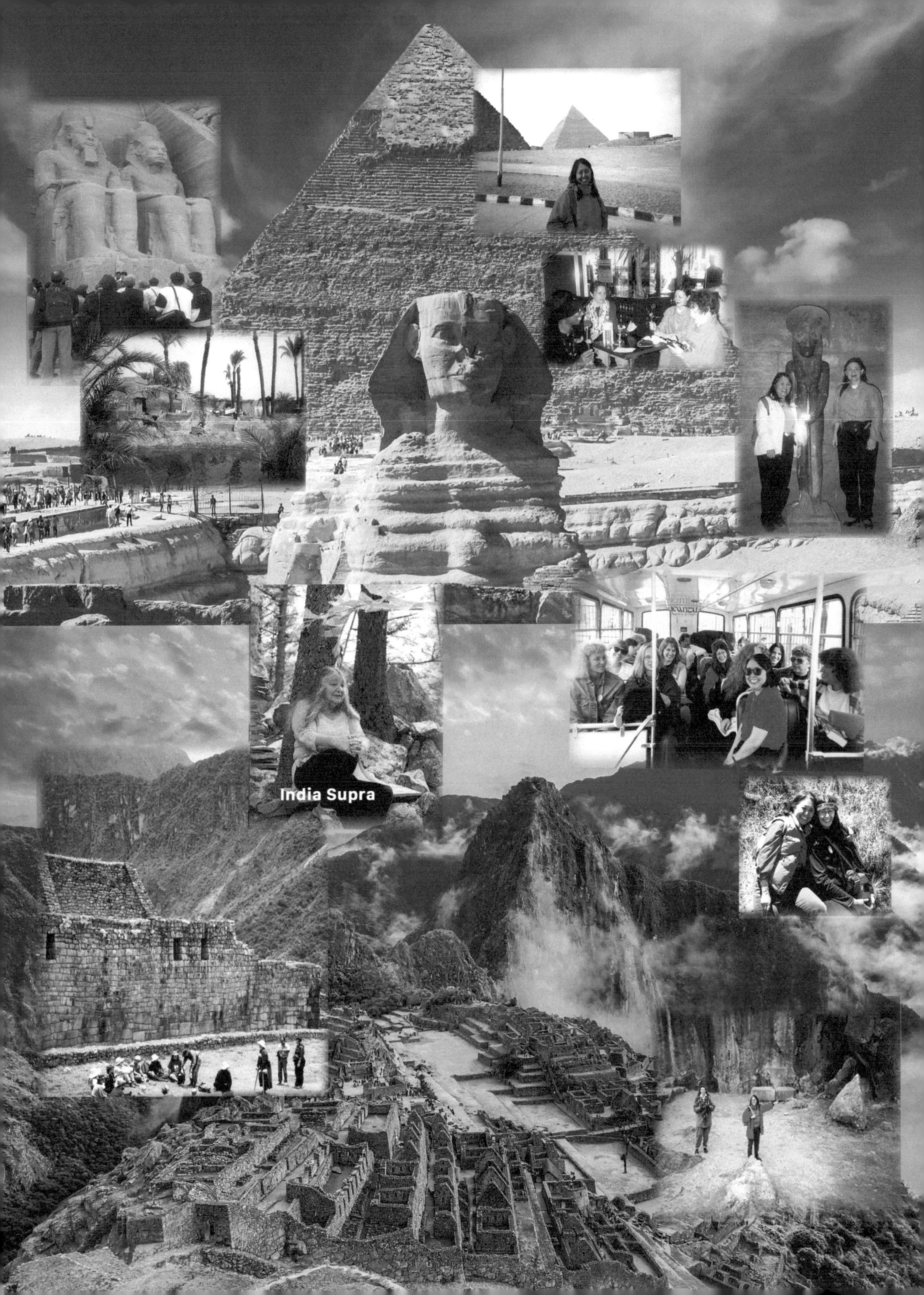
India Supra

Drinking Deeply from the Chalice Well:

A Women's Journey to the Realm of the Goddess

Monika Wikman

Jan Lovett-Keen

Chapter 26

Home – Four Corners – Labyrinth

My internal clock stirred me to think about moving, and the Sunday open houses that realtors have in Marin was an opportunity to check out what there was out there. The real estate bubble was a long way off and, at the tail end of the recession, it was a buyer's market. My books and bookshelves were overflowing in the condo that had been a refuge when I left my marriage seven years before. I thought about where I might want to live and looked for "open house" signs. I discovered that I had an internal compass as well as an inner clock. On my first Sunday out, I found a lovely house with a view of the Golden Gate Bridge and then felt a clear inner "no." I am a morning person; I like sunrises. I wanted a house with a view that faced east. With this clarity, the area to look would be Mill Valley, which had east-facing houses in the hills.

I found my house. There wasn't an open house, but there was a realtor's sign. I called and made an appointment to see it. There were redwoods on each side of the house, and a huge, beautiful Monterey pine in front of it. I saw the tree before I saw the house. (Later when I couldn't prevent it from being cut down, it inspired me to write *Like A Tree: How Trees, Tree People, and Women Can Save the Planet.*) The realtor unlocked the door to show me the house. I walked in, looked around, and had the thought "I could live here the rest of my life." It had been on the market for eight months and, even with the price reduced, it had not found a buyer. I was very glad that it had waited for me. I'm being fanciful—and grateful, such good fortune can't really be explained (karma, synchronicity, angels?).

This was at the beginning of the 1990s, the last decade of the twentieth century. The Gulf War was being waged in the Middle East, the Cold War had ended when the USSR dissolved, the World Wide Web debuted as an internet service, Bill Clinton was elected President, and the World Trade Center was bombed. And, from the mid-1980s into the 1990s, a worldwide AIDS epidemic had been growing.

In 1995, the first highly effective treatments (protease inhibitors) were developed, but not in time for my colleague and friend, David Stockford, MD, who died in October 1995. David and I had been residents at Langley Porter together—he and Michael Steele, MD, were Jungian analysts as well as psychiatrists. They were a couple, and friends I had stayed with at their place up the coast in Mendocino. Together and individually, they were my friends. In November 1995, a month after David died of AIDS, I went with Mike to the house they had built on sacred land in the Utah corner of Four Corners, where Utah, Colorado, Arizona, and New Mexico come together. It was the first time I would go there, and the first time Mike would close the house down for the winter without David. Mike brought David's ashes with him.

The house that David and Mike built looked as if it belonged in this land. It was a simple, one-story stone building. The stonework walls and fireplace with its raised hearth had been done by Navajo men from recycled Anasazi stones. The beams were large spruce logs. Whatever they could do, the two did, putting in sweat equity. David, who had found the property, poked around and found the furniture and objects that were probably made and used decades in the past. It was like being in a time capsule. Mike and I were compatible companions, as we both valued having time to ourselves and as well as time with each other for some company.

I wandered out on the land on my own. I explored an area east of the house and down the slope where there were some rock formations, juniper and pine trees. I came across what once had been a small fire pit with rock walls and was drawn to clean it out, find new stones, and rebuild it—a outdoor Hestia ritual, in the spirit of the goddess of the Hearth and Temple, archetypal hearth keeper and maker of sacred space. In my search for right sized stones, I discovered a wind-shaped juniper tree growing out of a rock shelf. When I sat on its lower branch or stood upon the rock, there was a vista of sky and land before me. The place felt sacred. I made a stone circle and circumscribed the boundaries of this temple space. It was a place to meditate and pray. And so, I did.

My thoughts and prayers went to my son Andy, who was now living with me in Mill Valley—and living with tumors growing on his auditory nerves. He was taking courses that interested him at the College of Marin and getting around in the red Mustang convertible that had been mine, then Melody's, and was now his. He, actually, was the only one of us who knew its workings and knew how to take care of it well. As the tumors affected his hearing, high-tech hearing devices became available as had Apple computers, both of which helped compensate for the handicaps. He could be absorbed reading technical instruction books or in figuring out problems that arose—problems that my intuitive, symbolic mind was completely at sea about. He was my live-in technical help. He was a night owl and I was an early bird. We lived compatibly together with Pierre, the gentleman tuxedo cat.

My thoughts and prayers also went to my close friend Patricia Ellerd Demetrios, PhD. She as president and I as a board member of the International Transpersonal Association had participated in the international conferences in Prague, Killarney, and Santa Clara. She also had joined me to go to Ireland and Egypt on Feathered Pipe trips. We were in a women's circle together. Our discussions of Richard Wagner's *Ring* Cycle led me to write *Ring of Power* (1992). She had been diagnosed and initially treated for breast cancer over a decade before, had a mastectomy and underwent chemotherapy, but with metastatic nodal involvement, the prognosis was not good. She had been determined to see her daughter Gina through high school and into college. As the years went by, the breast cancer seemed to be a thing of the past. Then, in 1991, she had a biopsy done on a lump in the reconstructed primary site. It was a recurrence of the same cancer which was now inoperable.

Patricia explored alternative treatments as well as what could be done by Stanford doctors. She went to the Kushi Institute in Becket, Massachusetts for a month, to live there and study, adopted the macrobiotic diet and was bringing teachers to her home so others could learn the principles and how to cook macrobiotic food. I had my first Thanksgiving tofu turkey at her house. By now, Gina had graduated from college, and our daughters were friends. I had been worried about Patricia when her spirit dimmed, and I saw her become disheartened by the criticism leveled at her as ITA president at a board meeting. I think she had lost her meaning to live and her belief in what she was doing that had sustained her—from seeing her son and daughter grow into adults and from her conviction to go into transpersonal psychology. Her very conservative image as an Atherton wife who had achieved everything her own mother wanted changed when she picked up a brochure about a new non-accredited school: the first Institute for Transpersonal Psychology. Going against negative family judgments, she enrolled, got her PhD, became Board chairperson of this fledgling school and got it accreditation. (I tell her story in *Close to the Bone*). All this before being asked to be the president of ITA.

I made my second trip to Four Corners in May 1996. It was good to be there again and feel outside of ordinary time. I took in the landscape by going out on the land where I could gaze around for a 360-degree perspective. Before I had stayed close in, mostly had looked down, making my way among the trees and rocks. Now, I looked at the horizon and as I turned I could see sacred mountains and mountain ranges in all directions, and the expansive sky above them. This land was in the midst of where the Hopi and Navajo hunted, made camp, and left shards and arrowheads behind. In the far distance was where the Anasazi once lived; the people who had built pueblos into huge cracks in the red stone mountains, leaving behind their ruins and the mystery of who they were and why they left. I felt as if I was at the center of a sacred medicine wheel.

I went back to my sacred space, to the tree. I found it as I had left it seven months before. Four Corners is high desert country. The air is very dry, and there had been no rain. I cleared away some dead branches, smoothed the sandy soil of small animal tracks, made the circular stone perimeter a little higher. Then I created a spiral out of flat white pieces of stone in the floor of this space. In my outdoor temple, the branches and the scale-like leaves of the Juniper provided a roof, with its one large horizontal branch over the space its main beam. Light filtered through branches and leaves, without the color of stained-glass windows but in providing dappled light, created much the same effect. Putting it in order was a Hestia meditation, a personal spiritual practice.

The spiral I had created was a miniature. I had on many occasions created spirals of many sizes—at Muir Beach which was close to home, and in faraway places, like Samothrace. Wherever I went, when there were empty beaches, time, and stones, I had been creating spirals. I did not keep track of the time or the number of turns in the spiral. One stone at a time, it was finished when it was finished, often after I had found just the right stone to put in the center. This is why I knew—without using the sand tray myself—why sand tray work tapped into the unconscious in creative ways and could be healing. This is what I had been doing. Creating spirals in this meditative way as I had been doing centered me. I dropped into the archetype of meaning, the Self, which brought me home to my center. In sand tray work, after it is completed, it can be observed and analyzed. The spiral is the shape of the path we take in life. By pattern or fate, by karma or the imprint of family and culture, by repetition-compulsion, or, as I think, to have a different outcome this time around, we attract an opportunity to heal what we could not in childhood or exercise the choice we now have.

Between my first trip to Four Corners in November and now here in May, my life had taken a turn in the spiral—I took Patricia into my home. When I came back from a week away at the beginning of the year, I called to say hello and see how she was doing. I was alarmed by how weak her voice was, drove from Mill Valley to Atherton and called her oncologist to have her admitted to the Ambulatory Care Unit. I stayed at her bedside through the night, held her hand and talked to her—using imagery and suggestion, reminding her of how she had gone into remission before, and silently prayed. I intuitively felt that she could have died otherwise. Obviously, she could not stay in her house alone, so something else was needed. I came back early the next morning to Mill Valley, stopped to get some groceries and there ran across Rachel Naomi Remen, MD, who recommended David Gullion, MD, as an oncologist in Marin for Patricia. I called him and found he could see Patricia later that same day, which we did.

Patricia moved into the library-TV room of my house. The care she needed was, as it turned out, easy to mobilize once I knew who to call (which Dr. Guillion's office staff provided). A home care service coordinated nurse visits, drawing blood and daily deliveries of IV nourishment and fluids that could go into her venous port via a pump while she slept. She needed injections which helped create more red blood cells, and had a transfusion as well. A month later, after she had rallied, she began once-weekly chemo. I went with Patricia and while we could watch the colorful IV anticancer cocktail drip, I added an invisible additive, visualization: as the chemo was selectively weakening the cancer cells, she could visualize and thus direct her white cells to gobble them up (like Pac-Man, the then-popular game). I had learned about the effectiveness of visualizations from the radiologist-oncologist, Carl O. Simonton, MD. Patricia's daughter Gina and son Mike came often, and visits from friends others who helped her were scheduled. I went about being a Jungian analyst with an office practice and an occasional lecture, as usual.

In March, I went away for ten days to do a Feathered Pipe Women's Wisdom workshop in the Bahamas. The house was full of good energy, it was a sunny place, and it had a happy feeling. Andy, Patricia, me, and Pierre the cat were a fine combination of housemates. The setup of my house helped, too. In my hillside house, Andy's bedroom-cave, with his array of musical equipment, computer, books, and collectibles, was downstairs, as was mine—including the room where I did my writing. Our women's circle met in the living room next to the library-TV room—Georgia Johnson-May, Nancy Ramsay, Elizabeth Ostermann, Grace Dammann, Patricia and me.

As smoothly as all of this was going, it was for me a metaphoric combination of being on call like a doctor and being a mom with her antennae up to hear the slightest sounds from her baby. Concern for Andy (and what the neurofibromatosis was doing) and for Patricia meant that I was never fully at rest—which takes psychic energy.

It was good to be back at Four Corners. Mike was there, missing David. We were compatriot-friends, getting through a rough stretch of life. One of his ways was to do as much physical work as he could on the property. We were both born in June under the astrological sign of cancer, feeling-intuitive types, whose work it is to listen to others. Neither of us needed to talk, though from time to time we'd bring up a memory or an update.

Patricia died on June 25, 1996. She was fifty-six. I waved goodbye as I left to see my mother in Los Angeles over the weekend. When I came back on Sunday, I learned Patricia was in coma at Marin General Hospital. She had visited her home in Atherton while I was away, taken a turn for the worse, and been brought back to MGH by her son and daughter. When I saw her in the hospital she was initially semi-conscious. She was clear enough by the next day to say that she wanted to go back to Atherton. We had a short, sweet conversation that didn't acknowledge that she was ready to leave this life. She died peacefully in her own bed at her home the next day, with her son and daughter present.

Patricia died three weeks before my third visit to Four Corners. I felt as if she accompanied me. When I got to my tree sanctuary, I rolled and tied a copy of her poem protected in plastic ("I, Matter") to the large branch over the space. Her poem with her photograph at the top of it were from the celebration of her life and memorial held outdoors at her home in Atherton. Tied parallel with the branch, one could clearly see her face as if she were looking out, seeing through the same opening in the trees—the vista I could see when I sat under the branch.

I was again drawn to the area that felt like being in the center of a medicine wheel, one that stretched to the horizons where mountains were its edge. As I meandered over the natural contours of the land mostly covered with desert grasses, the idea of creating a labyrinth entered my mind. Not the complex pattern of the Chartres labyrinth, but the seven-circuit labyrinth, the oldest design which is at least five-thousand years old and found all over the world. Using whatever it is that provides information—which is like being a dowser and dowsing stick together—I found where it should be.

This was not an undertaking for this trip, but remained as something important to me to do when I next returned. Out on the land by myself, I followed this inner sense, laying it out in the direction that felt right, tracing the pattern with a stick, its length serving as the measure for the width of the path through the labyrinth. I altered the design by making the center a circle where several people could sit. I had found one standing stone that I placed at the corner of the entry path. Once into the stone gathering and placing phase, Mike helped by finding and lugging stones into a pile for me to use.

Later, when Toni D'Anca came with me and had a real compass, we found that the opening of the path and the direct line with which it began aligned exactly due east. My reaction was "Wow!" I thought about Stonehenge and Newgrange, about being in the cairn at the Hill of Witches on the Winter Solstice when it was lit up and glowed at dawn on the summer solstice, about assumptions that there had to be astronomical knowledge and devices, and wondered if instead, it was an instinctual or inner knowledge in the body-psyches of the designers. If I could align this one labyrinth, I could entertain this far-out possibility.

To me the spiral path and the labyrinth path are both symbols and images of our life journey or soul path: of going in and coming out, of being changed as we walk these paths, of not giving up when we were close to what we thought was the goal, only to have the path move in another direction.

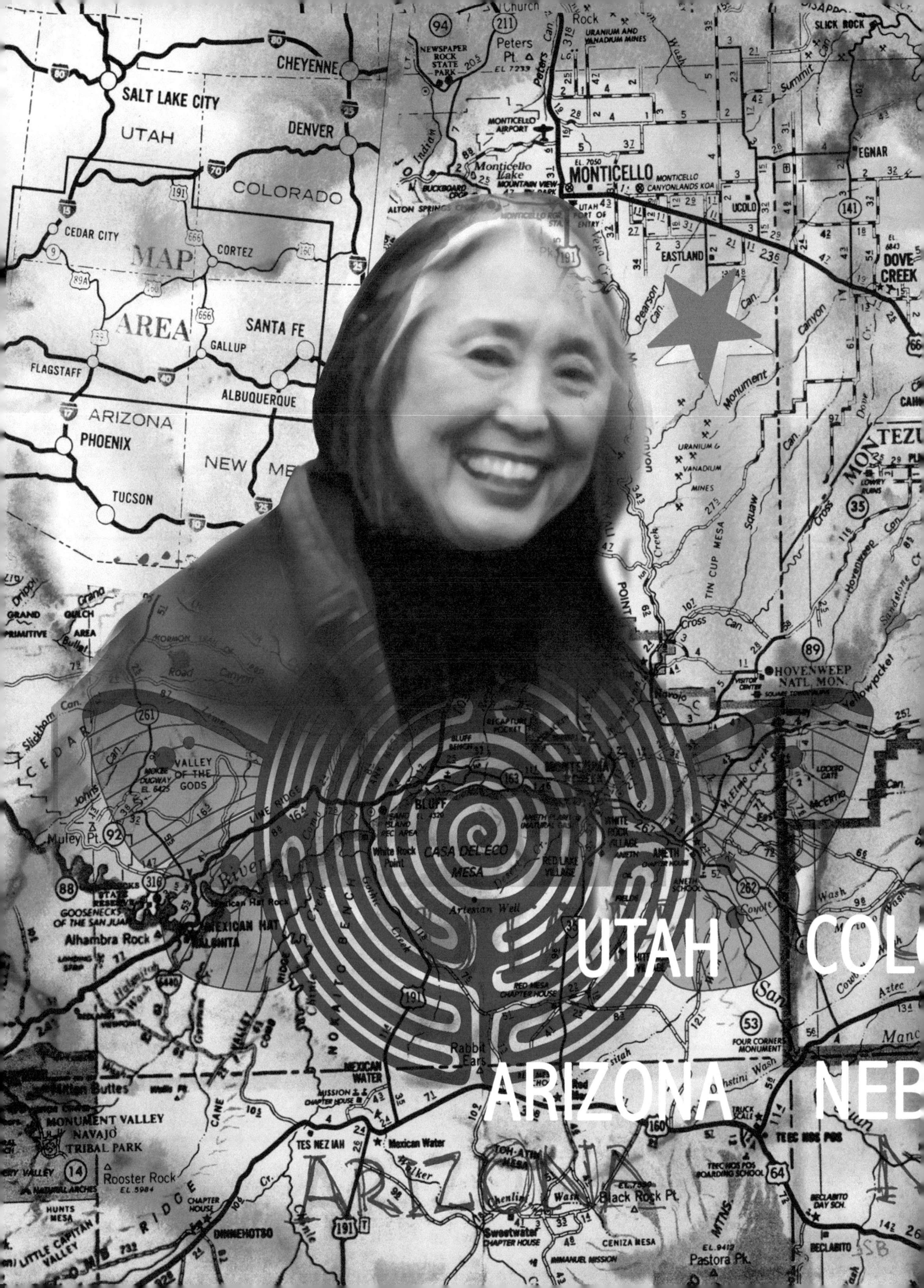
SALT LAKE CITY
CHEYENNE
UTAH
DENVER
COLORADO
CEDAR CITY
MAP
AREA
CORTEZ
SANTA FE
GALLUP
FLAGSTAFF
ALBUQUERQUE
ARIZONA
PHOENIX
TUCSON
NEWSPAPER ROCK STATE PARK
Peters Pt.
URANIUM AND VANADIUM MINES
SLICK ROCK
MONTICELLO AIRPORT
Monticello Lake
MONTICELLO
MONTICELLO CANYONLANDS KOA
UCOLO
EGNAR
EASTLAND
DOVE CREEK
Monument
URANIUM & VANADIUM MINES
TIN CUP MESA
HOVENWEEP NATL. MON.
VALLEY OF THE GODS
Muley Pt.
BLUFF
CASA DEL ECO MESA
White Rock Point
Artesian Well
MEXICAN HAT
GOOSENECKS OF THE SAN JUAN
Alhambra Rock
UTAH
ARIZONA
RED MESA CHAPTER HOUSE
Rabbit Ears
MEXICAN WATER
FOUR CORNERS MONUMENT
MONUMENT VALLEY NAVAJO TRIBAL PARK
Rooster Rock
TES NEZ IAH
Mexican Water
TEEC NOS POS
Black Rock Pt.
Sweetwater
CENIZA MESA
DINNEHOTSO
Pastora Pk.
BECLABITO

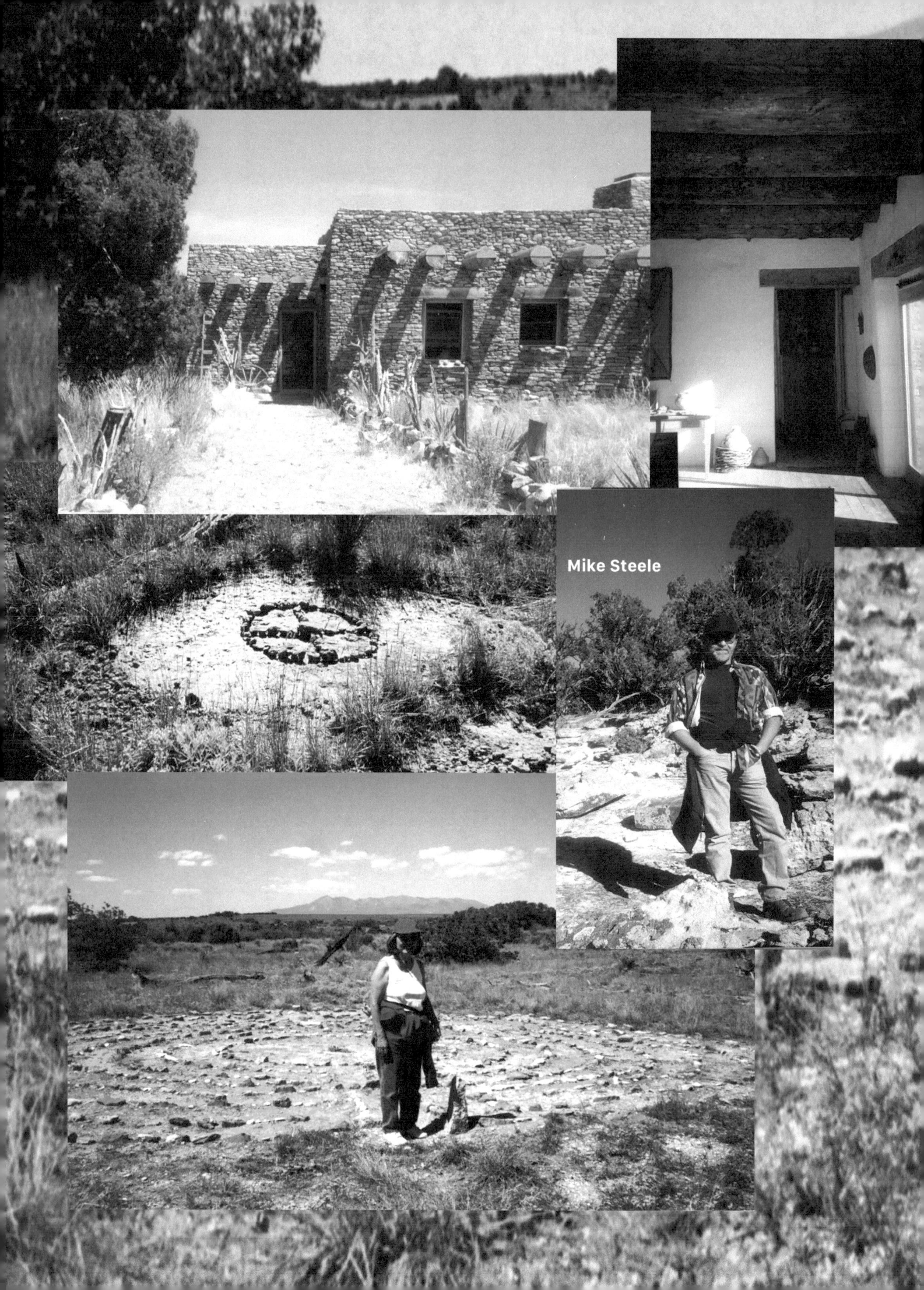
Mike Steele

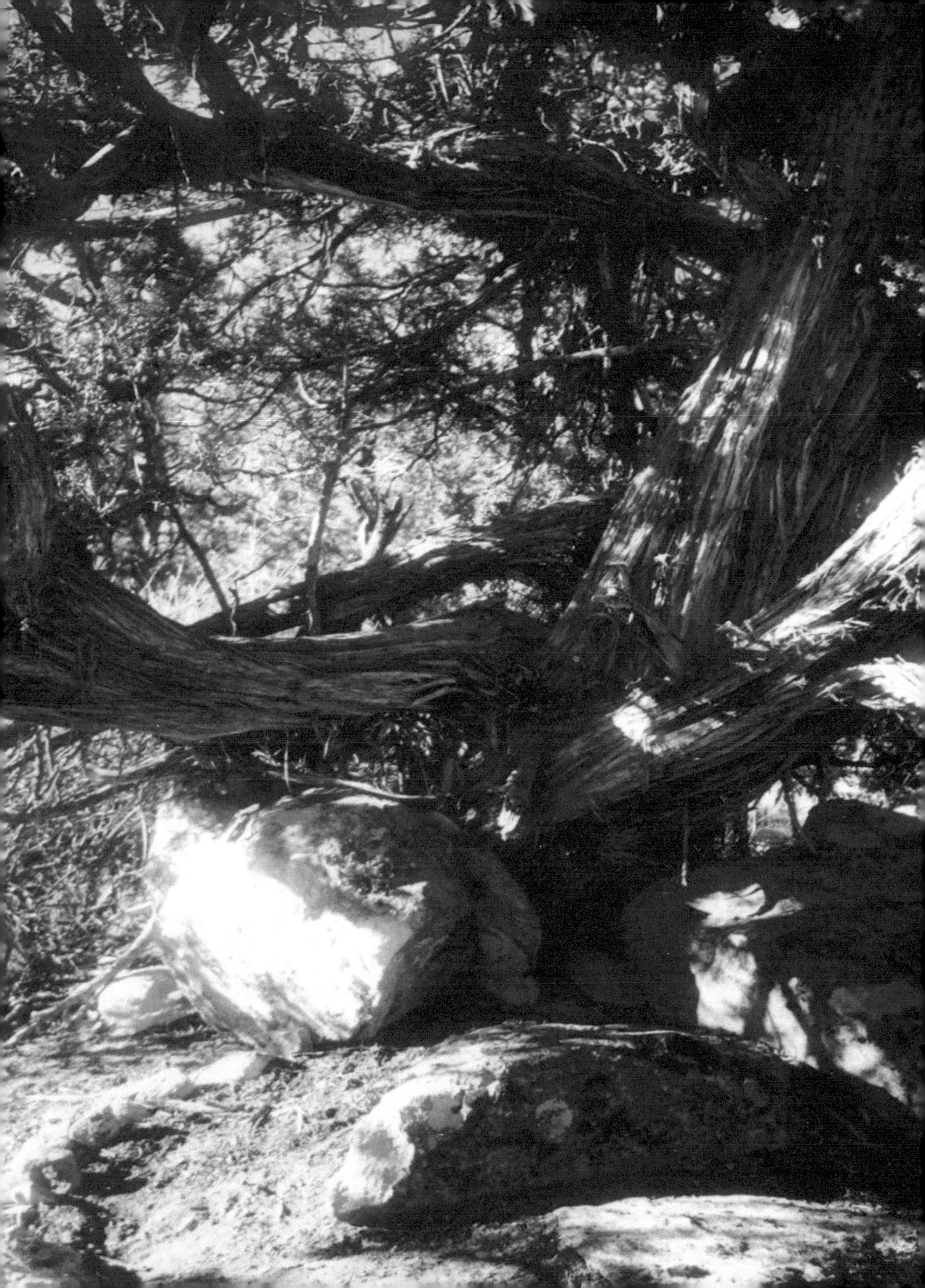

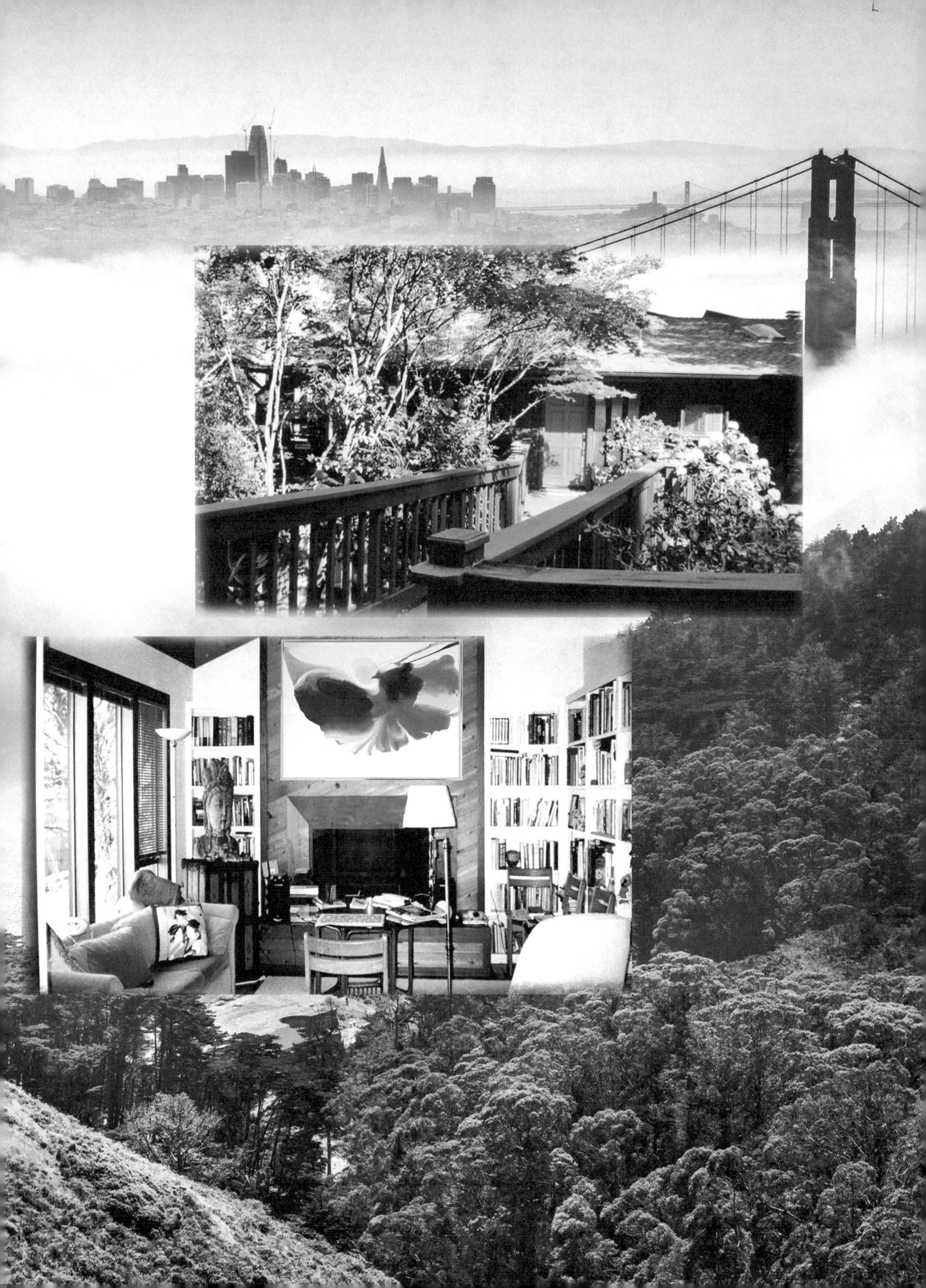

Chapter 27
Andy's Message – Close to the Bone

"I'm okay. I'm really okay. Tell Mom I'm okay." These are words that every Mom has heard or wanted to hear under a variety of circumstances. This particular message came to Jim the night after our son Andy died. Jim had gone back to his apartment, was alone in his grief and on the edge of sinking into depression when he heard these words. Andy was pleased and surprised that his dad could hear him from the other side; he exclaimed, "I didn't know you could do this!" He proceeded to tell Jim what he was experiencing. When Jim relayed Andy's comments, the words he used and his observations sounded just like Andy.

The morning he died, I had heard him call "Mom," loud and clear, not long after three in the morning. I was asleep on the sofa in the library-TV room, where he slept in a hospital bed. At this point he was a quadriplegic. Whenever he needed something, he called "Mom" in a whisper, which I always heard. I slept with one ear listening for him, since he could not speak above a whisper after an NF2 tumor (by now specifically identified as a schwannoma) had paralyzed one of his vocal cords. It startled me to hear him call me with his old strong voice; my first thought was, "How did he do that?!" I went to his bedside, expecting that his eyes would be open as usual when he called, but this time, his eyes were closed, he was breathing irregularly and with difficulty. I went to the rheostat to turn the light up and as I did, I heard him take his last breath. He had let me know he was leaving. I wouldn't wake up in the morning to find him dead.

Andre Joseph Bolen (February 16, 1972–June 4, 2001) died at age twenty-nine as heroically as he lived, enduring with grace and even humor the multiple physical losses and disabilities that was his fate. His warrior marks were the surgical scars on his body from the major and minor surgeries that his rare disease required. His journey did not fit Joseph Campbell's model, *The Hero with a Thousand Faces*, which begins with a call to adventure. There is another model of the Hero's Journey, which is usually unheralded and often even unappreciated by the person whose story it is, or by those near and dear. It begins with loss and pain, with unchosen circumstances and suffering that life can bring. I have long thought that we needed another designation other than "heroic" for the courage, patience, and forbearance that such journeys take. I have spoken of such journeys as "heroinic," fitting for women whose stories are also heroic. "Victim" and "survivor" are inadequate and simplistic.

In January on a sunny afternoon, Andy and I left the house, and were on the sloping path up to his car when he lost his balance and fell backward. He grabbed at the railing to break his fall, missed it, spun around, and fell hard. He managed to get himself into a sitting position and had a lot of pain in his neck. When he said that it felt like a whiplash and he was afraid to move, I called his neurologist to alert her and for an ambulance to take him to the emergency room at St. Mary's Hospital, where she would meet us. The paramedics came and strapped him into a cervical spine board, which relieved his neck pain considerably. His color returned and there were initially no signs of spinal cord damage: all extremities could move and had feeling. I went in the ambulance with him. I had called his father who followed us over the Golden Gate Bridge to San Francisco. At the hospital, a CT Scan showed a line fracture at the C4 vertebra. He had broken his neck. He was admitted overnight, lying flat and fitted with a cervical collar. At the end of this traumatic day, he was comfortable and even had his dry humor back.

He had had an intense year before this. Since we learned that he had tumors on both auditory nerves, he routinely had audiograms as well as MRIs, with Dr. McAuliffe tracking the unpredictable course of NF2 and Mark Renneker, MD, staying on top of current knowledge, and experts. One of the auditory tumors had grown to a size that it was dangerous to the brain around it. There were now two new cutting-edge work being done for NF2 auditory tumors. The gamma knife had been developed and was being done at UC Irvine in Southern California. Here, the tumor could be removed without surgery. Surgical removal of the tumor and placement of an Auditory Brain Implant (ABI) on the midbrain during the same surgery had been developed at the House Ear Institute in Los Angeles, which offered the possibility of hearing afterward.

We got information and perspectives from Mark Renneker, MD, and then Andy and I made appointments to meet and hear directly what each of these approaches involved, and to also get an intuitive sense of them as people. With Andy's technical mind and ability to grasp of the situation, and with it being his disease to live and treatment to endure, the decision would be up to him. He chose the House Ear Institute, which was by far the harder course, but the one with more potential, but no promises. The ABI had gotten FDA approval only two months before this. He talked with the technical people about how the ABI worked, would be tested and programmed. Andy's course and certification in audio mixing made it all understandable to him.

In October 2000, the two surgeons who had developed the treatment, Dr. Brachmann and Dr. Hitselberger, removed the tumor and placed the ABI. The operation took between six and seven hours, required a transfusion, and he was placed on a respirator for the first twenty-four hours in ICU. Six weeks later in mid- November, his ABI was tested. It was a twenty-one bulls-eye placement; every single one of the twenty-one electrodes responded, which was a first for any subject. When given an audiogram to test hearing pure tones, the results were in the borderline-normal range. From stone-deaf to this felt near-miraculous. Andy described the sound of voices as if created by "a synthesizer through a cheap amplifier." The plan was that he would be returning to the House Ear Institute to tweak the ABI—he had been using it and had begun classes at the College of Marin. He drove and had a note-taker provided by the Disabled Student Program.

Now, all progress was stopped. When he fell, he fractured a vertebra in his neck, with surrounding soft tissue bruises. With the risk that further movement would cause more damage to his spinal cord, he was put into a "halo" to immobilize his neck. He was missing the lamina bones in his neck which shield and protect the spinal canal with its vulnerable cord and nerve fibers. They had been removed during the operation to take out the dumbbell shaped neurofibroma when he was eighteen. He also had a problem with balance and a foot drop, and he had learned to eat with his left hand, all disabilities from NF2. The halo was secured with screws that went into his skull, anchoring the metal rods that were attached to a neck and shoulder apparatus that kept his neck from moving. Seeing Andy in it hurt my heart then, and remembering how he looked does so even now.

The halo crossed his forehead. It looked like a torture instrument and at the time it was put in, the local anesthetic had not been effective, so it really had been. It reminded me of the crown of thorns that Jesus wore at his crucifixion, and Andy's thin unshaven face as the days went on made the resemblance even stronger. The halo also had disabled the Auditory Brain Implant which meant Andy was once again deaf. He had a very heavy "cross to bear."

A month in the acute rehabilitation unit followed. The halo was removed when the line fracture had healed, but as it turned out, even without severing the cord, swelling at the site had resulted in his becoming a quadriplegic. Only motor function was affected. It could have been worse. His mind and personality remained as good and stable as ever, as did all other major body systems. I was not being a Pollyanna, and he was not feeling himself a victim.

Andy came home in March. Autumn and winter had come and gone and now it was spring in Marin. Everything was green. He was happy to be home again. The library-TV room now had him as occupant. I knew what he would need from having had Patricia here, and I knew which home care services to call. Andy needed skilled nursing care, someone who was strong enough to lift him, and since he would be around us a lot, someone compatible for a daytime shift. An introverted, able-bodied male nurse who fit our needs manifested. I think that a clear image of who or what is needed is like having a clear intention, and that an intention, like a visualization, or prayer, invites a response from the invisible realm. This then can be called synchronicity, or magic, or angels.

Andy settled into a routine that gave him inner time for himself as well as company. In the months before his death, I think he may have been doing a life review: once when Melody was over, she asked him what he had been doing. He said that he was going over every trip he had ever taken. I noticed that he was saying "thank you," for every little thing anyone did for him, and in a note I asked him about this. It wasn't something he used to do. He said back, "I always was thankful, I just often didn't say so." He also was receptive and appreciative for the healers, prayers, ceremonies, that were done for him. I had gone back to work—I have had limited office hours for a selective practice for years now, and had book events scheduled during the end of March into the beginning of April for *Goddesses in Older Women.* Betty Karr, my longtime assistant came and stayed during the ten days I was on book tour.

From his first after-death communication when Jim heard him say, "Dad, I'm okay, I really am okay, tell Mom I'm okay," his words were primarily caring and reassuring support for Jim, and through Jim to me. He found himself in a place where there were lots of people who had died, and lots of helpers. Many others were having difficulties adjusting to where they were. It sounded like a temporary reception area. This initial communication was heartwarming, "I am very much alive! Tell Mom I am very much alive!" He once said, "I can eat anything I want, and I don't even have to poop!" The words were so much him. The fact that he would take such delight in this in particular added to my sense that it really was Andy. (His inactivity made bowel function a daily concern.) He said he had a new body, he could move freely, and that at this stage, he could have anything he wanted by thinking about it. He reiterated to Jim how much all the love and prayers for him helped him, and continued to help him now. Just as Andy often made humorous, pithy comments in the midst of his multiple disabilities, he did so after he died. For example: I went to the crematorium to be with his body as it went into the furnace that would transform it into ashes. Jim had not wanted to do this and was aware of the time and feeling badly when he heard Andy say cheerily: "Hey Dad. I'm not there, either!"

Another such moment was when Jim and I went to Andy's bank to close his account. We had to bring his death certificate and a notarized form that he had died without a will, and that according to California law, we were his beneficiaries. It was a depressing task. The two of us sat across a desk from the banker, who had turned away to look at text on his computer. Andy's death certificate was on the desk in front of us. This is when Jim heard Andy say, "Think of it as my diploma!"

I think that Andy graduated from life *summa cum laude.* NF2 was his soul-testing curriculum in non-attachment and non-comparison with others. Leaving his body was graduation from earth school.

Months after Andy's death, Terry Tempest Williams called. We have a bond that hasn't to do with time spent together. My life and hers take place in different parts of the United States. I got to know her first through her book, *Refuge* and most recently, *When Women Were Birds.* In between reading each other's books, we occasionally crossed paths—the last times had been at the World Parliament of Religions and the Bioneer conferences where we took time out together. We met and recognized each other as heart-motivated advocates and activists, who are fired up by what we love. Alice Walker's title *Anything We Love, Can Be Saved* is an operating principle for Alice's activism, and for Terry and me.

I told Terry about Andy, and before we hung up, she told me that she and her husband, Brooke, were living in Castle Valley, Utah, near Four Corners and that there is a natural rock formation outside of the house which is a natural altar. She said she'd light a candle for Andy. Later, she told me what had happened. She lit the candle and introduced herself to Andy as if he were there, and told him she had just talked to me. Then she said, "I wonder what it is like where you are?" He replied—she heard him speak, audibly, through her whole body. He said to her, quite matter-of-factly: "You'll find out, soon enough."

Whereupon, Terry became very alarmed; she told me that she poured out all of the many, many things she had yet to do and wanted to accomplish.

Her alarm had to do with the lump she had discovered in her breast, which she feared was malignant, joining the "one-breasted tribe" of female relatives who had died of breast cancer. She wrote in *Refuge* about learning that the image she had in her mind since she was a little girl, of a huge mushroom shaped cloud, was not a dream or imagined. She had been in a car downwind from the atomic test grounds and had seen the huge mushroom clouds in the sky. When she finished telling him all that she had yet to do, Andy spoke to her again and said, "You have as much time as you need." His words were like a promise, even before she learned the lump was benign, the words sunk in.

Terry wrote to me: "The biopsies were fine. I am healthy and whole. My conversation with Andy was a big part of that, realizing in dialogue with him, how much I wanted to stay, how my work was not done, how much I wanted to live. 'You have all the time you need' was like a breath that entered me from the other world. He showed me what a fine line it is—how we do have access to both. Bless him. Bless you. We are family."

Andy's words "You have as much time as you need" are true when why we are here and what we do here matters to us and to others. I believe that this depends upon being motivated from inside out—which is having a passion or a calling, motivated by your heart to follow a path of service, or creativity, or relationship. Those of us who can choose a path that is meaningful are privileged.

But, what about Andy and other individuals, for whom fate—as a disease, or as a consequence of an accident, or war, or even deliberate cruelty—increasingly limits health, mobility or length of life? I believe that how Andy played the hand he was dealt was a more intense version where the choice can become limited to how we respond. To be on a soul-path depends on our response to the life we have and the physical death that comes soon enough—at the end. Andy is a role model for courage, humor, adapting as long as it is possible, and being ready to leave his body behind when it was time.

I included some of Andy's communications after he died in the revised edition of *Close to the Bone* because I wanted to add this information to the book that I had written about finding meaning and becoming a protagonist in your own story once you are diagnosed with an illness that is considered terminal, or where the odds are against survival. I drew on myths, psychological, spiritual, alternative-integrative choices people had made and remissions.

When I revised *Close to the Bone* in 2007, AIDS was no longer a terminal illness. It was an example of how a disease that is supposed to kill you can be changed by a new treatment. AIDS had devastating effects on the gay culture and on individuals when their lives went from "gathering flowers in the meadow," to finding themselves in the underworld of fear and debilitating deaths. AIDS matured individuals and gay culture from an emphasis on youth and play (archetypal Peter Pan and Wendy, the Lost Boys, and Never-Never Land) into caretaking and social activism. It was a boys into men shift, a coming out and fighting back movement. The Stonewall riots in1969 were an expression of this. It was about valuing themselves and not accepting oppression and being defined by patriarchal men. It was liberating as feminism is for women.

The original publication of *Close to the Bone* was October 2, 1996. Andy was in the audience at the book launch at First Unitarian in San Francisco. Michael Steele was at the piano, music flowing through his fingers, reminding me of listening to him play in their home, before David died of AIDS a year before. Patricia Demetrios had died that June. I received the first hot-off-the-press author copy of *Close to the Bone* on August 27, which was Patricia's birthday. What we know "in our bones," is soul knowledge—not what we have been told, but inner knowledge-*gnosis*. When we consciously face death or disability, it can bring us close to what we know in our bones. I liked that October 2 was Guardian Angel Day, and not a saint's day, because I feel that those of us who sense the invisible-liminal realm know in our bones, of presences, spirits, angels, ancestors, people who love us and look after us from the other side. Andy is now one of my guardian angels and it seems to me that he also now can be many places at once, and that helping others who ask him is all that it takes.

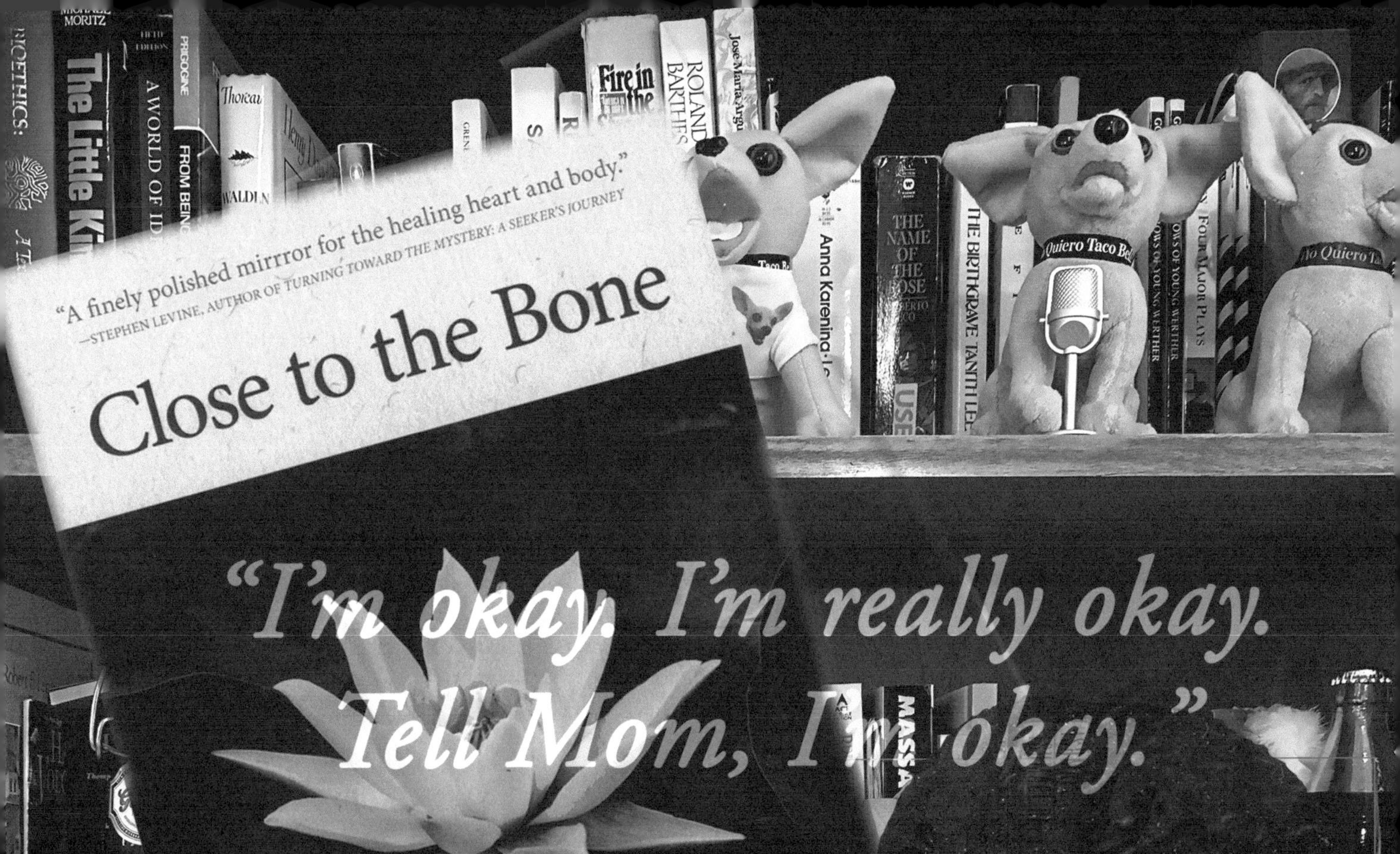

"I'm okay. I'm really okay.
Tell Mom, I'm okay."

Life-Threatening Illness as a Soul Journey

JEAN SHINODA BOLEN, MD

André Bolen

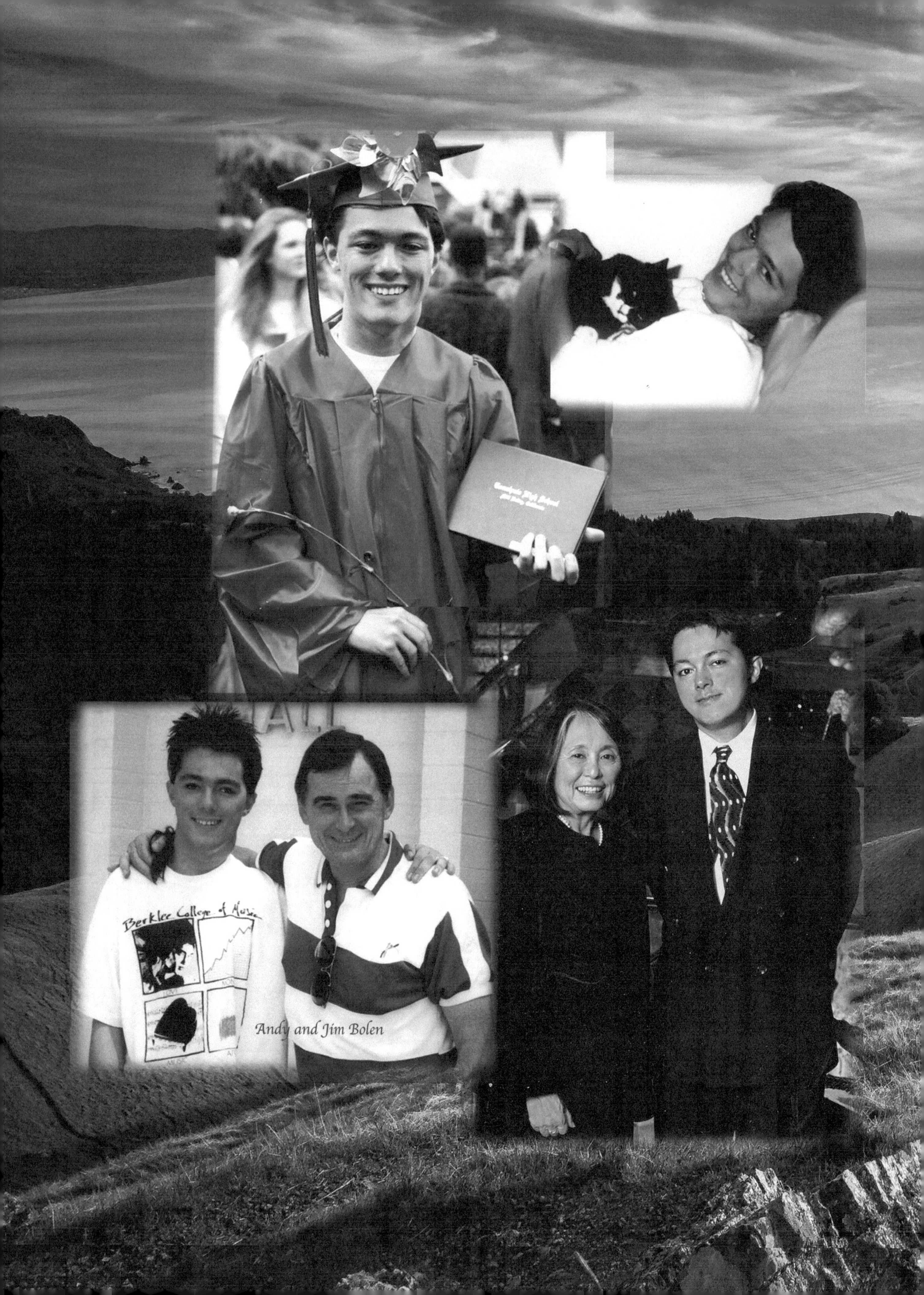

Andy and Jim Bolen

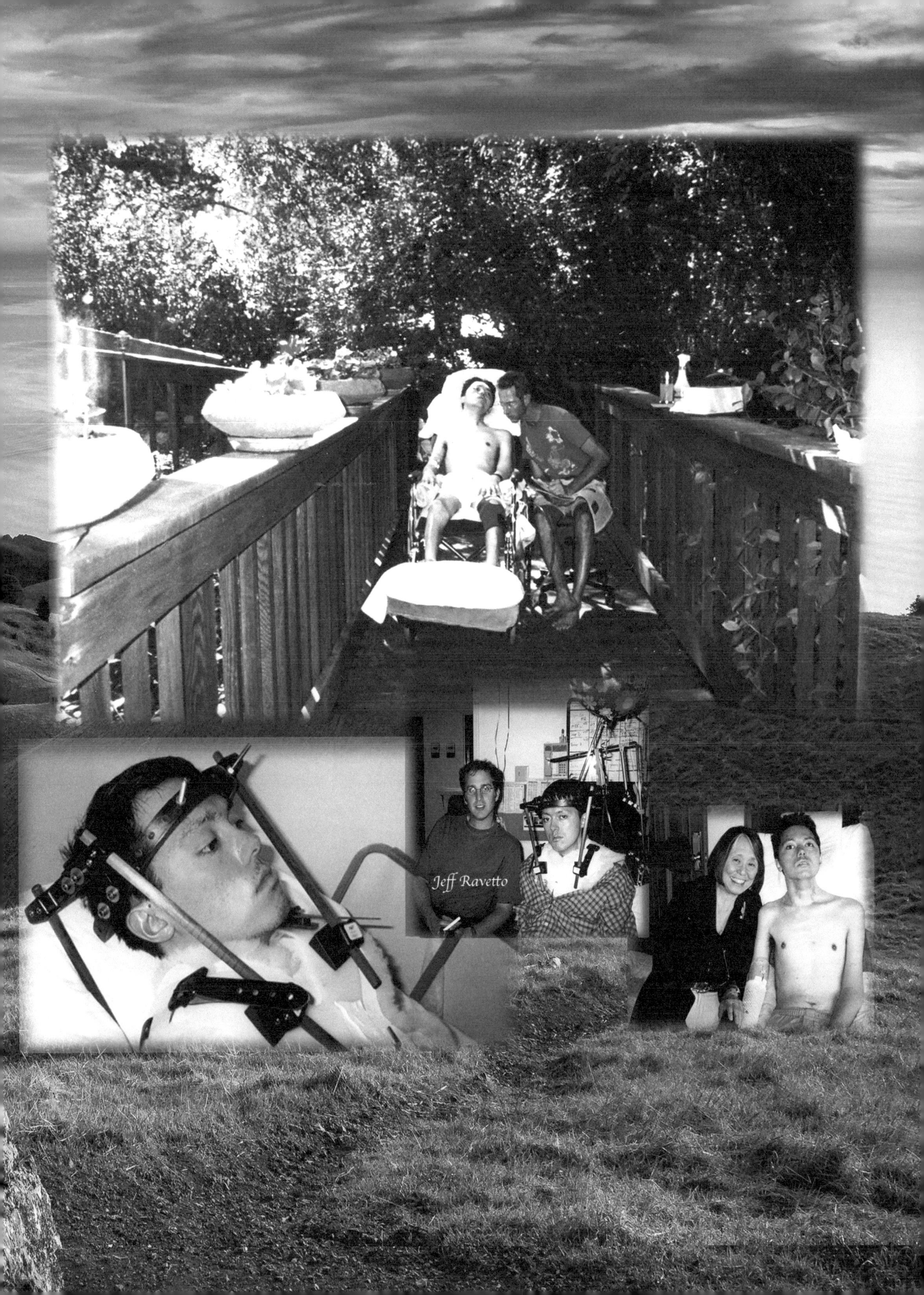
Jeff Ravetto

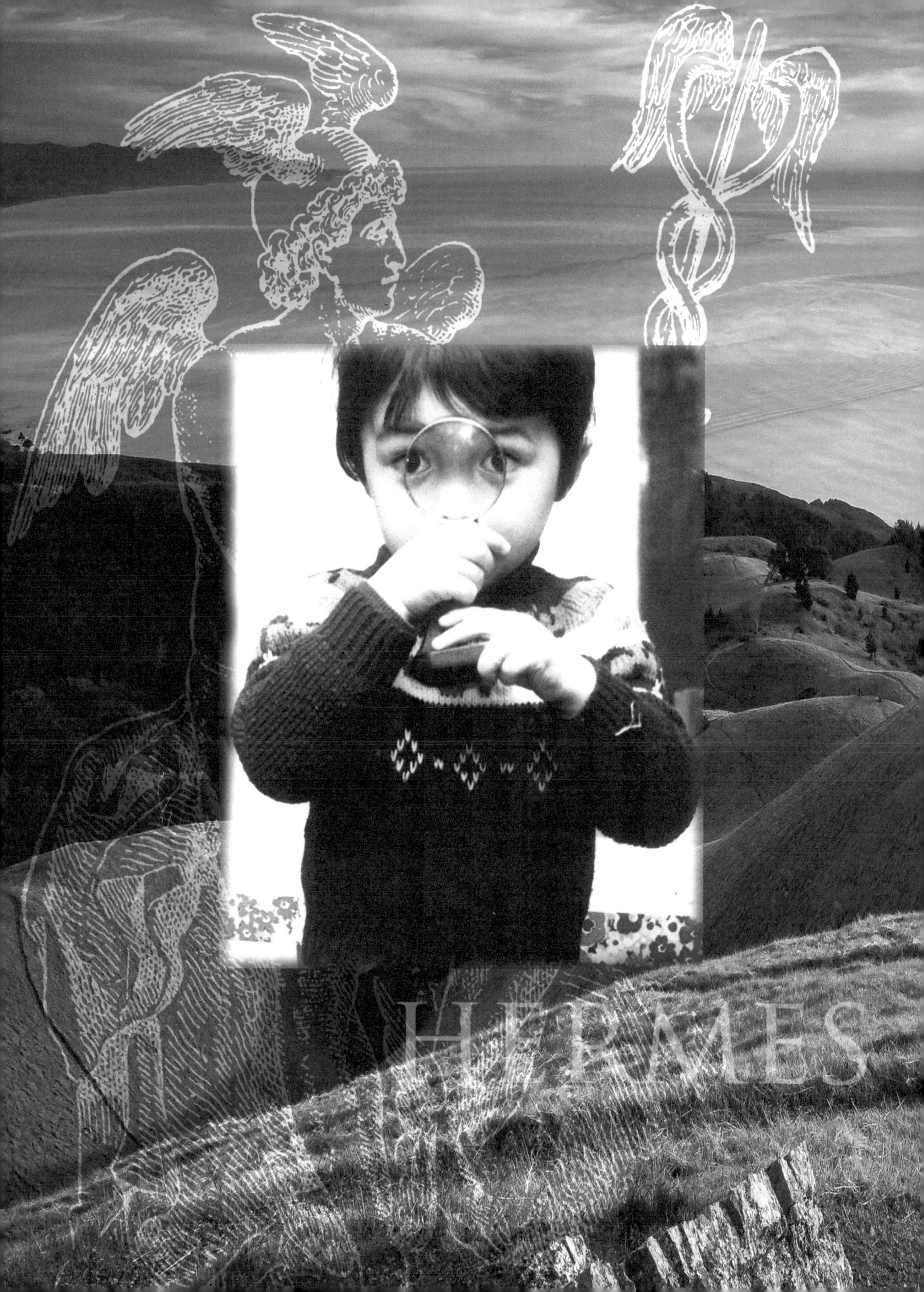
HERMES

Section 6

Liminal Circles, Spiritual Activism, Author, Cancer

Chapter 28

Those on the Other Side - Soul Friends

Muir Woods lies nearby, just over the hill from where I live in Mill Valley. I often walk there in the early morning among the tall redwood trees. It feels like a green cathedral with its soaring trees, which are the tallest trees in the world. A few are more than 360 feet tall, and may be over 2,000 years old. Walking among these old-soul trees when it is quiet is to be in a familiar sacred space. I often find my way to my chapel space, which is between the trunks of two large trees, one of which is scarred from fire, the other with a growth recalling the anatomical human heart, which I see when I lean with my back against its trunk and look upwards across to the other tree. The clear space between the two trees forms a circle with room for two, though I am almost always there by myself. Only once or twice have I shared this *liminal* space with a close friend. It seems to me that it can be a threshold between the physical world and the realm of spirit, soul, and whatever angels are.

Each of us is the "one and only threshold of an inner world." Thus begins an observation from poet/philosopher John O'Donohue, which I find obvious as a psychological statement that others may balk at accepting because of how education and science separates the mental realm of thought and measure from what we perceive with intuition and feeling.

> The Celtic mind was not burdened by dualism. It did not separate what belongs together. The Celtic imagination articulates the inner friendship that embraces Nature, divinity, underworld, and human world as one. The dualism that separates the visible from the invisible, time from eternity, the human from the divine, was totally alien to them.

Beyond this non-ordinary reality, I think of metaphoric others in concentric circles who contributed to who I am. Many are names beyond my memory, names beyond my lifetime—bloodline ancestors and spiritual relatives who went before me. I think of C. G. Jung and the words that first drew me into feeling that this is how I work as a psychotherapist: for one person, the patient, to be affected by the work, so must the other—the doctor. There are different ways of saying the same thing that applies to significant relationships: for one person to be transformed in the relationship, the other must also. Or, a meeting of two souls is like a chemical reaction, for one substance to be affected, the other is also. I have met many people soul-to-soul, including my patients and analysands, participants at events, those I influenced or mentored and vice-versa, friends and colleagues throughout my life, members of my family who were close at times in my life, and the teachers, writers, poets and musicians from whom I learned from in person or through their work.

The family members I was close to who are now on the other side are my son (Andy/Andre Joseph Bolen) and my father (Joseph Shinoda), whose last moments I witnessed, and my mother (Megumi Yamaguchi Shinoda, MD) who was ninety-nine (February 9, 1908 - May 1, 2007) when it was her time, and my uncle (Mits/Mitsuya Yamaguchi, MD) who had walked me down the aisle and with whom I spent time, often going to the movies, after my mother was tucked safely in bed. I had been with both of them the weekend before she died. She had recovered from the devastating effect of my father's long cancer illness and death in 1963. This was when I took a leave of absence at the beginning of my psychiatric residency during which my father died, my brother needed to be placed where he would be cared for, and my mother's depression required her to be hospitalized.

When she recovered, my doctor mom moved her office from Little Tokyo to a professional building in Hollywood, where she practiced psychotherapy, hypnotherapy, and could use her knowledge of internal medicine to diagnose and refer. She took courses at UCLA, studied the stock market and charted stocks—this was before computers. She was fine living alone, and enjoyed her office practice until she no longer felt she could keep up with what she needed to know about psychiatric medication. She closed her office when she was eighty-eight. And then, it was if she had no need for her mind anymore, and gradually ceased using it.

I marvel how the help she needed—competent, loving help—materialized to see her through a lengthy dementia decline. I was so grateful that it happened and wonder if this is how the invisible world works to take care of people who have done good in the world as she had done. She was the first physician in the Los Angeles Japanese-American community doing obstetrics and family medicine. Then, when she opened her office in Hollywood, she had a large transsexual practice. After she had treated a transsexual patient with her usual consideration, compassion and competence, the word went out in that community of marginalized people about her. Some patients who had seen her in her former office who now travelled across Los Angeles to see her in Hollywood.

When she needed help, help arrived: her brother, Mits, the youngest of the Yamaguchi siblings had become a widower, and it worked out well for both of them for him to live with her while he went to his office. Then Alicia Santiago materialized. She had been with her previous patient as primary caretaker for five or six years and had become available at just the right time. Uncle Mits lived in the house and was there every night. Alicia arrived in the morning to take care of my mother's morning ablutions, and the household had a cheery late morning breakfast in the big familiar kitchen. My mother regressed and was like a cherished, spoiled child, easily made to smile. Ice cream could bring her joy, or sitting outside, absorbed reading the Los Angeles Times, and not be able to recall any of it. Alicia was not only competent, but she also loved her patient. The saying, "it's never too late to have a happy childhood," may apply to my mother. Linear time was immaterial. When I was with her, she had no sense of time since I was last there or what it meant or tell her when I would be back again.

Meanwhile, Mits was also getting older, and was seeing fewer and fewer patients himself. He had a consulting room in a younger colleague's office and had lunch at the hospital where he still had admitting privileges. In 2007, a month or two before my mother died, Mits shut down his practice. He, like my mother, had been a loved physician. His son Ken Yamaguchi and daughter-in-law, Monica, lived in Scottsdale, Arizona, in a retirement community comprised of many multi-storied apartment buildings, each with its own underground parking. The apartment next door to theirs became available at this time, so that when Ken and Monica came out for my mother's memorial service, they rented a truck to take Mits and his belongings back with them. He moved next door and had their company, and his privacy, and as he became more in need of care—there they were, his bedroom separated from their apartment by only a thin wall. He could not have stayed in my mother's house after she died because half of the house was in a bank trust. There could not have been a better situation than this. He stayed next door to Ken and Monica until he died at age ninety-nine on January 27, 2016.

I look at how my mother and uncle had circumstance and people work out well in the end of their physical life—truly as if looked after. I wonder: is this how things can work out? Was this synchronicity? For Mits, the coincidences were uncanny, and seemed more than good luck. The availability of Alicia for my mother, also. I live by myself, feel privileged to be able to do so, and think this is likely to continue. But if I should have a cognitive decline or become physically disabled, then what? By looking to my mother and uncle, I am encouraged to trust and have faith that whatever happens to me at the end will turn out well.

At my mother's burial service, my brother Stephen's ashes were put with her in her casket, and his name is carved on the headstone with both my parents. He died in 1999 at age fifty-six. That and this memoir is where memory of him will be. The circumstances of his life were bleak and seemed meaningless. I was a teenager at Forest Home (Presbyterian) church camp when it struck me that I could have been him. As an adolescent, the thought which I had heard church leaders say, "There but for the grace of God go I," made me thankful. My good fortune was an insight through which I acquired soul lessons in gratitude and humility. In what I call a conversation with God, I asked in prayer, "How can I say thank you?" The answer that came was to help less fortunate people—which I could do by becoming a doctor. I think of the medical school classmates I had who had intellectually and physically disabled siblings, who (as far as I could know), came to a similar conclusion or calling, without the conversation. But I suspect now that I have words and understanding for such things, that spared siblings have some survivor guilt and can be found in greater than average numbers among the helping professions.

Even then, when I felt spared and was full of gratitude, I wondered, what about Stephen? Which made me wonder about God. What kind of God would give me what I had, and let him be the object lesson? Stephen was my close-to-home example of meaningless suffering. I remember the logical quandary that I came to think of as simplistic: "Either God is all-powerful, and He is not good, or He is good but not all-powerful." It was like a question for debaters, and led me to allow for ambiguity, to go outside these parameters of "good" and "powerful", and continue to think from time to time about divinity and soul, both of which are beyond the grasp of mind because they are known through *gnosis* not *logos*. I was attracted to a book with the title *Your God is Too Small,* by J. B. Phillips, which helped stretched my then-Protestant mind several years later.

I realize how good it is to feel fortunate and to have gratitude—to feel blessed. It makes my heart center expand, to feel loved and more loving; it leads me to have the following thoughts: Love is a subjective feeling, as is joy. The sense of presence, of divinity, of bonds that are invisible yet felt, are dimensions of spiritual reality that are also subjective and no less real because they remain outside of measurement. Love makes us happy; love looks at others through the lens of compassion; love allows us to see beauty as a soul attribute and as a soul perception. Beauty as seen objectively is compared to a standard or to others. With age, objective physical beauty diminishes, while subjective beauty can grow when the soul shines through and is perceived by the soul of another.

The friends who are in my virtual-liminal circle were beautiful to me in my life as are others who are still alive. Jananne Lovett (Keen), Patricia Demetrios, Anthea Francine, Elaine Fedors Viseltear, and Myrna Cramer (known after she married as Marriam Ring) were longtime friends who crossed over the threshold between this life and what comes next. They were sister-pilgrims, witnesses to my life, "soul friends" or *anam cara* in the Celtic tradition, which I learned of and immediately understood from John O'Donohue. I met John O'Donohue at an early Jung in Ireland Conference, thanks to Aryeh Maidenbaum, a Jungian analyst whose creativity is expressed through who, where, and what he brings together with Jungian themes in the world.

Elaine Fedors Viseltear came to an early Jung in Ireland Conference with me. She and I traveled to hill towns in Italy and France, to Igazu Falls and Buenos Aires, to the Omega Institute and Jung on the Hudson in New York, to Boston and Kripalu in the Berkshires. We became friends when I was a psychiatric resident and she was an occupational therapist at Langley Porter; we were housemates in Sausalito until meeting our respective husbands at a Thanksgiving dinner. She and Arthur moved to the east coast. My two children and hers were born around the same time. She became the editor of the *Journal of Occupational Therapy.* I divorced and she was widowed when we were in our fifties. She (Elonka/Elaine) had a "Russian soul," which I could sense, but which she rarely put into conversation—a comment now and then sufficed to know what was troubling; to talk about spousal difficulties in any detail would have been disloyal. This was an ethic we each had. We knew significant people in each other's lives, some of whom no one else in our current lives would know. Companionable silences and curiosity made us good company for each other as we explored new places in the world. Getting around physically became increasingly difficult: her spirit may have been willing, but her body gave up. *Crones Don't Whine* definitely applied.

Anthea Francine led and inspired Women's Quest, the women's spirituality organization in Berkeley. She was a figure upon whom women projected priestess and the archetype of Demeter. She had been born and raised in England, and so spoke British English rather than US English. And when she spoke to audiences it may have been literally from a pulpit—if the event were being held in a church. She had gotten a master's degree from Graduate Theological Union in Berkeley and had come to the United States via Zurich where she had studied and absorbed Jungian psychology.

She carried her six-foot height gracefully and lived in a little house that had a fairy-tale quality. She became an issue in my marriage when I increasingly spent time and found depth in myself with her, as described by Ntozake Shange in *for colored girls who have considered suicide/when the rainbow is enuf*: "I found god in myself and I loved her fiercely." Anthea was not the reason for leaving; a strong individuation instinct propelled me out of the marriage. She had her own internal psychological conflicts, medical problems, and dramas. We lost contact for a number of years, a combination of going separate ways and me not wanting to be drawn back.

The day before she died, we had planned to meet. I was at a nearby conference, she was going to be free at a time that looked fine for us both—when this didn't work after all, we had a long, good catch-up phone conversation instead. Later, I learned that she had died that same night. She had gotten up during that night, then fell to the floor, dead. Anthea had feared dying alone—on the streets as a bag lady, from which she had been spared. I don't know if she had a sense of completion, of doing what she had come for, and if this was a good time to cross over, which she did while still in her fifties. I intuitively feel that this last conversation could have been a completion she needed. I know it left me at peace for her and about her.

I have thought about John O'Donohue's description of *anam cara*—soul friend—and quote the following from his book *Anam Cara: A Book of Celtic Wisdom* that is within the scope of my understanding.

> In the Celtic tradition, there is a beautiful understanding of love and friendship. . . the idea of soul-love; the old Gaelic term for this is *anam cara*, *Anam* is the Gaelic word for soul and *cara* is the word for friend. So *anam cara* in the Celtic word world was the "soul friend." . . . With the *anam cara* you could share your innermost self, your mind and your heart. This friendship was an act of recognition and belonging. . . . Where you are understood, you are at home. Understanding nourishes belonging. When you really feel understood, you feel free to release yourself into the trust and shelter of the other person's soul.. . . Real intimacy is a sacred experience . . . Real intimacy is of the soul, and the soul is reserved.

Each person in my liminal circle "on the other side," is someone with whom I felt a soul connection; they are *anam cara* friends and close to my heart family members still, though not here on earth anymore. One might ask what I am doing when I call the circle together. The simplest answer is that I imagine and remember them, and feel the connection which still remains in my heart. There is more to it if what I am doing is standing on this side of the threshold between this world and the other side, and if I am in a circle with their spirit and presence. And that this is real.

Presence is real to me. One example: I had a felt-sense that Patricia Demetrios was in the house for a short visit—was here and then not here, just days after she died. I have felt that angels had my back on many occasions and thanked them. Presence is "when two or more are gathered in my name, there shall I be also." Presence is "Yea, though I walk through the valley of the shadow of death, you are with me." Presence is what others sensed when someone who was loved lay dying peacefully. It is what Katherine Collis wrote about her mother June's passing: "What was striking was first, the growing sense of the house being full of presences, the room was filled with a deep quiet and peace." It reminded me of what India Supera told me many years ago when she sat with a dying friend and felt the house fill up with spirit-presence and afterwards was empty—and of the celestial music that she could hear at the same time.

Prayer is another subjective reality. I have often heard that people who are prayed for feel supported by the prayers of others. I think that it is similar to sensing rooms filling with presences, or angels, in the operating room. Invisible energies, some call them angels, are mobilized by prayers, and can be sensed by some people.

An I-Thou connection is yet another subjective reality that is invisible and felt. We know when we are treated, however politely, as an "It," versus when we are received as a "Thou." When we are most vulnerable, we know.

What if invisible support is readily available, but must be invited? When I imagine my liminal circle, it is an invitation, as are prayers, meditations, and rituals. I think they go out to angelic beings that may be as small as photons, as recognizable to us as Andy would be to me, or may be beyond our imagination. Might help come from them only when asked because human beings otherwise would not have the free will of choice and agency? I wonder if our invitations-prayers are then like pebbles thrown into a still pond, which create concentric rings that ripple out to responsive angels.

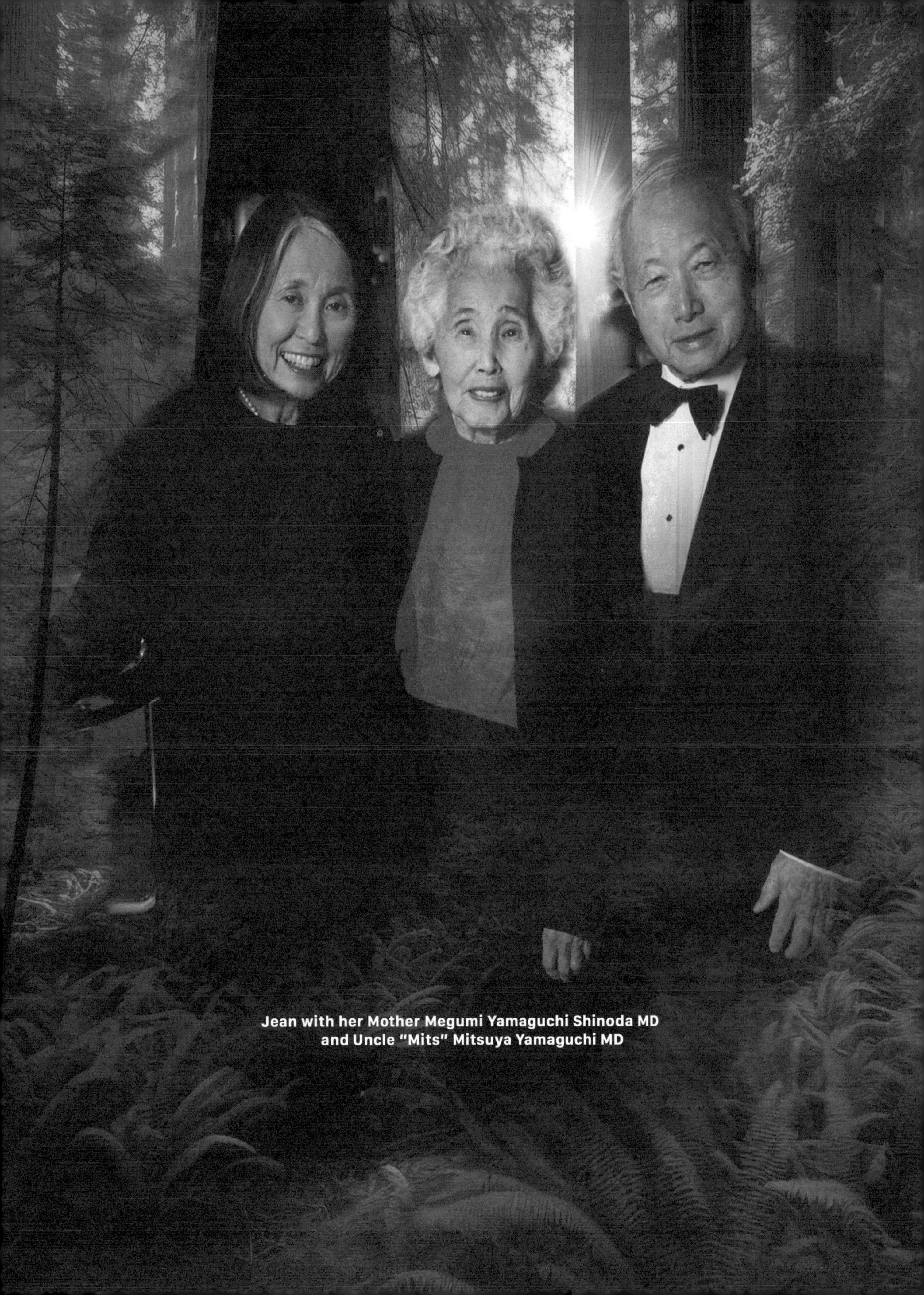

Jean with her Mother Megumi Yamaguchi Shinoda MD
and Uncle "Mits" Mitsuya Yamaguchi MD

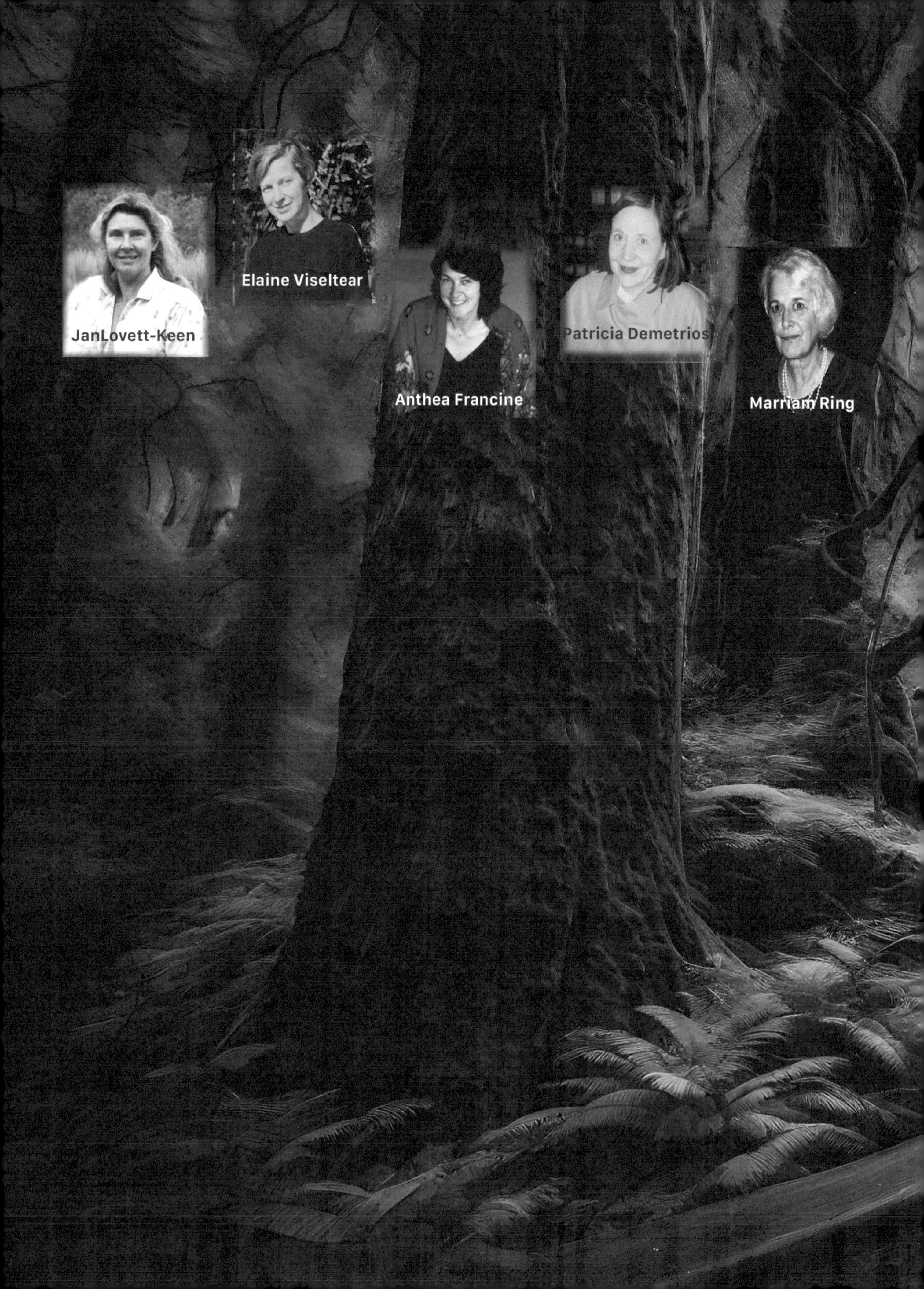

Elaine Viseltear
JanLovett-Keen
Patricia Demetrios
Anthea Francine
Marriam Ring

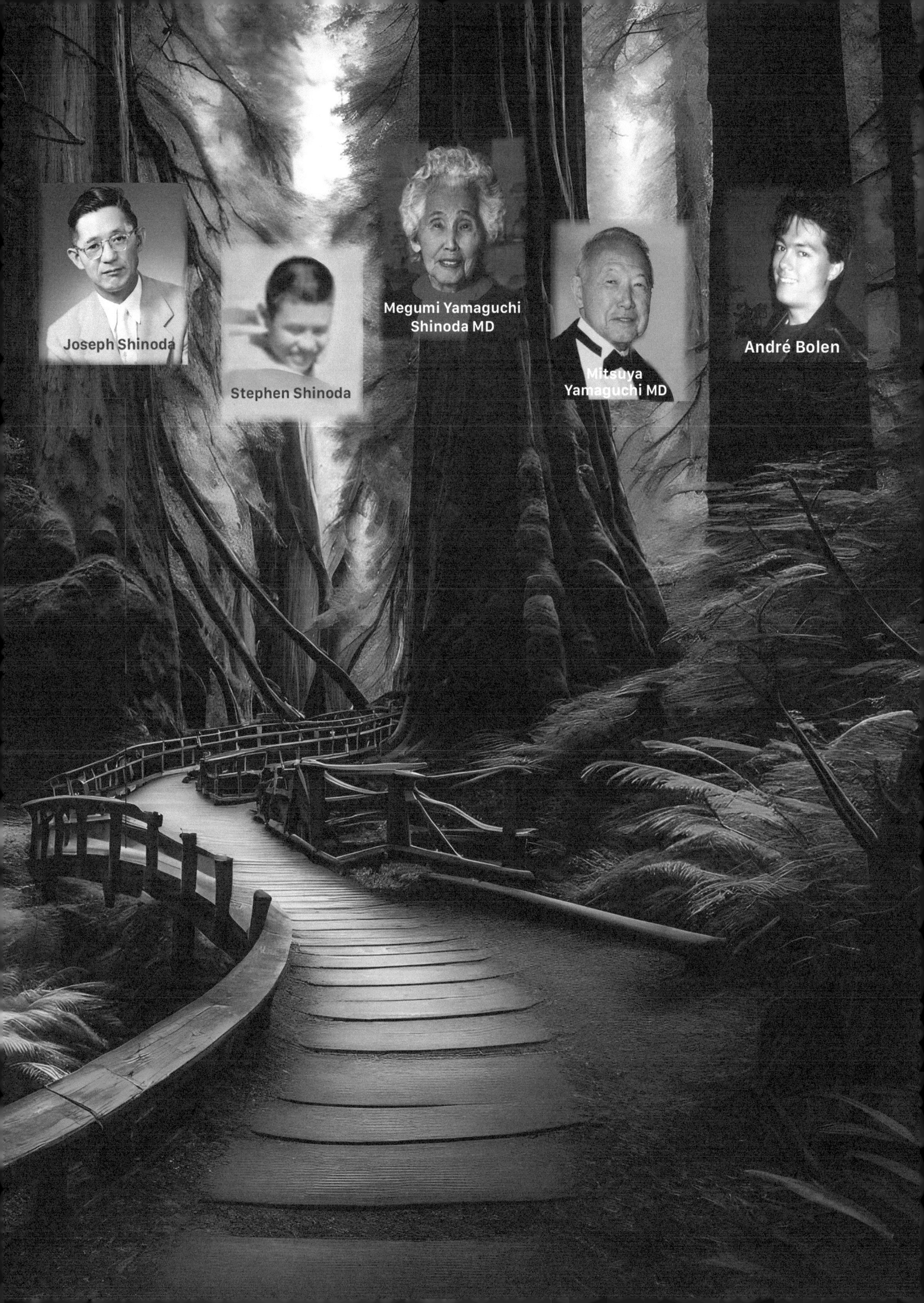
Joseph Shinoda
Stephen Shinoda
Megumi Yamaguchi
Shinoda MD
Mitsuya
Yamaguchi MD
André Bolen

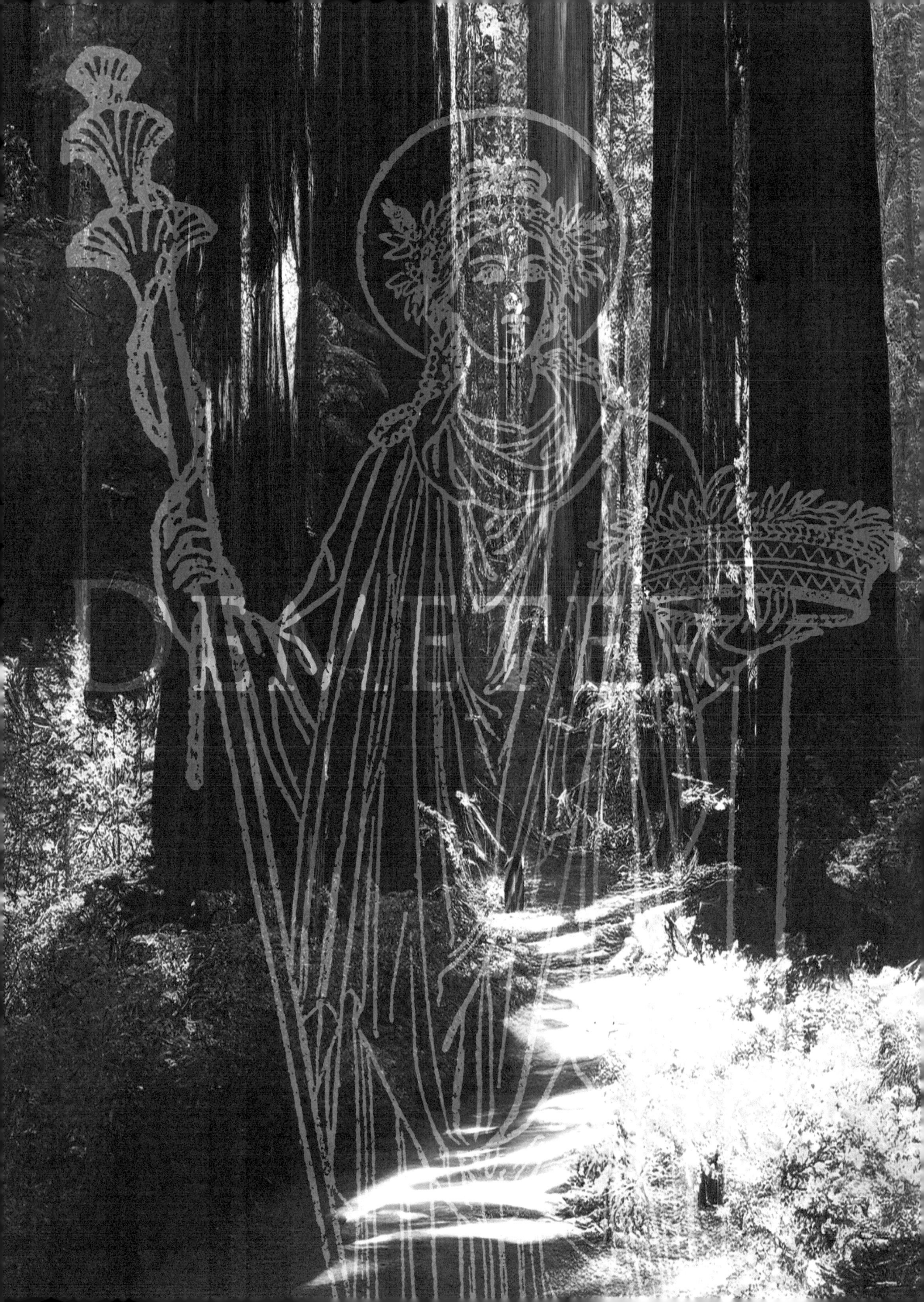
DEMETER

Chapter 29
Author-Activist – Millionth Circle

Once *The Millionth Circle: How to Change Ourselves and The World* was published in 1999, it was as if it had a life of its own and pulled me with it. The book was taken to the Parliament of World Religions in Cape Town, South Africa, where it became the seed idea that inspired the formation of The Millionth Circle Initiative and circle advocacy at the United Nations. It was what brought me to the UN, where I became a major advocate for a UN Fifth World Conference on Women (5WCW) for the next decade and a half, until I became convinced that it still would happen through efforts "on the ground" in India and not through the United Nations with the influence of the presidency of Donald Trump.

However, with the global pandemic and sheltering in place to avoid infection, circumstances changed—and my sense of possibility increased as I also sensed the increasing numbers of circles being formed, usually through women and with women.

We were now speaking and seeing one another or holding meetings through the visual and auditory gift of the internet. Friends who had gone to schools together or been at conferences or travelled together in the past, often had moved far apart. Now, they could meet online and catch up with one another. When no one person dominates this kind and quality of a gathering, it resembles a circle, not a hierarchy when people share their real lives (which women tend to do naturally and some men do as more and often younger men do). Families also began to meet together regularly in circle, getting to know one another's spouses and children—if each person who wanted to be included did participate, relationship-bonding and mutual support likely happens. Circles with a spiritual center are called together initially in silence by the sound of a bell or musical sound followed by a short silence. In this simple procedure, the heart chakra (heart level at the center of the chest between the breasts) can be felt and a sense of linking with others also occurs. To speak from feeling—from the heart—tells what matters and when support is needed. In a circle with a spiritual or heart center, there is the presence of love. I've felt the value of ending circles with a brief silence, followed by the sound that ends it.

The Millionth Circle

The "millionth circle" is a metaphoric number. It is the title of a slender book that I was inspired to write. It is related to the formation the number of women's circles that one day would reach critical mass and become the tipping point. Its antecedents were what I had learned from two social movements. First, the women's movement, which had grown out of consciousness-raising groups, brought us a new vocabulary (sexism, feminism, patriarchy) and values (gender equality, sisterhood). That, in turn, affected politics and American culture in the late 1960s and made the 1970s the decade of women. And second, the grassroots anti-nuclear proliferation movement that had drawn upon theoretical biology (Sheldrake), and applies to changes in the archetypal layer of the collective unconscious (Jung). My own experience of women's circles had shown me that circles with a sacred center can be a transformative vessel for personal change when they support the women in them to believe what they know to be true (their feelings and perceptions), and to act with courage and wisdom. What then can be intuitively grasped is that each circle also contributes to changing the world—through morphic fields and resonance—which I see happening as it becomes easier and easier to form circles and more and more of them are forming. In *The Millionth Circle,* I wrote:

> Start with women's circles
> each one is like a pebble thrown in a pond.
> The effect on women in them,
> and the effect women in them have,
> send out concentric rings of influence.
> There is no "always was, always will be"
> in human affairs.
> Something like a teeter-totter effect happens
> at certain points in time.
> and history changes.

The teeter-totter effect is how I explain "*enantiodromia*," a Greek word and a principle introduced by C. G. Jung in *Psychological Types* as "the emergence of the unconscious opposite in the course of time." It is the tendency seen in natural cycles of things to change into their opposites, which he saw in the philosophy of Heraclitus.

The UN became the major site for my activism after I went there with conveners of the Millionth Circle in 2002 and heard first-hand about what was happening to girls and women from women who represented NGOs (non-governmental organizations) who spoke at the parallel NGO events when the UN Commission on the Status of Women meets. I was appalled by what I was learning and inspired by the stories and the leadership of women who had themselves suffered from having been collateral damage during conflicts, or were trafficked, or endured deprivations based on gender (such as lack of food), or suffered female genital mutilation (FMG), or were forced into childhood marriage under patriarchy. It was because I went to the UN and the UN affected me, raised my consciousness, and made me want to share what I was learning that I wrote *Urgent Message from Mother: Gather the Women, Save the World* (2005). It was a message to her daughters from Mother Earth, Mother Goddess, Mother archetype. It was also about the invisible and visible power of women's circles and had questions that women in circles could use to deepen connections with each other.

Synchronicity and Origins of *The Millionth Circle*

I came to be at the UN through a series of events or synchronicities that led to writing *The Millionth Circle* and then for its immediate acceptance for publication. I had been invited to attend The State of the World Forum in San Francisco as a guest of an organization that I had known as "Beyond War." They had changed their name and focus with the signing of the nuclear non-proliferation treaty between the United States and Russia. I had been a speaker at their events and now was attending this conference as a participant. I spent the morning in Grace Cathedral's main sanctuary that had been transformed: there was music from the rainforest with its sounds of birds, images of the forest were projected onto the walls and columns, the height and architecture of a gothic cathedral, and dimness within it, all contributed to the feeling of being in the forest. I was in my own cocoon, my heart and mind in an altered state of receptivity—in timelessness. Then the program began: in each of the four directions, there was a shaman who, with one exception (the one from Hawaii) stood with a translator. Each spoke or prayed or drummed in their native tongue, and became for me, the indigenous human inhabitants of the rainforest. The forests make life possible for us on Earth; they are the lungs of the planet. Trees take in carbon dioxide and give out oxygen while we breathe in oxygen and breathe out carbon dioxide. We have a reciprocal relationship with trees, but as the human population grows and the forests are cut down, life on the planet as we know it is threatened.

"The Hundredth Monkey" was a major concept that sustained the anti-nuclear activists. It was an allegory told as if it were scientific observation about how a species can learn something new, and that when critical mass is reached, it becomes a tipping point for members of the species (in this case, monkeys) after which, the species does this new thing as if instinctual. The non-nuclear proliferation movement had been a grassroots one. Individuals opened centers, participated in citizen diplomacy, and raised awareness in schools and neighborhoods. One that I knew was Vivianne Verdon-Roe. She had been a school teacher in the Midwest who became an activist after she saw the film *The Last Epidemic*, which showed what would happen if one of the superpowers instigated a nuclear war and the other country retaliated. The result would be "nuclear winter," as the debris from all the destruction created a barrier through which sunlight would no longer reach the earth. Vivianne moved to Berkeley, California, opened a storefront anti-nuclear center, and learned about documentary filmmaking. She created *Women for America, for the World* which was a powerful statement that used newsreel and other footage and interviews with women (of which I was one) that she filmed in her living room. Her film was nominated for an Oscar and won. Between the nomination and the Academy Award, she and her partner had acquired a puppy which they named "Oscar." I was amused to learn that they would call him saying, "Come here, Oscar!" They were intentionally invoking the award.

When the rainforest event at Grace Cathedral ended, we all left to walk from the cathedral to the hotel where lunch would be served. When we got to the hotel lobby, we were joined by others attending other events. It was a crush; we were jammed together, moving slowly to where the lunch was held. The crowd was dense, had high energy, and many conversations were going on—literally over my head (I'm five feet tall). I'd hear snatches of conversation, but I was not paying attention until there was an excited conversation about getting "a million signatures!" My mind went from "hundredth monkey" to "millionth circle"—BINGO! That which I had thought, felt, and experienced as I was sitting in the cathedral came together. It was like what happens in a chemistry flask as various salts are added and dissolve into the solution; nothing appears to be happening, until one last addition causes a whole structure to precipitate out. In this case, ideas came together and formed a book.

I went home, opened my computer and wrote the beginning pages, the premise of *The Millionth Circle*: "How to Change the World." Then came insight and serendipity, as I wrote about what I knew of women's circles, how circles change the women in them, support them to find their voice, gain courage, and on adding a sacred or spiritual center gain invisible support through prayer or meditation as part of the circle experience. I realized I needed to provide "how to" information, which I had never done before. How to form a circle: the who, what, where and how basics, including when and how circles get into trouble. This is where serendipity came in, a happy accident in which I had intended to write a usual paragraph, but had the cursor centered, so that the next sentences came out looking like verse. Verse also takes up more space as white space expands as in poetry. Even better, I found that the result was condensed information.

When I finished writing, it didn't resemble any proper book manuscript. It would be enough to put into a fat brochure. I thought of Conari Press, because they seemed to specialize in small, wise books. I had the phone number of the editor because I had recently contributed to *The Fabric of the Future,* an impressive (and very thick) anthology of articles by fifty women: "Visionaries who Illuminate a Path to Tomorrow." I dialed M. J. Ryan, who answered at the first ring (never happened again), talked very briefly: "I have written a sort of a book—calling you because it would make a small book and Conari publishes this size books. I may have said a little more when M. J. asked: "What is it about?" I said, "It is about women's circles." Whereupon, she said, "Send it right over. We are working on our Fall Catalog right now, we have one blank page, and we have been actively looking for a book on women's circles."

This little book found her way into the bigger world. I received a call from Peggy Sebera to ask about using the name "The Millionth Circle" and inviting me to come to the initial organizing meeting which would be held in Petaluma, California, just up the highway from my home, in March 2001. Among those who came were the founders or executive directors of UN NGOs: Avon Mattison of Pathways To Peace, Elly Pradervand of Women's World Summit Foundation, Ann Smith of Global Education Associates, as well as women from San Francisco Bay Area nonprofits, and members of the women's circle to which Peggy belonged who hosted the gathering, with the support of Elinore Detiger (whose invitation had brought me to sacred sites in Europe). It was an auspicious beginning. I was present for only the initial evening, since my primary concern was for my son Andy, who was now out of the hospital and had come home. I attended the second organizing meeting in October 2001 which led to major decisions and personal commitments about the formation and focus of the Millionth Circle Initiative. It was held at the Mother Tree Retreat Center.

In my walks in Muir Woods and at Old Mill Park in the town of Mill Valley, I noticed how redwood trees form circles. In Old Mill Park, unlike Muir Woods with over a million visitors, annually, it's still possible to stand in the center of such a ring of towering trees. When I do, I know that there once was a "mother tree" where this sacred-feeling space is now. When a redwood is felled or badly burned, a ring of new trees sprouts from burls around the base of the trunk or from the roots of the mother tree, or from fallen branches that take root, or from its seeds. When they form a circle, they are called "daughter trees." The multiple ways redwood trees grow resembles how women's circles proliferate by inspiring new circles to form from the seed idea, or how others are formed by women who have been in circles that ended, or on moving somewhere new, formed new circles.

Standing in a ring of trees, I thought about how human beings once saw divinity as Great Mother, and how her center of worship in Canaan was in sacred groves or rings of trees on mountains which were cut down when the Israelites came up from Egypt. The "the land of milk and honey" became subdued, goddess worship was called an abomination and obliterated, and women were no longer spiritual leaders or priestesses. History repeated itself in medieval Christian Europe, when women healers and midwives were burnt at the stake as witches. I think of how the seeds of redwoods are so tiny (it takes about 120,000 coast redwood seeds, each three to four millimeters, to make a pound) and yet, when conditions are right, a seed or a burl can grow into a redwood tree, which are the tallest trees on Earth and can be many hundreds of years old. How long I wonder, can such seeds and burls lie dormant? How long will it take for humankind to remember feminine divinity and for women to realize soul and sacredness exists in them, not just in the patriarchs and alpha males that claim father-rights because they (not women) are made in the image of God and lay claim to dominion over everything they see and name.

My morning walks in Muir Woods often also takes me past the UN Memorial in Cathedral Grove. On May 19, 1945, delegates meeting in San Francisco to create the United Nations came to

Muir Woods to honor the memory of President Franklin Delano Roosevelt. FDR had died twelve days before 268 delegates representing 46 nations had convened. The UN Charter was signed on June 26, 1945 in San Francisco. Nations that signed committed to maintaining international peace and security, developing friendly relations among nations, and promoting social progress, better living standards and human rights. I make a point of stopping there before I take off for the UN.

I had not been to the UN before 2002, except once as a visitor. I had learned about the UN in high school, when I took part in the Model UN as a presiding officer of the mock General Assembly held in the council chambers of the Los Angeles City Hall. I had missed going to the Fourth UN World Conference on Women held in Beijing in 1995, where Hillary Clinton had said "Women's rights are human rights, human rights are women's rights!" After I had heard women leaders speak about Beijing and how the experience changed their lives and inspired them to do what they do now, I looked forward to going to the Fifth World Conference on Women (5WCW). I mistakenly and ignorantly assumed that this would be held in 2005, until I learned differently: not only were there no plans for 5WCW in 2005, I was told that there are no plans for any in the future, that "the era of women's conferences was over." This was when I became an advocate for 5WCW as were the Millionth Circle conveners, several of whom had been at the Beijing conference, and all of whom recognized how important it would be for women from all over the world to learn about and form circles of their own to share what they feel and know. Women in circles share information, support and encourage each other. In doing so, they find their voice. In sufficient numbers, women talking, supporting each other, have brought about changes in the world. This is how the women's movement of the late 1960s through most of the 1970s began—with women talking, learning, and becoming activists through participating in consciousness-raising groups.

The Millionth Circle conveners form the mother circle of the Millionth Circle, (there are over twenty of us). We've met together once a month on a conference call since 2001, rotating who convenes each time. In between, there are group emails that keep us informed about each other, including personal situations in need of prayer, as well as suggestions and recommendations to keep us informed. There is no hierarchy, each of us "checks in," meaning each voice is heard, responding to whatever the convener has introduced as the theme, which can come as a question or a poem, or something else. Once a year we usually have had a "Deepening Gathering," which is our circle retreat. Those who wanted to and could formed a Millionth Circle contingent at Parliaments of the World Religions, Gather the Women Conferences, the Omega Institute, and most consistently at the UN CSW, where we have distributed round UN-blue 5WCW buttons, sponsored panels, and held events. Carol Hansen Grey, one of the founders of Gather the Women, created the Millionth Circle website and later the 5WCW & 5WWC websites.

The Millionth Circle's emphasis is on circles with a spiritual center which invites the invisible world of spirit or soul to be in the center of the circle and in the center of the psyche of each person in the circle. Through meditative silence or silent prayer, wisdom and courage grows. Circles foster both the ability to voice what matters and say out loud what is in the heart and mind, and an equally important ability, to listen with compassion. Women's circles evoke a sense of sisterhood, and also a feeling of being in a maternal space. There is a deep sense of being connected to one another, at an archetypal level. This is rather like redwood trees which do not have a central root that anchors them in the soil, but link roots together to form a broad matrix of roots that are in communication with each other as well as anchoring the trees.

In Jungian terms, the circle with a center is a symbol of the Self, the source of meaning that has the many names of divinity: God, Goddess, Tao, Holy One, all that is, Sacred Mother, the universe, and many individual names of divinity. For the Tibetans, sacred paintings are in the shape of a mandala—geometrically, it's a circle in the center of a square. Jung described the mandala as a geometric symbol of the Self. When we are in a circle, it's like each of us is on the rim of an invisible wheel, each connected like a spoke to the center, in touch through our hearts both to the center and to each other. Each person has an equal responsibility to be present and to be true to herself. In a circle, there is a level in which symbol and people come together.

After a decade of advocacy for 5WCW, with the support of many NGOs, it seemed on the verge of happening. On March 8, 2012, International Women's Day, the President of the UN General Assembly, H.E. Mr. Nassir Abdulaziz Al-Nasser and the Secretary-General of the UN H.E. Mr. Ban Ki-moon jointly proposed the convening of a United Nations Fifth World Conference on Women in 2015, twenty years after the last women's summit in Beijing. In their joint statement, they said: "Given that women compose the half of humanity and the inherent importance and relevance of women issues for the global progress, it is high time that such a world conference is convened, more so as the world is going through enormous changes in all fronts having both positive and other implications for women."

The President of the General Assembly and the Secretary-General hoped that the international community in general would welcome this joint initiative. They also hoped that the Member-States who have the final authority to convene the proposed conference would take the necessary step in that regard during the on-going sixty-sixth session of the General Assembly. Their hopes and the hopes of all of us who had been advocating for 5WCW were not fulfilled. A resolution did not even reach the floor. There were many nation-states that did support it, but when the United States and several strong European Union members came out against the proposal, there was no chance for a resolution to pass. Someday I would like to learn from Susan Rice, then the American UN ambassador, why the Obama administration opposed it.

Over the years of advocacy for 5WCW, there have been a great many twists and turns as prominent individuals and organizations and representatives of their countries supported it, as well as the strong grassroots support that was everywhere. In 2012, the goal was in sight, and then—disappointment! It reminded me of walking the Chartres Labyrinth, and how it often seems that the center is very close, and then there is a U-turn, and the path swings away. While each time this happens, the center (or goal) seems more distant than before—but appearances are deceiving, because if you continue on the path, each step does bring you closer. There are 28 U-turns in the Chartres Labyrinth.

The set-back or U-turn in 2012 did not change my mind about the need for 5WCW but it and the change in administrations in the United States in 2016 has shifted where I put my efforts. I keep sensing that forming circles has become easier and easier to do—which is how morphic fields work, and how geometric progression also does: the more there are, the easier and faster more and more will form.

Women's March: We Rise!

I went to the Women's March on Washington on January 21, 2017, the day after the Trump inauguration. A half a million people were there. It was the center of the largest protest in American history, one that spread to 673 cities in 92 countries, and estimated 5,600,000 marchers in all. The symbol of the marches, a sea of them, seen all over the world was the hand knitted pink pussy hats (bright pink caps with upright ears). Most of the women I talked to were participating in their very first march. Like me, they felt call to the March, with some stress and anxiety at not knowing how it would turn out and online advice on what to do if it turned into a riot. The reality was anything but this. There was togetherness and human warmth, humor and kindness. There were grandmothers, mothers, granddaughters and grandsons, young parents with young children, fathers carrying babies, high school and college friends, white haired older women, a diversity of ages and races—though predominately women and lots and lots of hand-lettered signs. Kindness and consideration were the norms. It was, to quote a man I overheard, "the nicest mob scene I've ever been in." There was hardly room to move, impossible to hear the speakers and no room to march, with so many of us packed into the Washington Mall, and yet, it was wonderful to be there.

Time to think about the meaning of this experience began in Patricia Smith's living room that evening, where women who had come to the march from past Feathered Pipe retreats and made it back gathered. It felt good to be with this quietly elated and very tired circle, and to hear each woman speak. We were from Montana, New Mexico, Alaska, California, DC, and responses were similar to mine: glad to have come and needing time to process. After each had spoken, we were silent together. The last thing we did was stand up, hold hands, and as I sometimes do in my women's retreats, I led a chant. "We Rise! We Rise! We Rise," we chant, our hands rising up together, and then after the last "We Rise!" everyone naturally shakes and waves her hands above her head, and amidst much laughter, the circle is over. I go back to this now, because "We Rise!" was the meaning—the hope that I felt in the march.

Millions of women all over the world had responded on very short notice to demonstrate peacefully on January 21, 2017. Each came as women do, usually with friends. I believe most hadn't demonstrated before and were doing so because it felt right to do, because they—like me, were moved to act by the Artemis archetype in them—which felt like a call.

At this time in human and planetary history, when evolution or destruction is in the balance, lonely men with their one-sided left-brain dominance—and use of power over others because they are afraid to be vulnerable— cannot make wise and compassionate decisions for us all. I think that we are in a race toward what could be the end of us, or the beginning of a new era. It's a race between the hierarchal model we have that is based on power, fear and scarcity, and an as yet not created new one that may be forming.

The Women's March on Washington could be one early and hopeful sign, as are the growing number of grassroots activists who are socially conscious, spiritual people, feminist women and men, environmentalists—people anywhere who try to make a positive difference wherever they are, whatever their age, whatever they are doing. If each person's actions and beliefs contributes to changes and shifts in the morphic field of our species, and affects patterns (archetypes) in the collective unconscious and collective consciousness, evolution of human consciousness naturally would follow.

Then came the #MeToo movement, which generated twelve million posts and comments on Facebook in a twenty-four hour period. Women went from marching to running for office in the 2018 midterm elections: 472 women entered the race for a House seat, fifty-seven filed for the Senate, and of the thirty-six gubernatorial races in 2018, thirty-five had women candidates. When votes were counted, the 116th United States Congress had 106 women of 441 members comprising twenty-four percent of the House of Representatives, and the Senate had twenty-five women of 100, or twenty-five percent. Nine women were elected governors. Every woman who chooses to march, speak out, or run, leads other women by her example. This is another Year of the Woman, harkening back to 1974 when more women ran for and were elected. It may precede another Decade of the Woman, which was said of the 1970s, or if it becomes the Century of the Woman, then real change could result and climate disaster to the planet could be averted.

I was energized by being at the Women's March on Washington. Everyone who came was "voting with their feet" to support women on the day after the Trump inauguration. The marches and the events that followed mobilized a sense of sisterhood with women and support from men who were friends, sons, partners, and husbands, men who are in egalitarian relationships with women—which is to say that we all were feminists, in that we all believed in the equality of the sexes. For this to be so, also means that Artemis is a strong archetype in all who came. Artemis was the Greek goddess of the Hunt and Moon, first-born twin to Apollo, who explored the wilderness with her chosen nymph-divinities (modelling sisterhood). She was protective of the young of all species and was the only Olympian to come to the aid of her mother. Archetypes are innate patterns of being and behaving, their symbols tell something of their attributes. Artemis is one of many archetypes in women, and a positive image in men who are attracted to independent, competitive women. I have much more to say about Artemis in *Goddesses in Everywoman* and the book *Artemis: The Indomitable Spirit in Everywoman.*

Misogyny and autocratic patriarchy on one hand, the marches and spirit of women rising on the other: I was feeling the tension between both when I went to New Delhi, India for the Women Economic Forum (2018) organized by Dr. Harbeen Arora and her husband Vinay Rai. There I also went to an Apne App Worldwide site and saw what they were accomplishing, met with the executive directors of several other NGOS concerned with women and girls, and met the head of UN Women in India. India has the largest number of NGOs of any country in the world and its women have had huge and effective demonstrations. In 2019, according to government estimates, between three and a half and five million women lined up on National Highway 66, a long stretch of road that runs along the country's western coast. They formed a "women's wall" that stretched out 385 miles as a continuous chain to express the need for gender equality and protest a religious ban that prevented women of menstruating age from entering a sacred Hindu temple even after the Supreme Court ruled in favor of their entry.

I returned from India in 2018 with optimism that the Fifth United Nations World Conference on Women would happen in 2022, and that such a conference would have been fertile ground to seed circles with a sacred center, tapping into the sister archetype of Artemis, making it easier and easier for women to form circles, to find their voice and bring about change in relationships, family, organizations, corporations, and governments. Culture changes when the tipping point is reached and a shift in attitude and organizations, even governments occurs. Quietly.

This is the vision I had of the "Millionth Circle," a metaphor that would end the pattern of male hierarchy and dominance, with power over women and racial superiority. Then Donald J. Trump became president of the United States and the United Nations lost prestige and financial support from governments. While it became obvious that there would not be a Fifth UN World Conference on Women, there has been a growing movement of engaging and empowering women in politics.

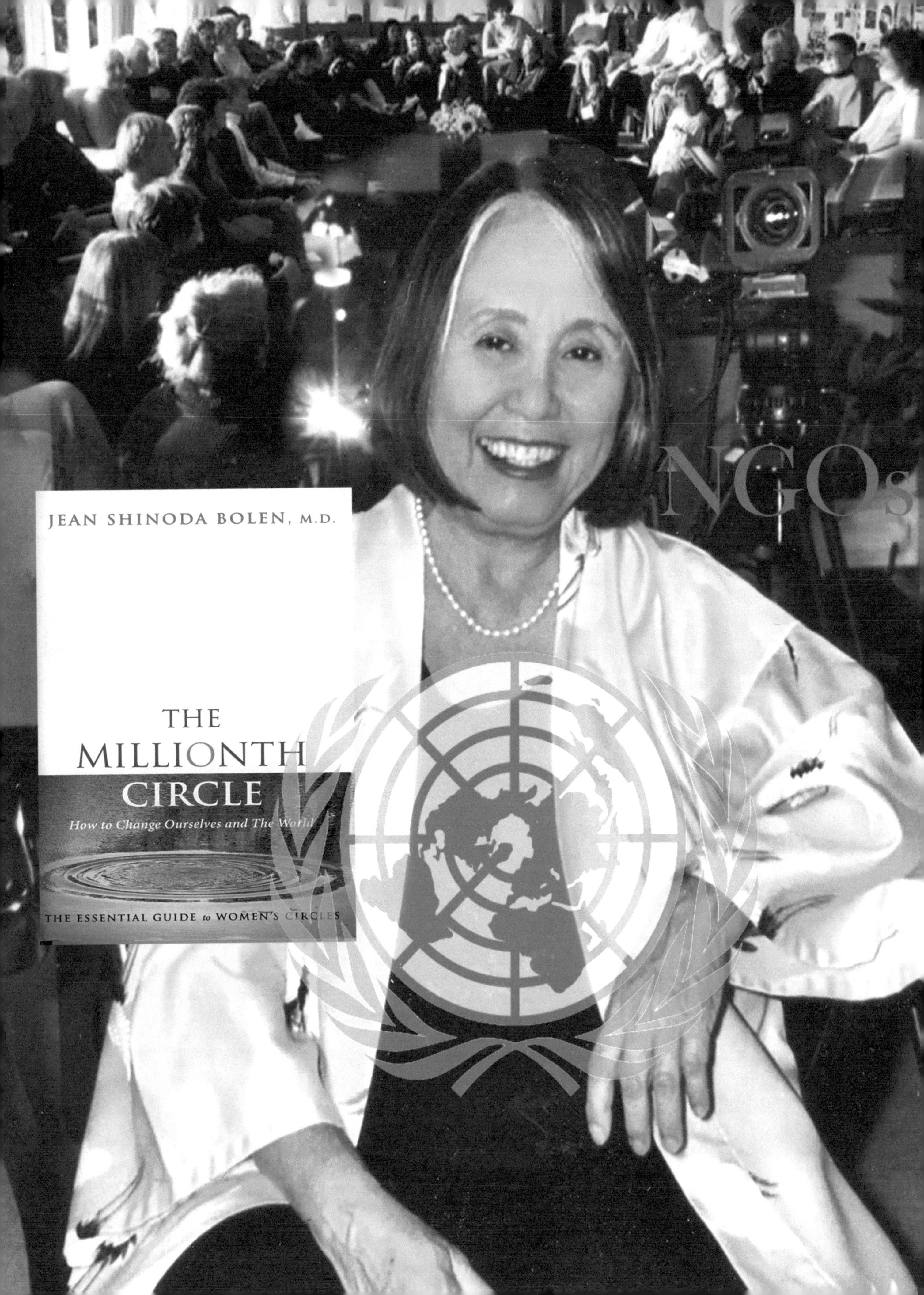
JEAN SHINODA BOLEN, M.D.
THE
MILLIONTH
CIRCLE
How to Change Ourselves and The World
THE ESSENTIAL GUIDE to WOMEN'S CIRCLES
NGOs

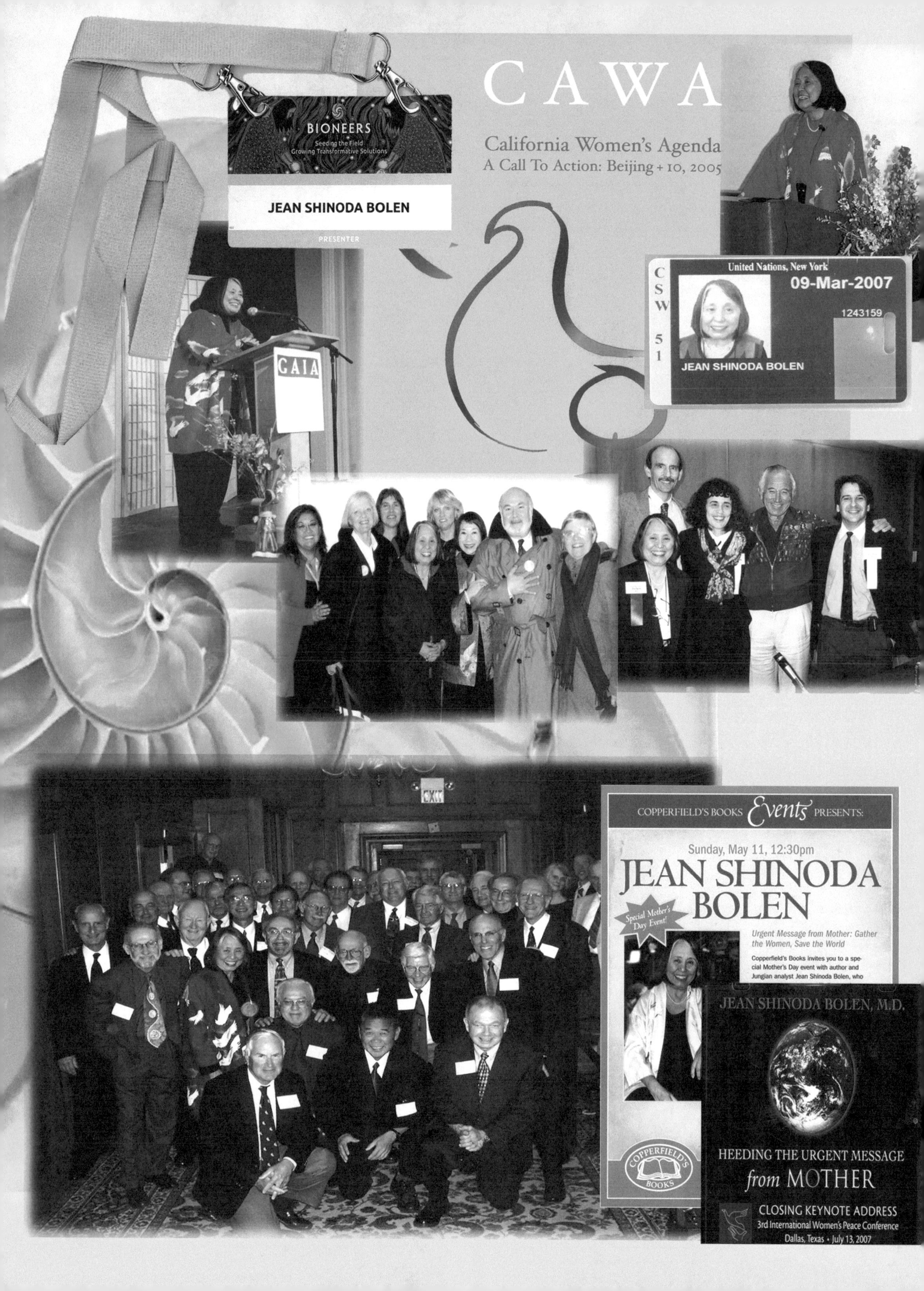

BIONEERS
Seeding the Field
Growing Transformative Solutions
JEAN SHINODA BOLEN
PRESENTER
CAWA
California Women's Agenda
A Call To Action: Beijing + 10, 2005
GAIA
United Nations, New York
09-Mar-2007
CSW 51
1243159
JEAN SHINODA BOLEN
EXIT
COPPERFIELD'S BOOKS Events PRESENTS:
Sunday, May 11, 12:30pm
JEAN SHINODA BOLEN
Special Mother's Day Event!
Urgent Message from Mother: Gather the Women, Save the World
Copperfield's Books invites you to a special Mother's Day event with author and Jungian analyst Jean Shinoda Bolen, who
COPPERFIELD'S BOOKS
JEAN SHINODA BOLEN, M.D.
HEEDING THE URGENT MESSAGE
from MOTHER
CLOSING KEYNOTE ADDRESS
3rd International Women's Peace Conference
Dallas, Texas • July 13, 2007

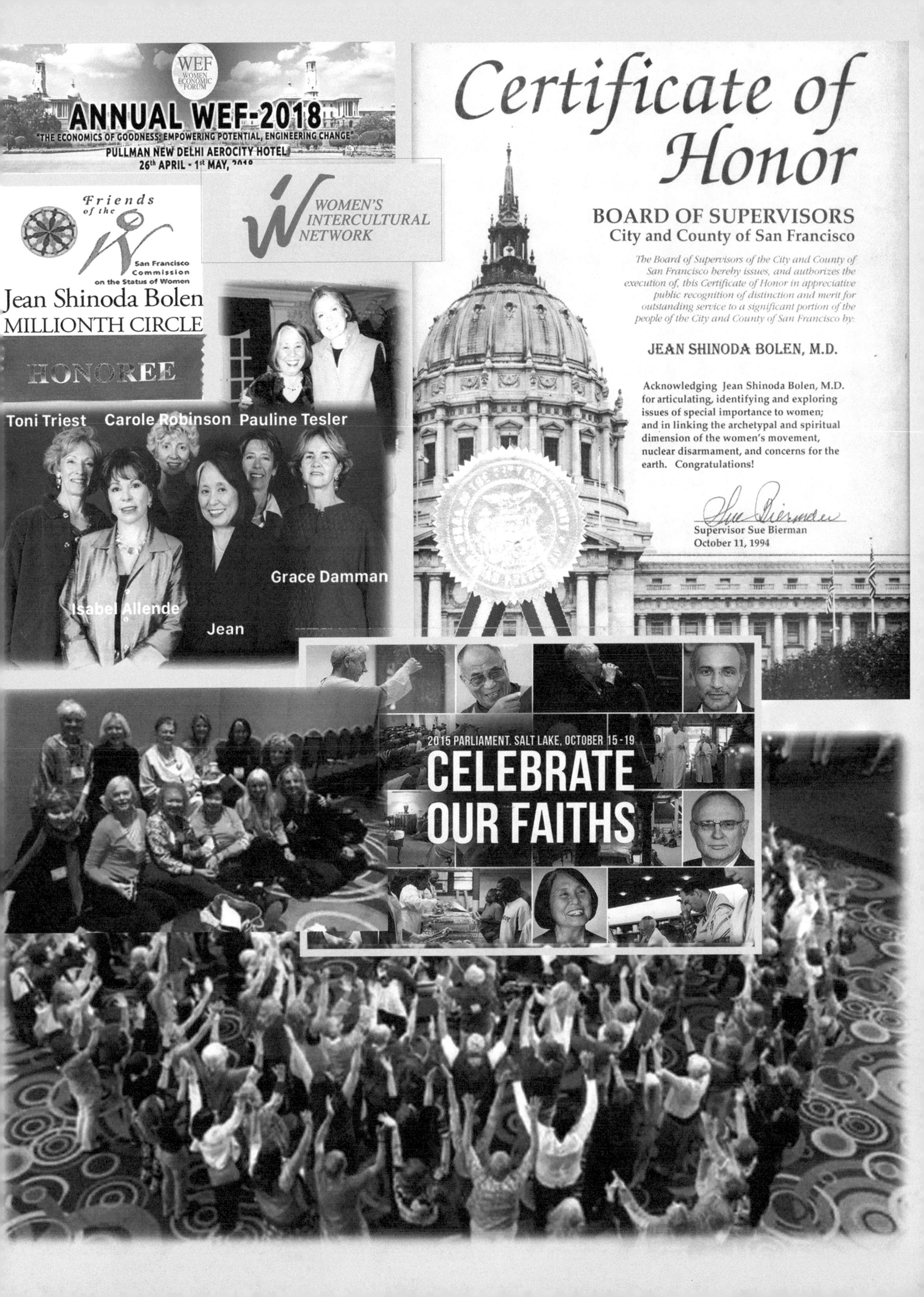
WEF
WOMEN ECONOMIC FORUM
ANNUAL WEF-2018
"THE ECONOMICS OF GOODNESS: EMPOWERING POTENTIAL, ENGINEERING CHANGE"
PULLMAN NEW DELHI AEROCITY HOTEL
26th APRIL - 1st MAY,
Friends of the
San Francisco Commission on the Status of Women
WOMEN'S INTERCULTURAL NETWORK
Jean Shinoda Bolen
MILLIONTH CIRCLE
HONOREE
Toni Triest
Carole Robinson
Pauline Tesler
Grace Damman
Isabel Allende
Jean
Certificate of Honor
BOARD OF SUPERVISORS
City and County of San Francisco
The Board of Supervisors of the City and County of San Francisco hereby issues, and authorizes the execution of, this Certificate of Honor in appreciative public recognition of distinction and merit for outstanding service to a significant portion of the people of the City and County of San Francisco by:
JEAN SHINODA BOLEN, M.D.
Acknowledging Jean Shinoda Bolen, M.D. for articulating, identifying and exploring issues of special importance to women; and in linking the archetypal and spiritual dimension of the women's movement, nuclear disarmament, and concerns for the earth. Congratulations!
Supervisor Sue Bierman
October 11, 1994
2015 PARLIAMENT. SALT LAKE, OCTOBER 15-19
CELEBRATE OUR FAITHS

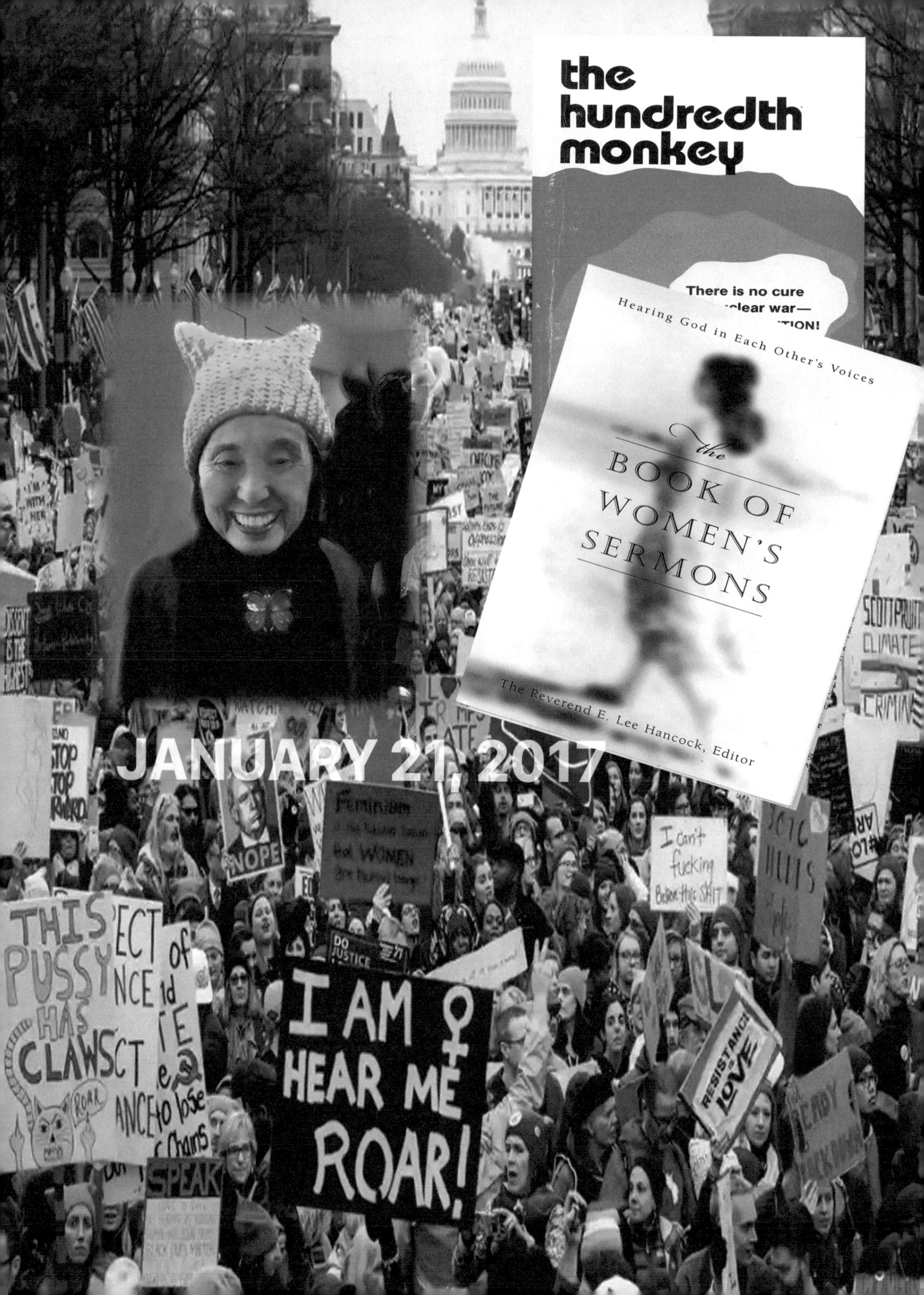
the hundredth monkey
There is no cure
Hearing God in Each Other's Voices
the BOOK OF WOMEN'S SERMONS
The Reverend E. Lee Hancock, Editor
JANUARY 21, 2017
NOPE
Feminism
WOMEN
I can't fucking Believe this SHIT
CLIMATE
THIS PUSSY HAS CLAWS
ROAR
DO JUSTICE
I AM ♀ HEAR ME ROAR!
RESISTANCE LOVE
SPEAK

Chapter 30

Birthing Books - Breast Cancer

When I wrote the slender book *Moving Toward the Millionth Circle,* I wanted the women working with NGOs who were doing soul work in the trenches of poverty, conflicts, and natural disasters to see themselves as I did without speaking in "Jungian." So instead of individuation or personal myth, I described what I saw them doing as having taken on an "assignment" that fulfilled three requirements that only they could answer: *Is it meaningful?* (Is it deeply felt personal work?) *Will it be fun?* (This is hard to say when the work is hard and people they care for are suffering, but there often is satisfaction, even joy, when something they are doing truly helps another; it also often turns out to be fun when done by hard physical or creative work and the doer is happy with the outcome.) Finally, *Is it motivated by love?* (Only the person knows.)

I told a story of the medieval stonecutters in which three stonecutters are asked, "What are you doing?" Each was chipping the edges of a stone to fit snugly into a wall. The answers went from "It's obvious—you can see what I am doing," or "I'm helping build a wall," or "I am doing my part to build a cathedral that will endure for a thousand years." As I mused on this, it occurred to me that many individuals who are physicians, psychiatrists, or therapists are like the first two competent stonecutters. They help patients adjust—or fit in. Sometimes, a person in therapy or a therapist has a sense of having had many lifetimes and feeling that there is a purpose beyond what they are doing now.

I believe that every individual and members of a circle can see or learn that what they do can be or is meaningful and helpful to themselves and to others they influence. While the visionary in them also believes that each of us can be contributing to evolutionary changes, by what we learn and do. The subtitles of all of my activist books envision big picture, big vision intentions: *How to Change Ourselves and The World* (*The Millionth Circle*); *How Trees, Women, and Tree People can Save the Planet* (*Like a Tree*); *Gather the Women, Save the World* (*Urgent Message From Mother*), *Energizing the Global Women's Movement* (*Moving Toward the Millionth Circle*). My hope is that these books help individuals realize that whatever meaningful acts or tasks each of us does can contribute towards our evolution as humans.

Whenever I have been inspired to write a new book, it feels like having been impregnated by an idea for it and once it starts to grow, the life of a book-to-be takes on energy and makes me attentive. This particular book is my fourteenth book and the first one in which I have ever focused on my personal life story. Whenever I become involved in writing a new book, it is a little like being pregnant. It's a creative process, as if a potential "new baby" is taking shape and growing in and through me. "She" doesn't come out of my head, like a full-grown Athena did from Zeus' brow. Intuitive-feeling writing comes through my heart-soul-body, like an inspired impregnation which I have often felt while I was walking in Muir Woods or on Muir Beach. It takes labor and delivery to birth a baby or a book—with the help of midwives (my editors have been women). Every new book is like a newborn baby who will need help taking her first steps into the world (publisher, publicists, endorsements and synchronicity make it possible).

Once out in the world, when a book of mine is meaningful to a reader who tells me how much it meant or how validating and encouraging, or what it led to, it is similar to hearing something wonderful about one's own child. It makes a mother's heart (and many a father's as well) proud in a similar way that a creative author or artist or inspired hardworking person feels when his or her work has touched feelings and evoked an emotional and often an intellectual response as well.

Birthing New Life: A New Baby Creates a New Mother

When my daughter Melody was born, I was a proud mom, awed that such a beautiful baby could come out of me! Through her birth, I participated in the miracle of new life and it's a girl! Through nursing her especially during the night, I felt as if as one with her. In some invisible way, we deeply affirmed each other as mother and daughter as we contemplated or gazed at each other when I held her in my arms. She was a distinct person even as a small baby. Her alertness and interest in what she gazed at, and later in her ability to focus on what she was doing was a strength. She didn't have to exercise her will or become dramatic to get her way—she just defined what she did or didn't do herself, smoothing tension with her astrological Libra nature. She was my first born and a daughter, which I think may likely be different from having a first born who is a son. A daughter comes with girl hormones, surrounded by her aura or feminine soul field. The urge to be one with mom which she experienced in the womb and in infancy pulls toward merger. Then when her archetype is Artemis or Athena (which are independent archetypes), merger may stir an opposing drive to differentiate from mom, to become herself—to individuate. I could see in Melody, and in the newborn nursery and later in pre-school, that babies come with their own energy patterns, personality traits—or archetypes.

Pregnancy, labor, and delivery with Melody was a profound initiation into motherhood and also feminism. I dropped into the archetypal-morphic field and was like every woman throughout time who had ever been in labor and had come through the transition phase. This is when pain is the most intense, and without surgical intervention, she will either birth her baby, or die in childbirth. This is when women in ancient Greece prayed to Artemis for help to deliver the baby or to deliver a swift death, with an unerring arrow.

Girls born at the beginning of the 1970s—the decade of the women's movement—were raised with *Free to Be... You and Me* as text. Such books, the culture of Mill Valley, California and a feminist mother supported Melody to value being a girl—which my mother consciously instilled in me and I honored in the dedication of *Goddesses in Everywoman*: "To my mother, Megumi Yamaguchi Shinoda, MD, who was determined to help me grow up—as she hadn't—feeling that I was fortunate to be a girl, and could do whatever I aspired to as a woman."

What I neglected telling Melody, though I thought it often, was, "What a beautiful child you are" and later, "What a beautiful woman you are," which I thought was obvious to everyone and was mentioned to me. James A. Michener, author of *Hawaii,* wrote about the beauty of the "golden children," whose lineage was a mixture of European and Asian genes. Much later, when writing this book, I mentioned regretting that I hadn't said this to her but assumed she was aware of her attractiveness. Not so. She remembered that when she was in middle and high school, the standard of beauty was Farah Fawcett (tall actress with long blond hair, long legs) whom she did not resemble. Melody and I had rare confrontations. When we did, it was over my exercising authority out of my maternal concern, which she felt insulted her judgment and integrity. I turned out to be a Sky Mother as my mother had been—though with the difference in generations, I was a huggy-expressive mom with Melody and Andy, until each reached adolescence and preferred that I not be demonstrative.

Challenge to Walk My Talk: Breast Cancer

In August 2016, I had a routine mammogram that I assumed would be fine. I had turned eighty in June, and had missed a couple of yearly mammograms. However, it wasn't fine. I was asked to come back which I did in September. On October 5, I had a needle biopsy of the suspicious mass in my right breast, which turned out to be cancer, followed by an appointment the next week with a surgeon, Leah Kelley, MD, and an MRI on October 19. Surgery was scheduled a month later, on November 18, 2016.

In between, I spoke at the Science and Nonduality (SAND) Conference in San Jose and went from there to the Millionth Circle Deepening Gathering at the Presentation Center in Los Gatos, which was about an hour away. Non-duality and the Jungian concept of holding the tension of opposites are two ways of saying the same thing. It seems to me that there doesn't have to be tension—two apparently contradictory ideas can exist together. When they do not compete, the psyche can tolerate paradox and hold them both. Otherwise, there is an either-or tension that often results in suppression of one (by the judgment of the other), which in turn can become a cause of anxiety or depression, or a spiritual problem, but when consciousness expands, both can be held, often in creative tension.

I was surprised by the mammogram and needle biopsy, since this was not a risk I thought I had. My first reaction was "Who, me?" Reality check: "Yes, you!" Dr. Kelley recommended a "lumpectomy" (the cancer is removed with a wide border of normal cells around it) and removal of a few lymph nodes under my arm. While I had an "of course" response to scheduling the lumpectomy, I declined having the sentinel and any other nodes removed, which is usually done. While it would be done at the same time, it is a second surgery and weighing pro and cons, I said no. Nodes are an important line of defense. Cancer cells are recognized and destroyed by immune cells in lymph nodes. Yet when they are found there, it also indicates spread and more aggressive cancer treatment is done.

Melody came up to see me through the surgery. As busy as she is, I can count on her to come through when I need her. Sensible, competent, trustworthy, loving are adjectives which fit her.

The lumpectomy went well. The pathology lab reported that there were margins around the specimen. When I saw my surgeon, she recommended the standard next steps: radiation (to my right breast—in case there were still some cancer cells there), and chemotherapy. Cancer cells are faster growing than normal cells and will die or be more weakened by radiation or chemotherapy because they take up or take in more of what poisons them than normal cells. Dr. Kelley respected my clear decision that I would do neither. Bilateral mammograms were scheduled in six months with follow up mammograms which remained normal in the years that followed.

What I now knew when the pathology report said invasive ductal cancer, it meant that my body's immune system had allowed cancer cells to grow instead of immediately recognizing and removing them. The body is continually making new cells to replace old ones. Different ones have different expiration dates, and some of them are abnormal and if they reproduce, they will turn into cancer. Patrolling through our vascular and lymph systems are immune cells with the job of identifying and taking out the bad ones. (There are different kinds that have different job descriptions, all of which can loosely be called our "white cells" to differentiate them from our "red cells" which are the red blood cells.) Cells age as we do and probably have less vigor and vitality. It seemed that my immune cells had slept on the job. I was surprised to learn that the incidence of breast cancer becomes greater with age—though tends to grow more slowly in the elderly. It was a mistake on my part to think that after eighty, I had a free pass. Then again, Medicare no longer recommends routine mammograms after seventy-four unless the woman has a specific concern.

Cancer was a challenge to walk my talk. I now needed to decide what I would do to be cancer-free. I had written about alternative and integrative, spiritual and mythological ways of healing of body and psyche in *Close to the Bone: Life-Threatening Illness as a Soul Journey.* The first step was letting others know and asking for prayers. Then the right book came (as with the Tao "when the pupil is ready, the teacher will come."). This was *Radical Remission: Surviving Cancer Against All Odds* by Kelly A. Turner, PhD. She based her book on conducting over a hundred direct interviews and analyzing over a thousand written cases. Of the nine factors that had contributed to their survival, one got my attention: "Radically Changing Your Diet." The rest had to do with psychological, social, and spiritual changes which included taking charge of your own health, following intuition, using herbs and supplements, releasing suppressed emotions, increasing positive emotions, embracing social support, deepening spiritual connections, and having strong reasons for living. Most of which I was doing, though I was learning more about supplements. Focusing on targets of my own choosing is so Artemis, and therefore, so me. I took in the information, understood the reasoning, and had the will and discipline to radically change my diet, including eliminating champagne, wine, (seems that cancer cells thrive or take up more alcohol than normal cells do) and other alcoholic drinks and drinking only bottled or filtered water. I was also learning about cancer fighting foods and supplements. Basically, diet change was the only one of the nine factors that I wasn't aware of or already doing.

Influenced by O. Carl Simonton, MD

As I experienced the challenges of my own cancer in 2016, I drew upon the important insight I gained back in 1973 from O. Carl Simonton, MD. He was a radiation oncologist who was a pioneer in the use of visualization in the treatment of cancer.

That cancer can have a major psychological component is one that I have held in my psyche ever since it became a big idea that I took to heart. In comic strips, it is the image of a light bulb turning on over a character's head. In words, it is the "Aha!" moment. This had come to me when I listened to Dr. Simonton describing the connection between beliefs, emotions, and outcome at a North-South Jungian Conference (1973). He told us about some of his patients with cancer who died and had seemingly welcomed cancer as a way out. Some thought they deserved the cancer, such as the man with cancer in his testicles, whose guilt about sex and what he had done, felt this was a justified punishment. Then there were his patients who survived their cancers. One in particular, whose cancer had spread through his body, was a man used to issuing orders—a CEO with a strong will to live—who took to the idea that the mind could direct the body, and visualized the immune cells gobbling up the cancer cells, like the then popular video game Pac-Man. Others who went into remission had reasons to live and did all they could to stay alive longer. (Simonton, *Getting Well Again*, originally published in 1978).

Up until I heard Simonton's talk and had an "Aha!" moment, I had a fatalistic but *not* gloomy philosophy, which went with the thought, "I could be struck down, anytime," or "I could be hit by a truck." I think it came from being the spared sibling, of realizing that "it could have been me," like standing next to my brother and having lightning strike him. Watching the news and seeing hurricanes or tornados or bombs suddenly change everything for some and spare others illustrates this premise. This philosophical mindset helped me appreciate everything that was positive in my life, to have gratitude, to enjoy the moment, because "tomorrow I could die." It leads me, still, to "stay current," to not leave unsaid positive words and feelings that I would have regretted not saying, to not owe people, and to have a living will and an advanced health care directive.

As I listened and took in Simonton's talk in 1973, I made a shift in my own mind. I did not substitute it for my fatalistic philosophy. Instead, I made room for an intuitive feeling, a certainty that even now I feel—that I will be around for a long time. At that time, a young mother with two-and-a-half-year-old daughter and a year-old son, it mattered that I be here for them, and after staying the course that led to becoming a psychiatrist, activist, and soon to be a Jungian analyst, to trust that this was what I was meant to do—and if so, faith that I'd have enough time. This had the effect of now holding two beliefs at the same time. I was experiencing the Jungian concept of "holding the tension of opposites." I now express this myself as "holding the opposites" or "holding the paradox," because there is no tension and I still hold both beliefs: I could die at any moment *and* could have time to do what I came to do.

In holding both ideas, either-or is not required. It seemed to me that holding both apparently contradictory beliefs was a conscious act that expanded something in me—my soul and heart became larger and could hold more. On pilgrimages to sacred sites, I had a "tuning fork" perception of where the energy was the strongest, something like a vibratory resonance in the center of my chest. Sometimes, the expression, "I feel your pain," can be literally so in me—as a diffuse ache in this same place which as I came to know as the heart chakra, and as I grew older seemed to grow larger. I also intuitively sensed—as soon as I read of it—that my body can be held in a soul field, as well as in and animating my body. Metaphorically, I thought of wave-particle duality in quantum physics about light: it can be either a particle or a wave, not either-or but in two apparently contradictory states, separately neither fully explains the phenomena of light, but together they do.

Soul Work: Psychotherapy as a Spiritual Practice

I am aware that when I am engaged in doing soul work—being creative, or listening with soul and heart, or writing when writing flows, or in a soul-to-soul conversation, or in reflection and contemplation evoked by ephemeral beauty—that while I am absorbed, I am in *kairos* (participating in time, rather than in *kronos* time, which is clocked time). I know that we differ in what absorbs us, and that this is a personal, individual indication of what deeply matters to us and what can fascinate and draw out what it is that is special in us. Only you know when you experience *kairos*—what is it you are doing when it happens? Is it with someone else, alone, in nature, with animals? Is it a physical activity, or to do with music, are you working with your hands, or when you use your mind? It's eternal time or being in flow, or in the mythology of Ireland, if you entered the Fairy world.

I think that individuation has to do with becoming who you were meant to be, doing what you have a gift for, becoming whole. It may take psychotherapy to become free of the inner critic that finds fault with everything, or free from unreasonable fears and guilt, or feelings of worthlessness or shame, which are usually related to parental and other authority figures in childhood. Or it can stem from being shamed as you got older by bullying peers, or by sensitivity to the contrasts in social class, manners, or experiences; or by betrayal of innocence sexually; or by bad treatment from others that got misinterpreted as being worthless. It's not enough to focus only on what is painful and inhibiting, or what triggers defensive, aggressive, or passive responses. It is even more important to discover what gives you joy: what you are doing when totally absorbed in doing it and finding how to incorporate what you love into the work you do, or who you are at ease with and when not, and why. Therapy that heals and is a growth medium goes much further than focusing solely on what is wrong, or how you were wronged, or problem solving—all of which has a place.

In my office when I am listening and responding, remembering, and seeing connections, making metaphoric links, seeing symbolic meaning, feeling privileged to be trusted, able to be genuine in my responses including laughter—then I am in *kairos*, and the fifty-minute session is also fifty minutes of spiritual practice for me. I think that keeping my appointments on time is similar to keeping my word while respecting and valuing the other person's time. This requires paying attention to clock-time (*kronos*) regarding when our sessions begin and end while being very much absorbed during the session as I take in what is being expressed and shared with me: such as emotions and feelings, thoughts and fears, significant dreams, people that matter, pain and hurt, courage to do something, and creative ideas.

Like a musician, I am responsible for keeping my instrument in tune—myself, ego in relationship to Self, soul and heart receptive, to be centered. To be so in the session is a spiritual practice. It also has an effect on the other person, like singing on key or off key in a duet. If I am centered, it has a centering effect on aligning the person in the chair opposite me. This happens in genuine relationships where there is love and trust; it's when people keep their word and love is genuine.

When talk shared has depth, there is a quality of timelessness (*kairos*) in the telling.

Initially I started my fifty-minute sessions on the hour, and found myself often running over, which meant I wouldn't have a break between people. It was much easier to end on time when a session ended on the hour by beginning ten minutes after the hour. Issues that arise in therapy over appointments stir up the same feelings in ordinary relationships, only they are supposed to be voiced in therapy. Dependability is a measure of respect and also of love. Children and adults get this. When you say you will do something, do you consider it a promise and act accordingly? Or, if something or someone more interesting comes along, do you forget and "stand up" the other person? Much pain is caused by this kind of thoughtlessness especially to children as well as to the child part in the adult. Therapy invites *transferences*—feelings toward "mother" or "father" as well as other significant figures that may be projected onto the therapist who, as a parental or important figure, can help heal or re-wound, by being there or not, on time or late, truly listening and feeling in response or not. Now that I also have an inner time sense as well as a clock, my sessions begin on time and usually end when they are supposed to, which gives me ten minutes in between sessions and works well.

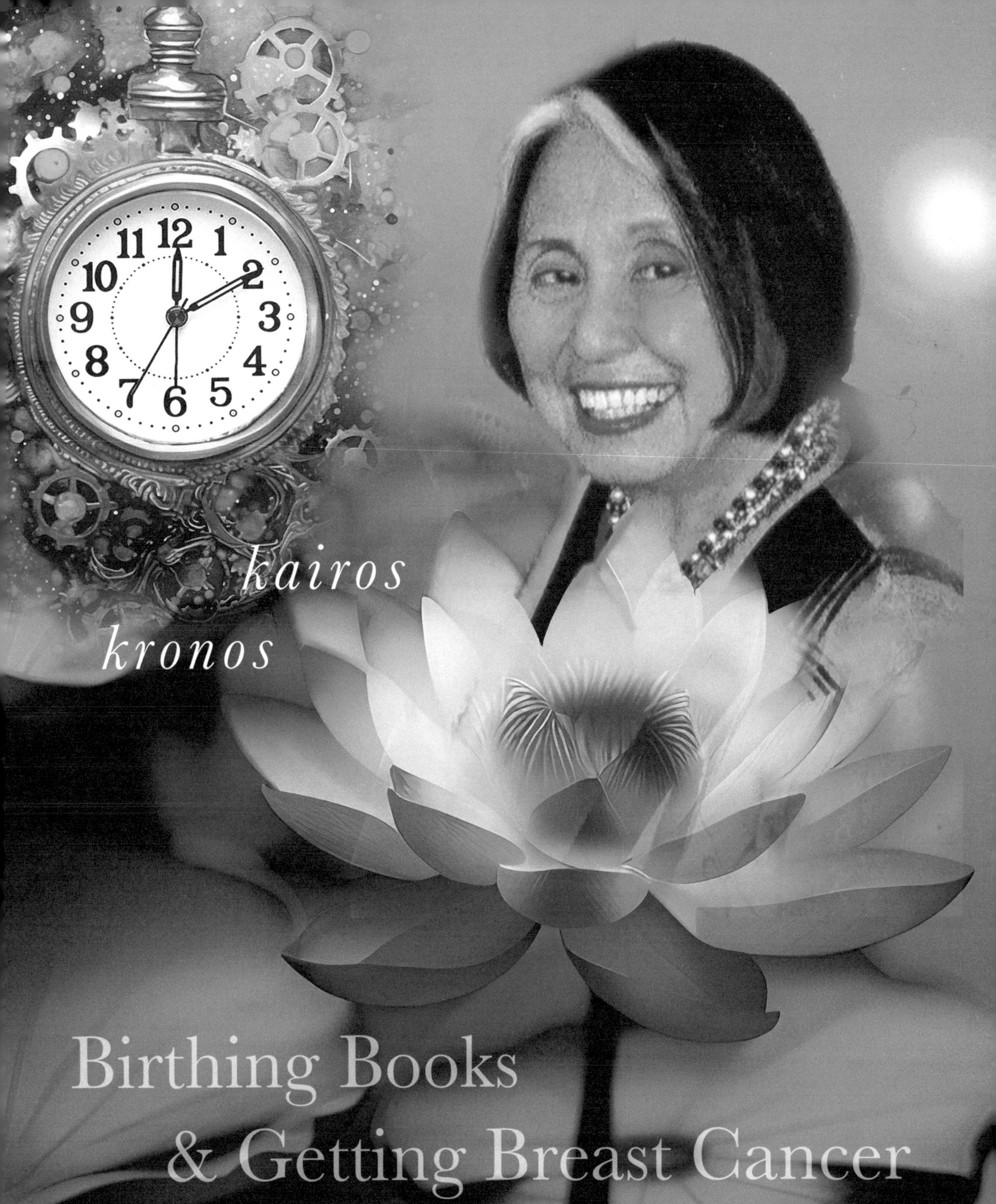
kairos
kronos
Birthing Books
& Getting Breast Cancer

Beautiful Melody

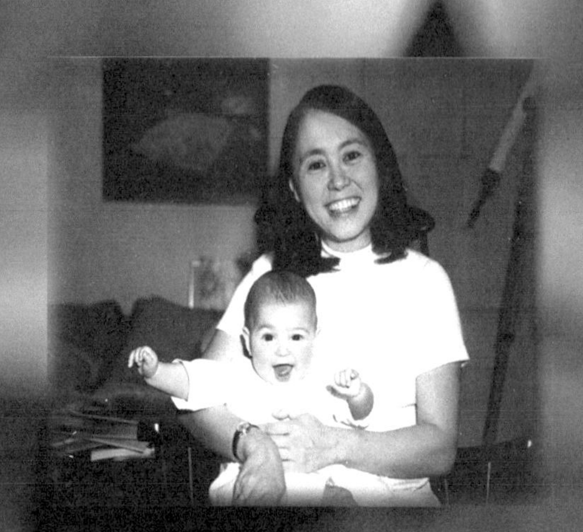

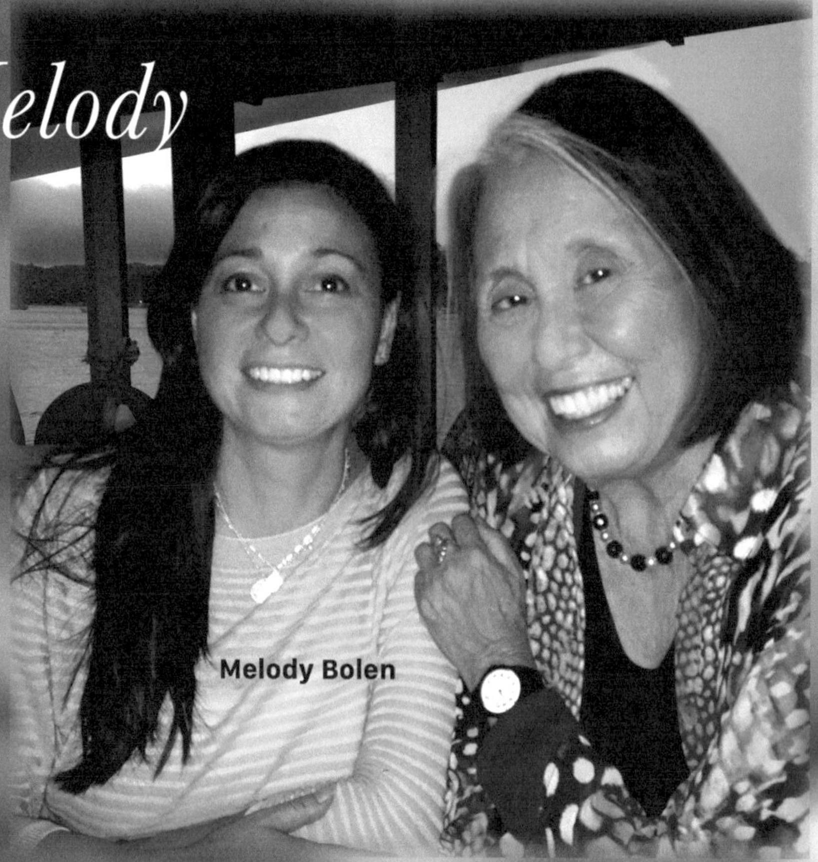

Soul Work:
Psychotherapy as a Spiritual Practice

Is it meaningful?
Will it be fun?
Is it motivated by Love?

Birthing Books

JEAN SHINODA BOLEN, M.D.
THE MILLIONTH CIRCLE
How to Change Ourselves and The World
THE ESSENTIAL GUIDE *to* WOMEN'S CIRCLES

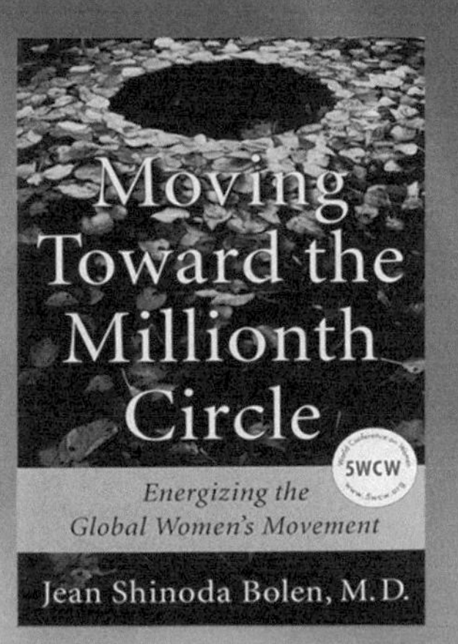

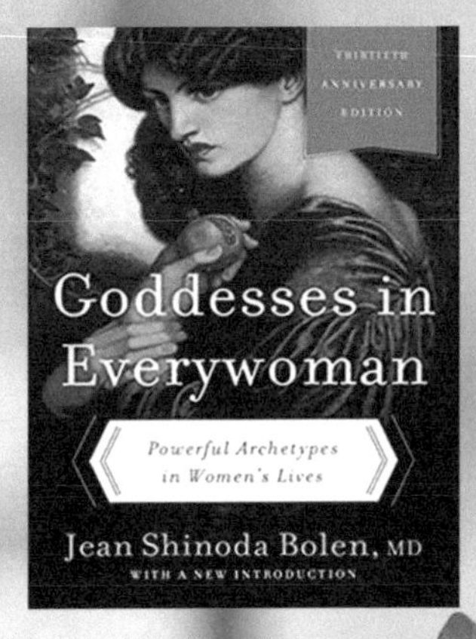

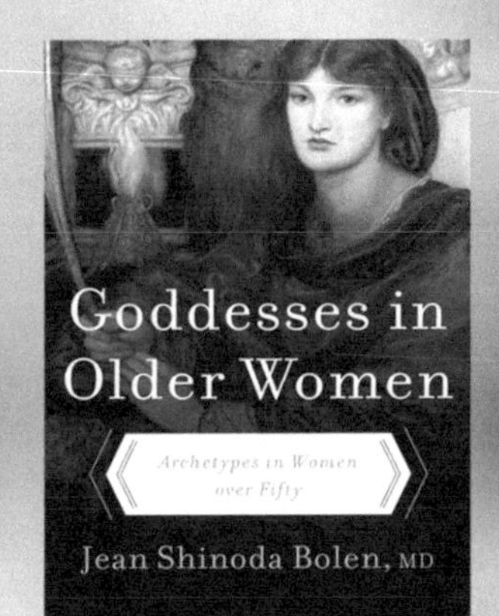

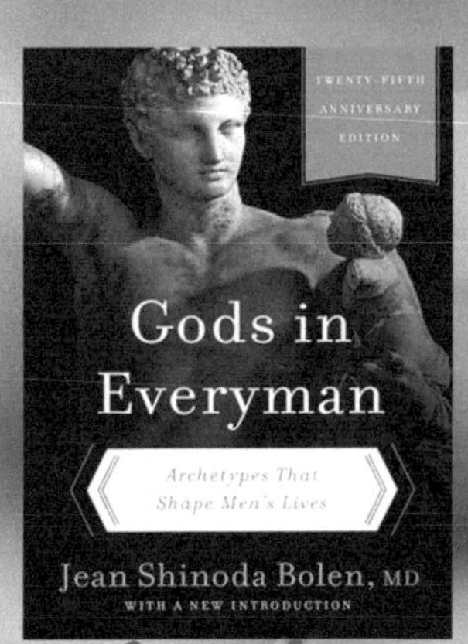

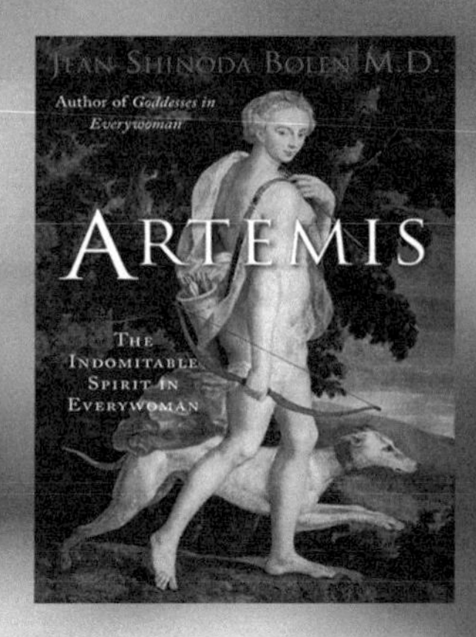

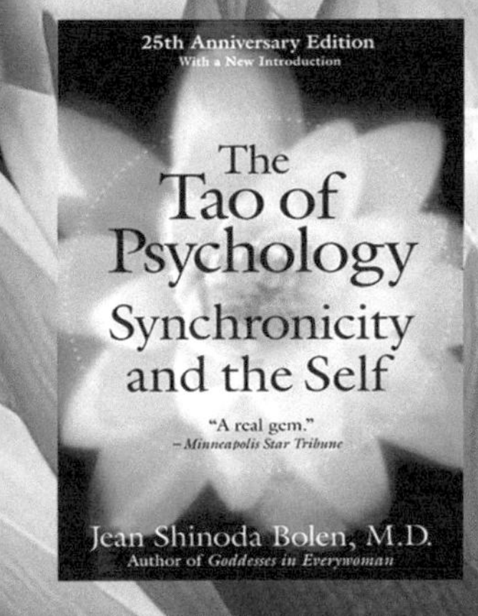

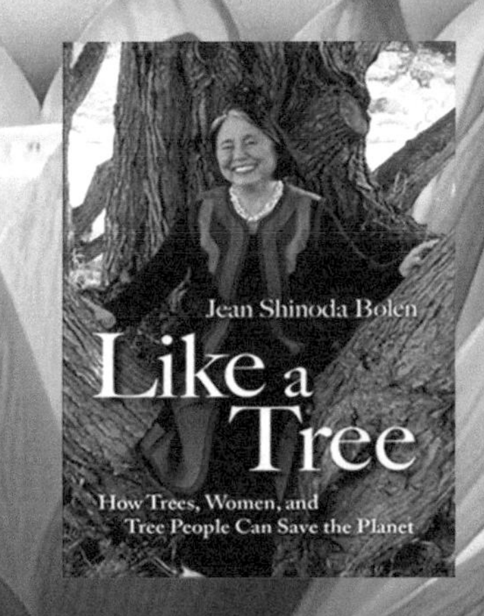

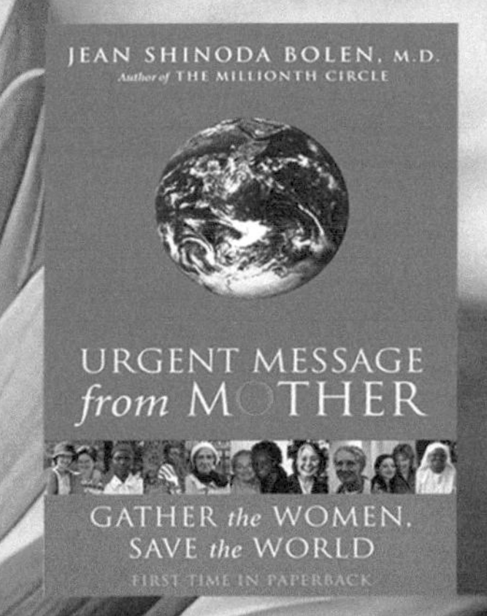

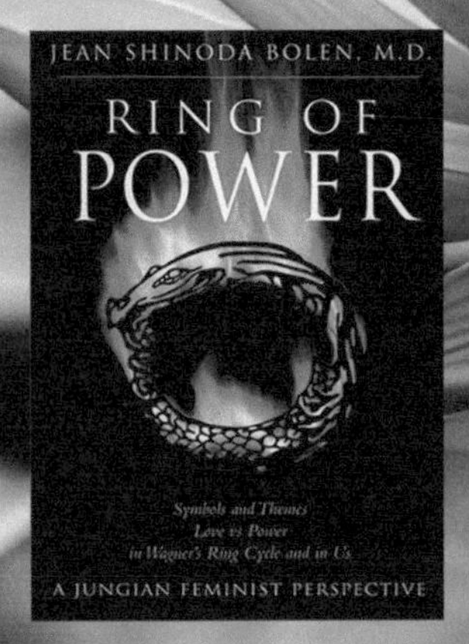

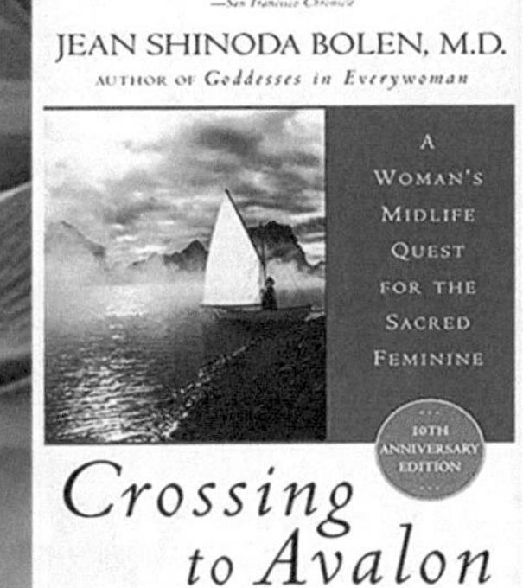

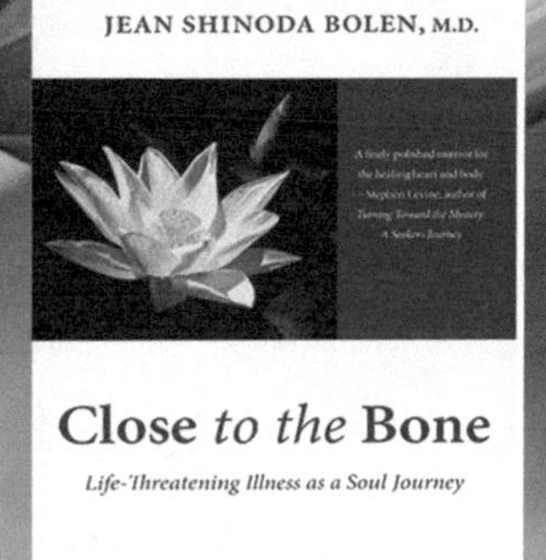

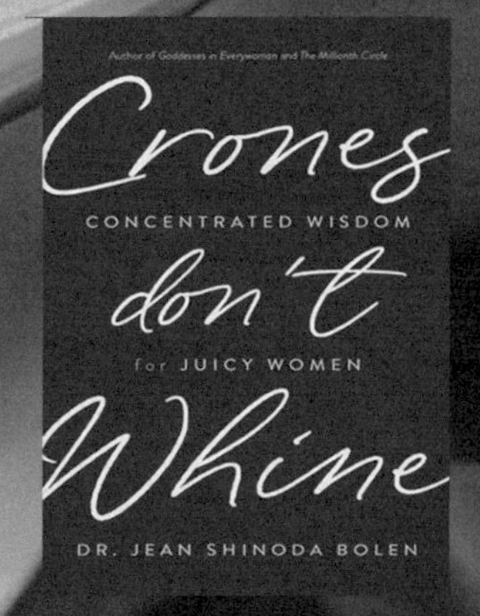

AHA!

Breast Cancer

audio Renaissance tapes, inc.

Dr. Carl Simonton's

Getting Well

A step-by-step, self-help guide to overcoming cancer for patients and their families.

Includes a 32-Page Self-Help G

by O. Carl Simonton, M.D.

Co-Author of the Best-Seller "Getting

Dr. Carl Simonton's

Getting Well

#450

Audio CD 2

©2005 Simonton Cancer Center

Additional inspirational audio materials, video programs and books by Dr. O. Carl Simonton and others are available from

O. Carl Simonton, MD

Kelly A. Turner, Ph.D

RADICAL REMISSION

The Nine Key Factors That Can Make a Real Differen

SURVIVING CANCER AGAINST ALL ODDS

Dr. Carl Simonton's

Getting Well

#450

Audio CD 2

©2005 Simonton Cancer Center

Additional inspirational audio materials, video programs and books by Dr. O. Carl Simonton and others are available from

visit our website at www.simontoncenter.com

or email us bookstore@simontoncenter.com

For patient retreat information call toll free, 1-800-459-3424

Carl Simonton, M.D.

Henson with Brenda Hampton

EALING

OURNEY

Kelly A. Turner, PhD

Chapter 31

Return of Cancer – My Dog – My Only Grandchild

Several years ago, I mistakenly thought I had finished my memoir and found it not so! It was just before I left for Cairo, Egypt to participate in the Women's Economic Forum founded by Dr. Harbeen Arora and held in many countries beginning in India. This was held March 4-9, 2020, at the Ritz-Carlton. I was delighted to have my daughter Melody join me and spend time together seeing sights as well as attending. I was an honored speaker and award receiver. I was very glad to arrive back home on March 10, especially after learning that President Trump, just a few days later, had cancelled all international flights to the United States for the next 30 days.

On March 19, 2020, California Governor Gavin Newsom issued a stay-at-home order to the entire state that more than half of the population could be infected with the coronavirus in the next two months and that all the non-essential working people should stay at home and work from home. After I returned from Egypt and had scheduled appointments, I spent only one day in my office seeing patients in person. From then on, I followed the directive to stay home and my work life changed. Ever since then, I have been doing therapy sessions from home on FaceTime and attending meetings, small circle sessions, and speaking at conferences including many international ones on Zoom while at home sitting in front of my laptop computer. The initial two months became three years where I live in California and many here remained as cautious as I did. For me and for many people in varied occupations, working from home and not going to an office made life easier.

Two Surgeons, Two Operations and One Patient (Me)

In 2021, toward the end of the first year of the pandemic, I had my annual follow-up to the breast cancer surgery that had been done in 2016, five years earlier. At this time, on palpation and then radiology, a very small sized lump was found at the edge of where the original cancer had been. Besides this, I had a slightly pouchy abdomen that led to getting x-rays of the area and as a result, another surgery needed to be done. Though it didn't seem to be a problem in that I had no pain or trouble with any of the organs in the abdomen, what was seen on radiology was described to me as a cyst with many small lobes or protrusions that had fit itself around the organs in my abdomen.

The decision was made for me to be operated on by two women UCSF surgeons in the same operating room in Marin General Hospital. Jocelyn S. Chapman, MD did abdominal surgery and had her office in San Francisco. Leah Kelley MD's office was in Marin. She had removed the cancer in my breast that was diagnosed and taken it out four years before this operation. Working together meant one surgery, not two separate operations. Dr. Kelly removed the small and simple growth in my right breast which was easily and widely excised and then Dr. Chapman did the more complex abdominal surgery assisted by Dr. Kelley. I had asked that if it were possible to not do a standard long vertical abdominal incision, that this would be my preference. A small initial incision was done and then parts of the long multi-lobed cyst was brought to the surface and opened. Fluid was initially drained out of the cyst and examined. It apparently wasn't cancer, and so four small incisions were made in places in my abdomen to remove the remnants of the cyst walls which had made its way where it could among the intestinal walls and organs. Transparent, Band-Aid-sized, very adherent tapes were then placed over each of the incisions on my abdomen. These "Band-Aids" would stay until they dropped off, which was enough time to heal the incisions. The cyst with its many lobes was a large benign growth. There also was no pain.

Because of the pandemic, this surgery was done at Marin General Hospital as an outpatient—unusual, but safer. I spent many hours that day in the post-operation area next to where surgery took place and could be followed closely. If my post-op recovery went well, I was to be discharged as an outpatient and not hospitalized.

The surgery was performed on December 3, 2021. I'd cancelled my office hours and the assumption could be that this was part of the Thanksgiving holidays. The surgeries went very well. I felt fine except that I got tired more easily. When I returned to my office practice and to the heavy schedule of online events as well, as the weeks went on, I felt physically more and more tired. I mistakenly assumed that I had taken on too much and didn't think it had to do with the need to rest and recover from the surgery. Most people do rest and take time to recover from their surgery because of the drain and pain which preceded the operation and hospitalization that followed.

After the surgery and ever since then, my weight became what it was in college.

My problem was that I was not paying attention to what my body needed to heal—like rest. What I hadn't been told and now have learned from experience is that when the patient is awakened after surgery, there will be a need to recover from the anesthesia, which apparently stays in the cells of the body for some time afterwards. More important, though, is the body's need to heal which will take time and energy. There were only four Band-Aids over small incisions to remove the multi extensions of the lengthy cyst that fit itself around the large and small intestines in my abdomen and had to be removed—the intestines would be bruised and need time to recover.

Nurses take care of post-op patients who usually stay in the hospital after surgery is done. Post-op nurses are likely to tell their patients to take time to recover and do less than usual while they are healing. There is a need to use a body's energy to heal and not do what I did on returning to work and taking on more. Instead, rest, take it easy, and give the body time to heal the incision on the surface and below, as the handling of organs in our bodies is probably physically traumatic. After taking anything out of the body with surgery, there will likely be tissues and small blood and lymph vessels and nerve fibers that are cut, and any oozing fluids are carefully stopped. The surgical incision on the surface is brought together with sutures that usually are absorbed in the body as the wound heals. Patients may not think about such matters if their surgery is like mine and done as an outpatient and there are no symptoms from it nor post-operative pain. If not for the pandemic, I would have been kept in the hospital and advised to give my body time and energy to heal. But since we were in the midst of a medical pandemic crisis, with seriously infected patients in the hospital, I could have been exposed to coronavirus and become infected. Thank goodness I was not.

My Little Dog Dani

Once the surgery was done and after I had my energy back, I was feeling fine. This was when it occurred to me that I could have a dog. I've always been a dog person but ever since going to college and medical school, there wasn't a place or time for a dog, except when I was part of a warm and traditional family and our two children were growing up. Then we acquired a large family dog. She was a Bernese Mountain dog that lived outside in her doghouse. She came into the kitchen from time to time, but as bedtime approached, she had to go out. I was used to having a family dog live inside, while their dad had grown up on a farm in Iowa where dogs lived outside and so she did.

As the pandemic continued with sheltering in place and wearing masks to go grocery shopping, it was obvious that stay-at-home replaced my life as an "up-up and away" airline passenger. I went online, saw and read about dogs that were available. They were in several different locations and situations. In reading about dogs and thinking about the dogs I had or knew when I was a child and being thoughtful about what a dog might need from me and how it might be for me to live with a dog, I felt I needed a small dog that needed a home and decided to visit the San Francisco Family Dog Rescue, which I did in March 2021. This was my second year of sheltering in place and doing my office practice at home or speaking to those I could see on my computer screen.

I learned that during the pandemic, reservations were needed to visit where the dogs were. I could select three small dogs and spend time with each one, trust my feelings and make a choice. Then came a sequence of events that changed the situation. I left with plenty of time to be there early. It was during the pandemic, and visitors had to have reservations, which I had made, and would not be with others who might also want to meet small dogs at the same time. I had directions on my iPhone and set out. Family Dog Rescue was south of the city of San Francisco and I learned later that they had recently moved but were nearby. It looked like it would be easy to go across the Golden Gate Bridge, get onto the north to south freeway that goes down the peninsula, and then change onto another freeway at a prominent intersection, go east and then take the off ramp toward where the new site of the Family Dog Rescue. However, when I followed instructions and took what I thought was the offramp as designated, it didn't work. I now had to go back onto a lengthy part of the freeway, with its very few off ramps that took me miles in the wrong direction.

When I finally got to the Family Dog Rescue and was in an upstairs office, I could look down and see the small dog yard and the large dog yard. People were there. I came too late. Then a big muscular woman holding a small dog that I didn't see clearly, came in and put the dog on the floor. In a flash, the little dog immediately went under one sofa, was lured out, grabbed the goodie, and was back under the sofa. She raised the sofa, and the little dog immediately then went under a second sofa in the room. This time, she lifted the sofa and grabbed the little dog at the same time. She then put the little dog in my arms. The dog was shaking all over and was terrified. It was easy to hold this little one and once it was obvious that I could, the large woman left and closed the door behind her. Time passed. It was over a half hour before she returned.

Meanwhile, the little dog and I got comfortable together. She had settled into my arms, and stopped shaking, her coat was mostly black with tan fur on her face, and minimal light-colored hair on her belly and legs. She had large stand-up ears, big dark eyes and a black nose. She was listed as a terrier and chihuahua mix. Then the woman who had left us together returned. It was getting toward closing time. She inquired if I wanted to meet the dogs I had asked to see, and if so, I could make an appointment the next day. As I held the little dog and thought, my mind considered but my heart was absolutely sure: Take her home with you! Which I did.

I am sharing my realization that it feels as if the invisible world of those on the other side who look after me brought me this dog that is a perfect match for me.

The little dog's given name on her papers was Danielle, which seemed too big and fancy a name for her. I called her Dani instead. She turned out to be a wonderful dog companion and is an introverted, polite dog. I didn't hear her bark until a couple of months passed. She gained a couple of pounds. Her coat of black hair grew thicker while light colored hair grew to cover most of her underside. Her trust and delight is to lie on her back, totally vulnerable, and let me pet her underside. She was from Central California, and about or over five years old, and weighed only about ten pounds when she came home with me. She has her own bed on a big leather chair in a front room with the television set, sofa, art and full bookcases. My bedroom is downstairs. The stairs have never been blocked, and I have never invited her to come down or forbidden her to do so. It is as if we understand one another, both introverts!

She doesn't care for dog toys or do tricks; she is curious and likes to explore while on a leash with me or sit in the car in the upholstered small dog box carrier which is attached to the passenger seat from which she can look around at the landscape as I drive. She avoids letting people or other animals get close to her. After she was comfortably settled in my home, I heard her bark if anyone came to the front door. She barks to let me know. She is curious and sensibly cautious. I now let her outside the front door on her own, which opens onto a wide wood deck entry area that becomes a wide walkway from my house to the hillside at the same level. She never bolts out, she always takes time to look around before moving into the unfenced sloped yard which has trees of many sizes, bushes, high grass which for a little dog must seem a bit like a jungle.

When I take her for a walk I put her on a leash, and while I walk on the paths and roads, she can explore while comfortably leashed. When I let her go outside and want her to return, I could blow a whistle but hardly ever need to use it, because she seems to read my mind and comes through the slightly open door.

I think of Dani as an "old soul" dog. Much as there are old soul and young soul people, it seems dogs fit into being one or the other as well. It felt like it took synchronicity for me to meet her and take her home. How did this happen? I can't know how but do realize that Dani and I may have been brought together because we both needed one another. Such is the mystery of synchronicity and sensitivity, in which there are very little answers to what, how, and why. My intuition and awareness senses those souls "on the other side" who care about, watch over, and help me—much like Dani on "this side."

A Change in the Weather

Just about everyone used to a normal life pattern was changed by the pandemic, and that was followed by the change in the weather in the United States, and certainly in California, where it rained and rained in the third year of the pandemic, filling empty lakes and rivers, with the rising ocean inundating towns and houses on seashores or riverbanks in other parts of the country.

People who could work from home did so for three years, more or somewhat less. There was very little socialization or attending events where lots of people used to be involved. While sheltering in place, I traveled only twice. Melody and Amar had found a large house with a lawn that went down to the beach on the west side of the large island of Hawaii. They invited Melody's dad James Bolen, Amar's mother Kusum Tankha, and me to join them. It truly was a vacation. This was soon after I had adopted my dog and while I would be away, I brought her to stay in a house on the hill above Shelter Bay in Mill Valley that took care of four or five dogs. I went to visit the house to meet Cheryl Shirley who, with the help of her mother, made this a place where a dog could have the company of other dogs who would go on walks every day, each leashed. My recently adopted Dani did not know that this was only a place to stay and so when I returned to bring her home, it must have been unexpected, like a repeat of previous experiences. She was quiet as we went home until she realized once we were home that this was her home. Within a month, I had a second reason to travel and took her to the same place. I was on my way to Feathered Pipe Ranch in Montana to lead a weeklong retreat with Monika Wikman as my co-leader. When I came back and went to pick her up, Dani came bouncing out to greet me and go home.

A Wonderful and Unexpected Surprise: Granddaughter Reiya

It was still the midst of the Covid pandemic in Winter of 2021 with a spike in cases and government urging people to not gather in large groups. Christmas plans of getting the two families together - ours and my son-in-law's- were called off. Melody and Amar still drove up from Los Angeles for Christmas Eve to see me and Melody's father, and as we sat around the dining table in my home, Amar and Melody gave each of us a card with a picture of a sonogram. Melody was now four months pregnant; they were expecting! Both were very happy about this. It was a surprise to me, I knew they had been trying on and off but hadn't heard anything in a while. On April 20, 2022, Granddaughter Reiya James was born in the hospital at UCLA. She came earlier than expected, and both Melody and her newborn were kept in the hospital after the delivery, with Reiya staying longer, until the happy day when Amar and Melody took her home. Her birth meant there would be continuity. Melody is my only direct descendent after her brother Andre Joseph Bolen died in his late twenties. Now there is a grandchild for me as well as for her grandfather James Bolen.

I met Reiya when she was little more than a newborn and again before she was a year old when Melody and Amar visited. Through FaceTime, Reiya and I can see each other face to face and thus we became familiar to each other. Reiya was walking before she was a year old and was fascinated with new objects and or new places and became used to seeing me face to familiar face with smiles and sounds and is very much cute.

Now I have a granddaughter, am active, and am writing this memoir with my little Dani dog for company. Reiya's birth felt like an especially additional good reason to live for more than another decade during which Reiya would be growing up.

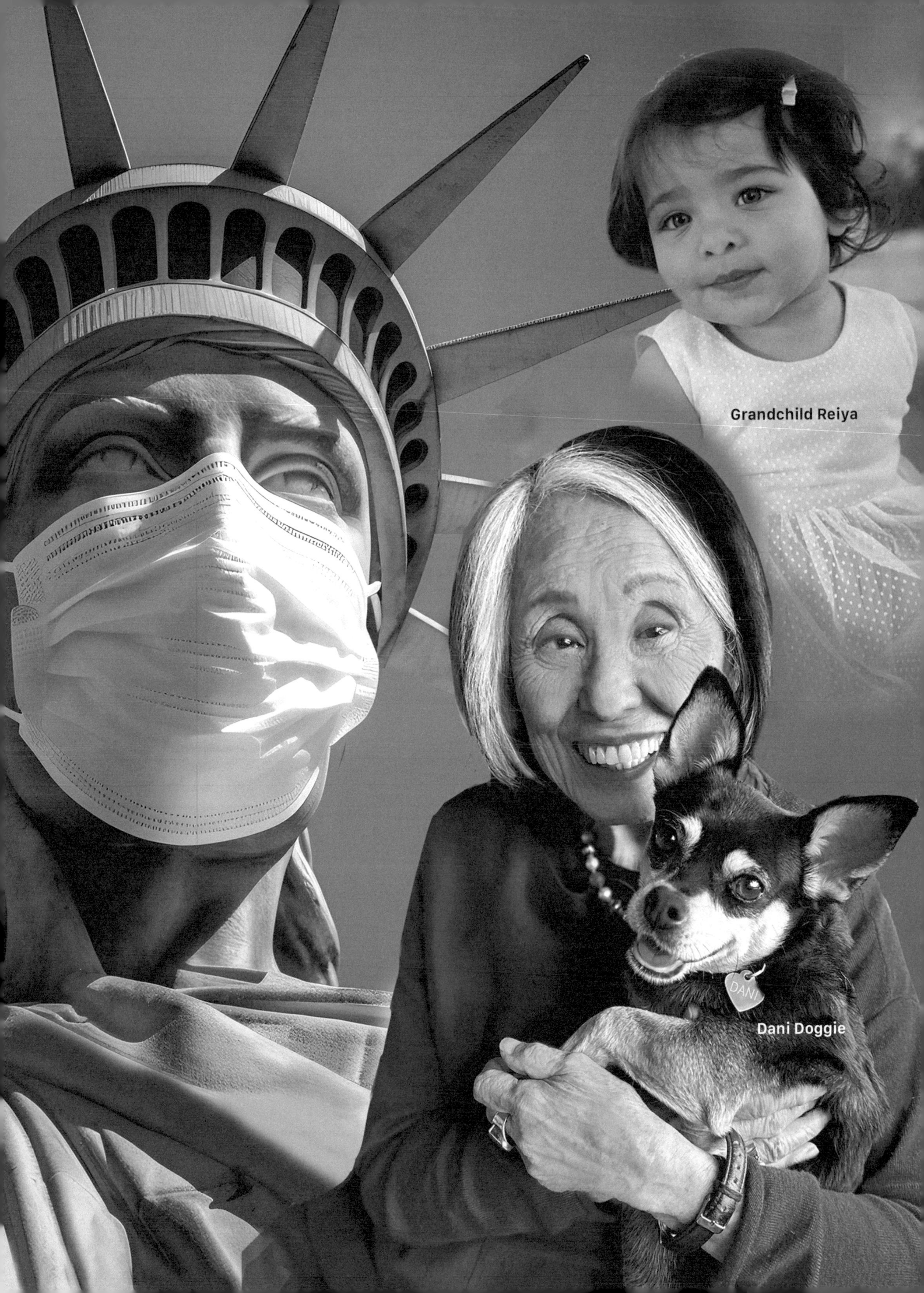
Grandchild Reiya
DANI
Dani Doggie

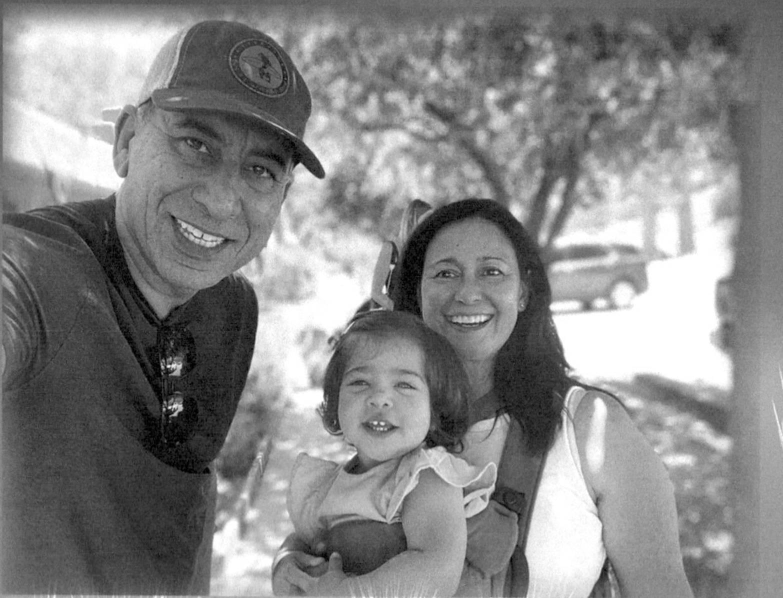

Amar Tankha Reiya Melody

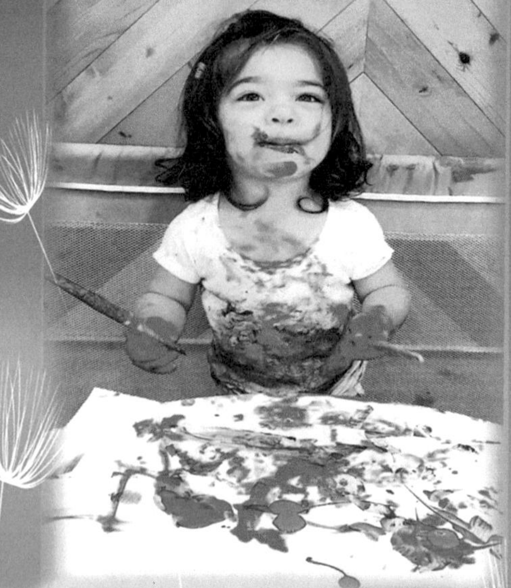

Reiya James Tankha

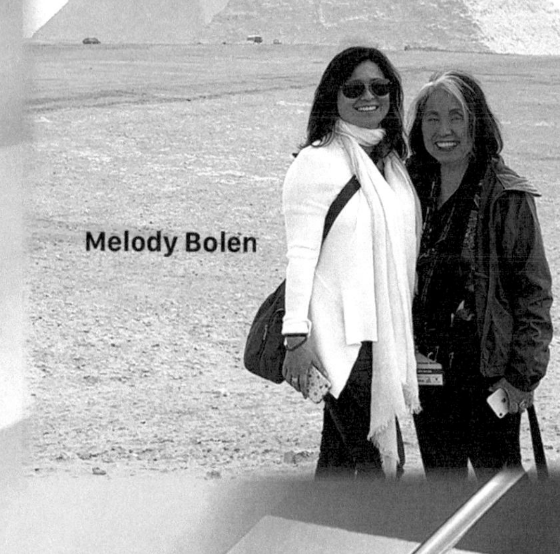

Melody Bolen

TRAVEL WARNING

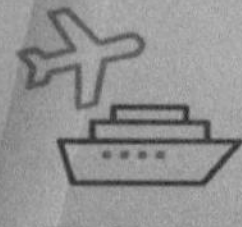

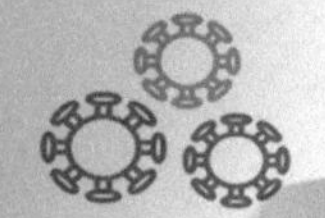

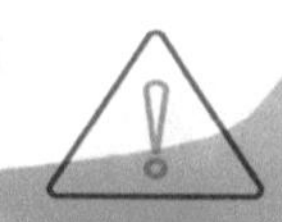

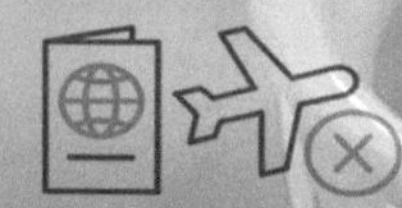

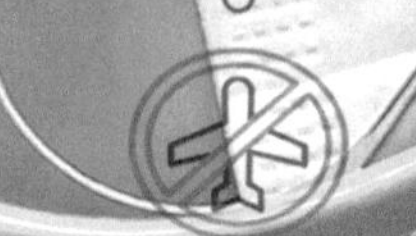

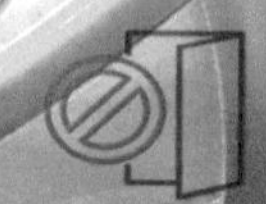

MARQUIS
Who'sWho®

Marquis Who's Who Honors Jean Shinoda Bolen, MD, with Inclusion in Who's Who in the World

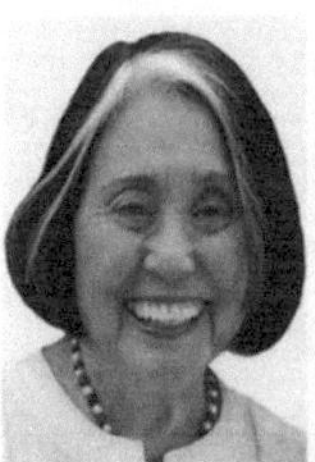

MILL VALLEY, CA, March 1, 2021, Marquis Who's Who, the world's premier publisher of biographical profiles, is proud to honor Jean Shinoda Bolen, MD, with inclusion in Who's Who in the World. An accomplished listee, Dr. Bolen celebrates many years' experience in her professional network, and has been noted for achievements, leadership qualities, and the credentials and successes she has accrued in her field. As in all Marquis Who's Who biographical volumes, individuals profiled are selected on the basis of current reference value. Factors such as position, noteworthy accomplishments, visibility, and prominence in a field are all taken into account during the selection process.

Dr. Bolen is a psychiatrist, Jungian analyst, author, and clinical educator celebrating more than five decades in private practice and teaching, The daughter of Joseph Shinoda, a Pomona College graduate and editor of the college newspaper, who headed a leading firm in the wholesale floral industry, a business started by his father, who immigrated to the United States from Japan, Her mother Megumi Yamaguchi Shinoda, M.D., graduated from Barnard College Phi Beta Kappa and Columbia University Physicians and Surgeons, Alpha Omega Alpha. Her mother was one of four M.D.s in a family of six, whose grandfather Minosuke Yamaguchi, M.D. initially came to the United States to study medicine at Ohio Wesleyan University and settled in New York City. Dr. Bolen was a pre-med and history major while an undergraduate at UCLA, Pomona College, and the University of California, Berkeley, where she graduated in 1958. She received her Medical Degree from the University of California San Francisco, School of Medicine in 1962, took a rotating internship at Los Angeles General Hospital (1962-63) and completed her residency in psychiatry at the Langley Porter Psychiatric Institute, University of California San Francisco Medical Center (1963-66), She became a diplomate of the American Board of Psychiatry and Neurology (1971) and was honored as a Distinguished Life Fellow of the American Psychiatric Association (2006). She entered the analytic training program at C.G. Jung Institute of San Francisco (1966), was certified as an analyst in 1974, and a member of the International Association of Analytical Psychology (IAAP).

In 1967, Dr. Bolen established her private practice in psychiatry and began her teaching career as a member of the clinical faculty at the UCSF Medical Center as s clinical instructor, then assistant clinical professor in 1969, associate clinical professor in 1976, and was appointed as a full professor in 1984, and continued to teach at UCSF until 2010. She is a faculty member and a supervising analyst at the C. G. Jung Institute of San Francisco. She was appointed as a member to the Council of National Affairs of the American Psychiatric Association and became chairperson. With Alexandra Symonds, MD, she co-chaired Psychiatrists for the ERA (Equal Rights Amendment). She then became a board member of the Ms. Foundation for Women. She has served as a NGO representative to the United Nations Commission on the Status of Women, representing Pathways to Peace (USA) and the Women's World Summit Foundation (Geneva). She has been a plenary speaker and honoree at annual Women's Economic Forum conferences in New Delhi and Cairo, and was the leading NGO advocate at the UN for a 5th World Conference on Women (5WCW).

She is the author of 13 books translated into over a hundred foreign editions beginning with the Tao of Psychology, Synchronicity and the Self, Goddesses in Everywoman: Powerful Archetypes in Women's Lives and Gods in Everyman: Archetypes that Shape Men's Lives. Her book The Millionth Circle: How to Change Ourselves and the World led to the formation of the Millionth Circle Initiative (www.millionthcircle.org), its conveners have been active at the UN and at the Parliament of the World's Religions since 2002, More recent books, Like a Tree: How Trees, Women and Tree People can Save the Planet, and Close to the Bone: Life-Threatening Illness as a Soul Journey addresses two current major concerns: global warming and the pandemic. While sheltering in place, Dr. Bolen maintains her private practice virtually, as well as speaking at international conferences and teaching widely on several continents. Her website (www.jeanbolen.com) lists her books, upcoming events, and archived presentations.

About Marquis Who's Who®:
Since 1899, when A. N. Marquis printed the First Edition of Who's Who in America®, Marquis Who's Who® has chronicled the lives of the most accomplished individuals and innovators from every significant field of endeavor, including politics, business, medicine, law, education, art, religion and entertainment. Today, Who's Who in America® remains an essential biographical source for thousands of researchers, journalists, librarians and executive search firms around the world. Marquis® publications may be visited at the official Marquis Who's Who® website at www.marquiswhoswho.com.

A Marquis Who's Who® Publication

Who's Who in Medicine and Healthcare

2021

Top Professional Series

Who's Who in Medicine and Healthcare

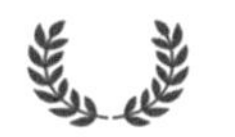

EXECUTIVE SPOTLIGHT

Jean Shinoda Bolen, MD

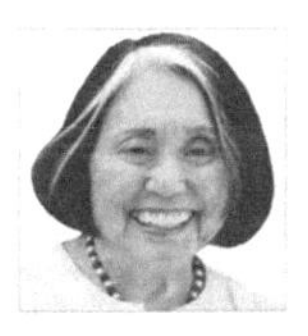

Psychiatrist & Jungian Analyst
Author
MILL VALLEY, CA UNITED STATES

XI

AWAKEN

Notable Living Contemporary Teachers
Notable Living Contemporary Teachers

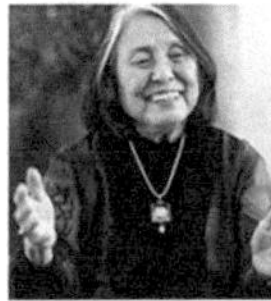

Home Base
Mill Valley, California USA

Foundation of Teaching
Archetypal Psychology, Love, Presence, Dream Work, Synchronicity

Jean Shinoda Bolen M.D.

Jean Shinoda Bolen, M. D, is a psychiatrist, Jungian analyst, and an internationally known author and speaker. She is the author of "*The Tao of Psychology*," "*Goddesses in Everywoman*," "*Gods in Everyman*, *Ring of Power*," "*Crossing to Avalon*," "*Close to the Bone*," "*The Millionth Circle*," "*Goddesses in Older Women*," "*Crones Don't Whine*," "*Urgent Message from Mother*," and "*Like a Tree*" with over eighty foreign translations. She is a Distinguished Life Fellow of the American Psychiatric Association and a former clinical professor of psychiatry at the University of California at San Francisco, a past board member of the Ms. Foundation for Women and the International Transpersonal Association.

Jean Shinoda Bolen is an Analyst-member of the C.G. Jung Institute of San Francisco and the International Association for Analytical Psychology. She is a past member of the Board of Governors of

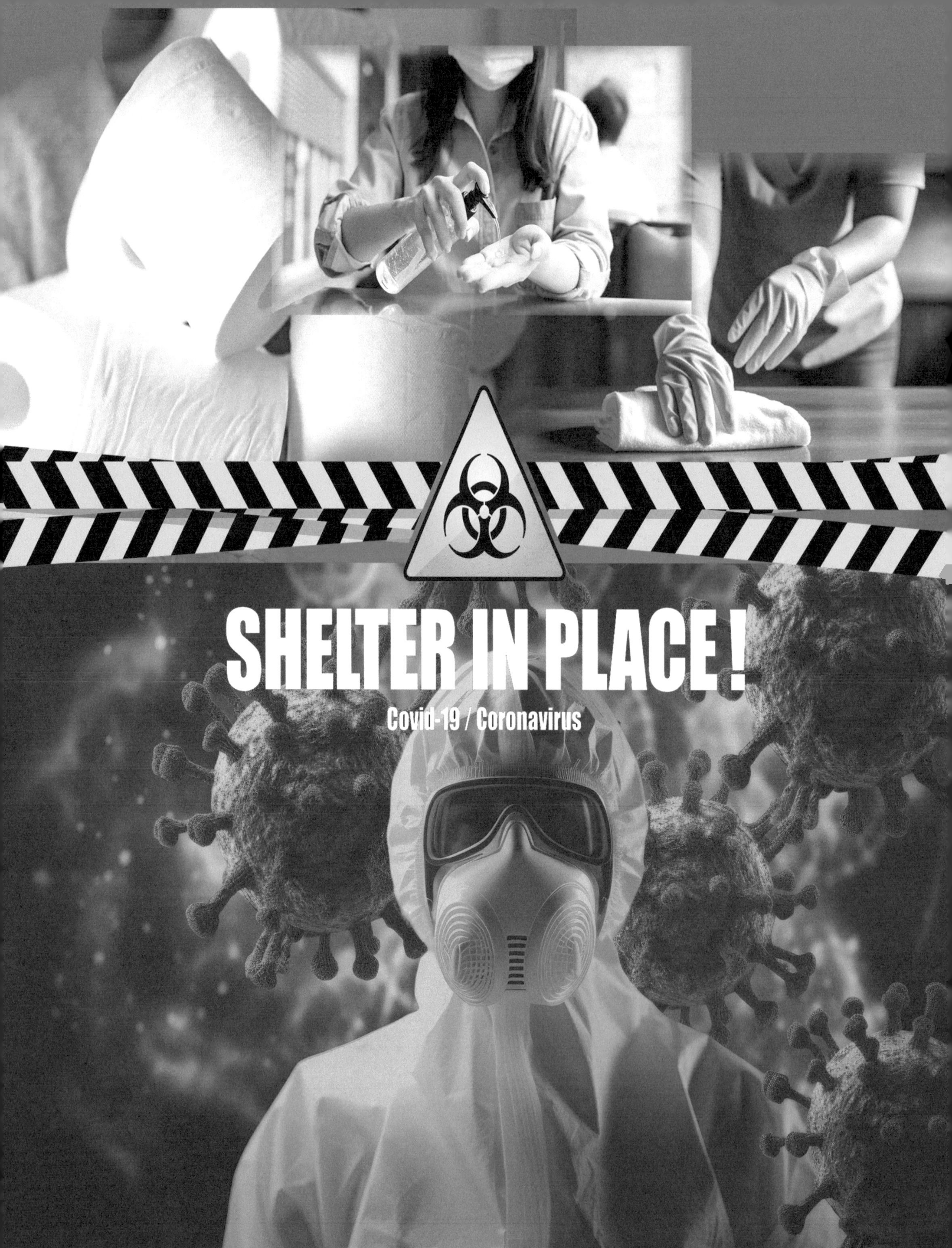
SHELTER IN PLACE !
Covid-19 / Coronavirus

Chapter 32

Honors & Recognition in Who's Who

Shortly after I returned home from Egypt and was sheltering in place, doing my Jungian analytical sessions and psychotherapy with my analysands/patients on my laptop computer screen, a photographer with his equipment and questions came to my home. His arrival and the interview was due to the unexpected honor I was learning about. I had been chosen to be a Distinguished Life Fellow in Marquis *Who's Who in America*, with an inclusion in *Who's Who in the World.* I had agreed to be interviewed and photographed for the books in my Mill Valley home. The interviewer came wearing vinyl gloves and a face mask so as not to cough out or breathe in an infectious virus, and as a result all was done under special circumstances as planned with the intention of taking still photos, motion picture filming, sound and video recording. He came prepared with a variety of professional equipment which included several cameras, lights, even a camera drone. He also had a list of questions, all of which focused on my professional and public life in my past to which I responded with thoughtful answers. Then came the final question: "What do you want your legacy to be?"

My immediate response was "I'm not done yet!" This statement resonated through my whole being. Little did I know when the pandemic began in 2020, that sheltering in place, not travelling, and instead using FaceTime and Zoom, I would be doing individual therapy sessions, as well as be a speaker at major conferences and attending regular meetings from home for over the next three years. Working from home on FaceTime for individual Jungian-psychiatry sessions and on Zoom for meetings or conferences was what I did from the time the pandemic began.

My photo and an entire page of information appeared in the seventy-third edition of *Who's Who in America 2020.* It was huge and heavy volume (2,694 pages). My page of information details personal, academic, professional information and achievements. It's in the beginning of the thick book in the Distinguished Listees section (p. 129).

Then followed in 2021 a thin volume titled, *Who's Who in Medicine & Healthcare 2021*, also published by Marquis. This volume opened with "Executive Spotlight' which began with my headshot photo and three pages of information about me. This was followed by 224 featured physicians. In addition, publicity was created by Marquis to honor those of us who were chosen to be honorees. I was featured with seven others in the *Wall Street Journal* and was one of four in *Fortune* magazine in June/July 2022.

I received a Marquis *Who's Who* plaque in 2022 with my photo and a beautifully framed text about me with a heading that reads: "Marquis *Who's Who* Honors Jean Shinoda Bolen, MD, with Inclusion in *Who's Who in the World.*"

Early in 2020, I was also interviewed to be an honoree by IAOTP, the International Association of Top Professionals, at their annual gala in New York City at the Plaza Hotel held the first weekend in December. While this was an honor, I was comfortably sheltering in place and did not want to travel. But as it turned out, I did not need to leave home. IAOTP decided to cancel their usual annual event because of the pandemic.

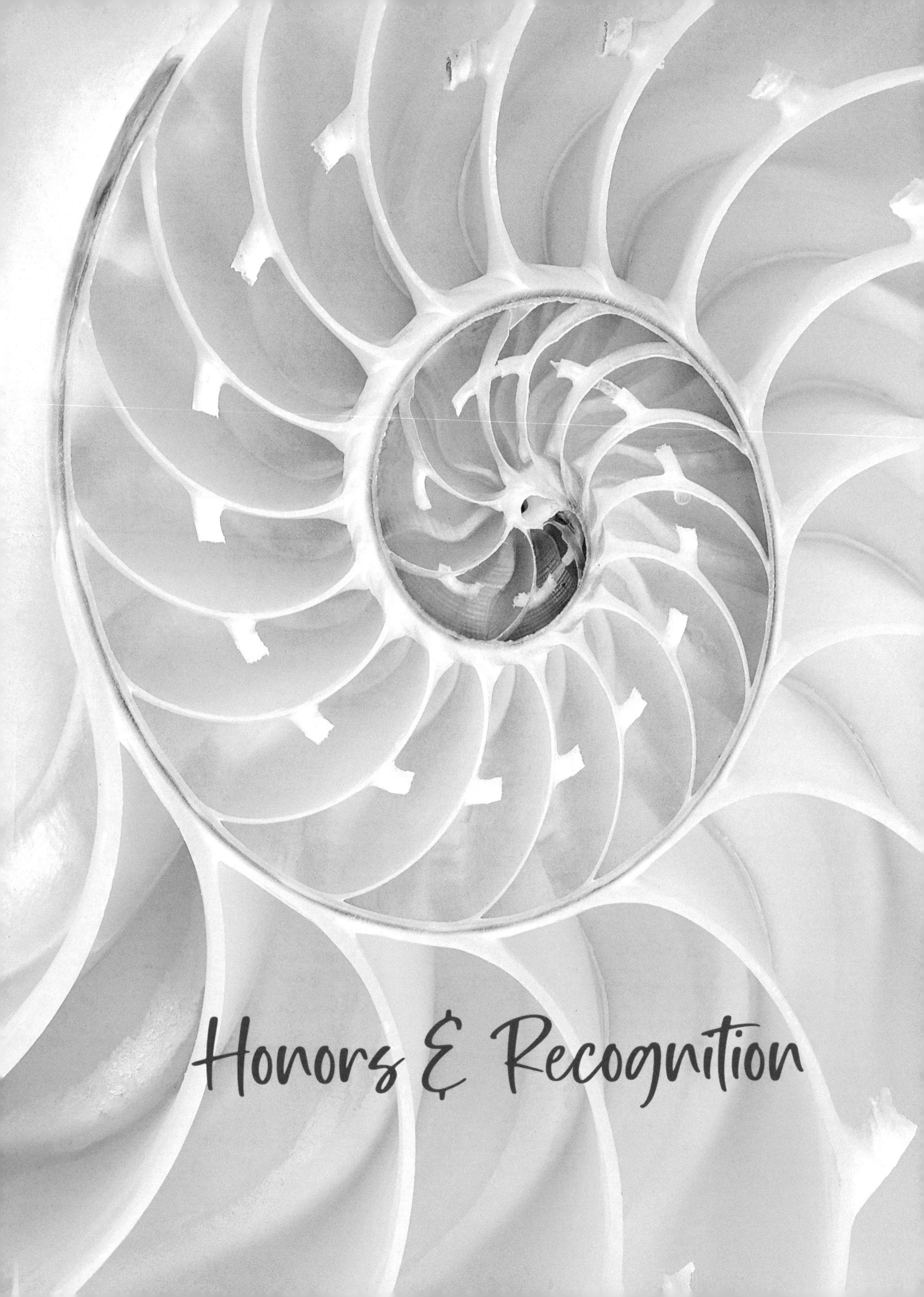

Honors & Recognition

THE WALL STREET JOURNAL.

JEAN SHINODA BOLEN, MD

MARQUIS Who'sWho®

Lifetime Achievement Award

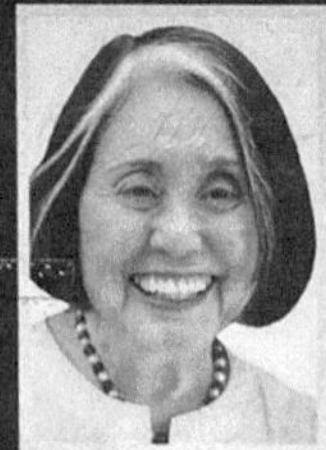

JEAN SHINODA BOLEN, MD
PSYCHIATRIST, JUNGIAN ANALYST, AUTHOR, WOMEN'S ACTIVIST

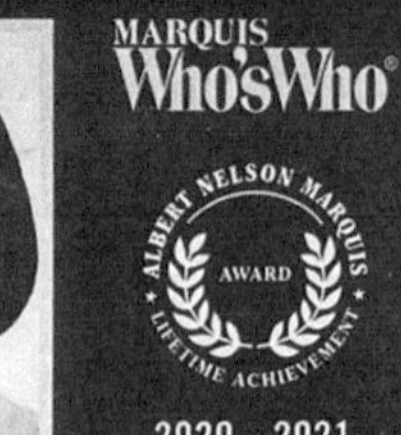

2020 - 2021

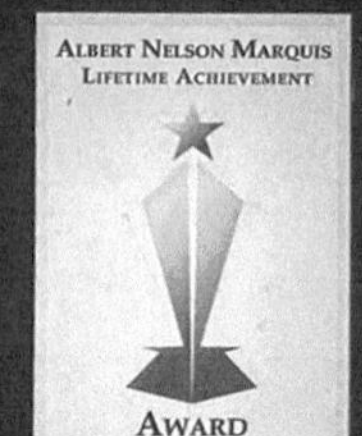

PAUL S. DUFFEY, PHD
MICROBIOLOGIST (RET.)
CA DEPT. OF HEALTHCARE SERVICES

Lifetime Achievement Award

Marquis Who's Who is proud to honor its most distinguished listees based on their career longevity, philanthropic endeavors and lasting contributions to society. Out of 1.5 million biographees, only a small percentage are selected for the Albert Nelson Marquis Lifetime Achievement Award. Among that prestigious group, a handful are chosen to represent Marquis in The Wall Street Journal. It is our great pleasure to present them here. Congratulations to our prestigious listees!

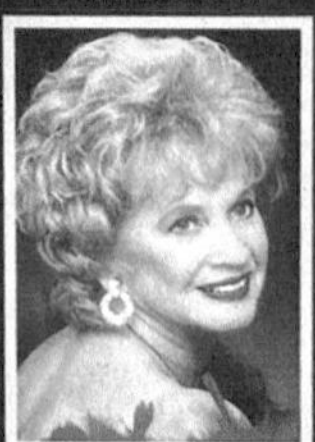
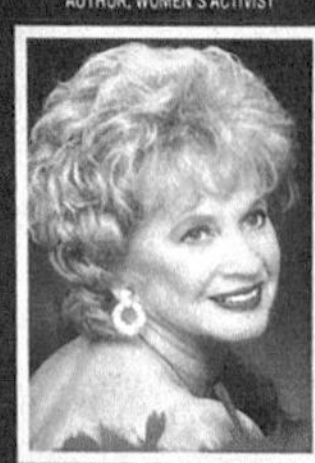

PHYLLIS DUKE
SCHOOL ADMIN., BUS. MGMT.
OAKWOOD ACAD.; DUKE PROPERTIES

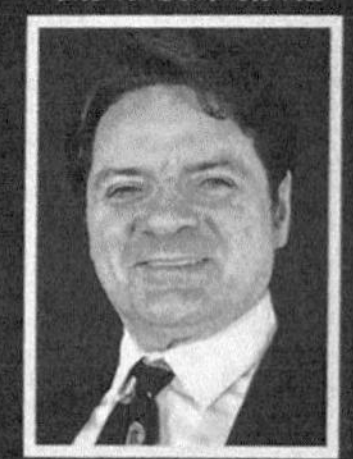

TOM HILLERY
EXECUTIVE PRODUCER
STARLIGHT PRODUCTIONS

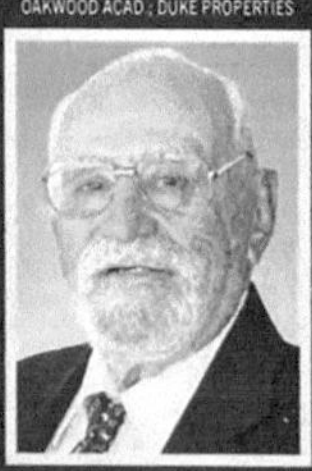

JOHN W. KRAUS
AEROSPACE ENG. CO. EXEC. (RET.)

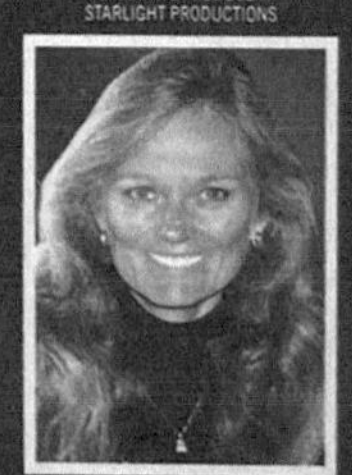

JENNIFER LENDL, PHD
PSYCHOLOGIST
PERFORMANCE ENHANCEMENT UNLIMITED

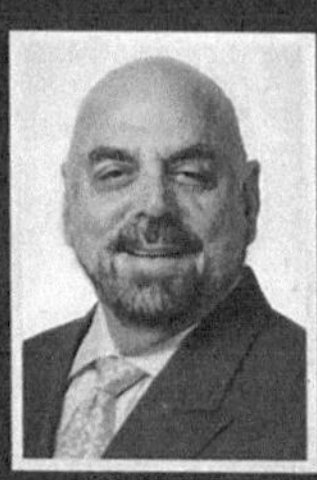

DAVID LYMAN, ESQ.
CHAIRMAN & CHIEF VALUES OFFICER
TILLEKE & GIBBINS INTL. LTD.

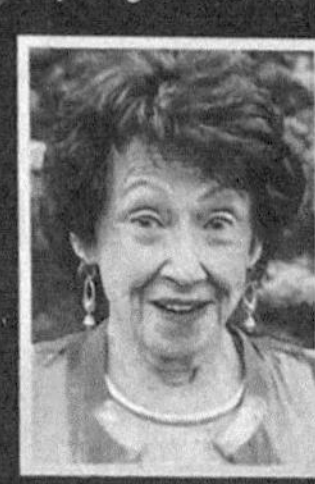

JAYDENE MORRISON
EDU. COUNSELING FIRM EXECUTIVE

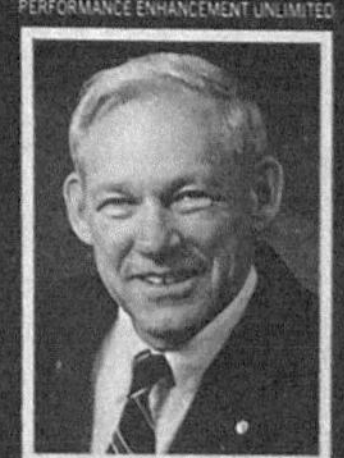

ROGER AUSTIN NEWELL, PHD
GEOLOGIST, MINING EXECUTIVE
CONSULTANT

MARQUIS
Who'sWho®

Marquis Who's Who Honors Jean Shinoda Bolen, MD, with Inclusion in Who's Who in the World

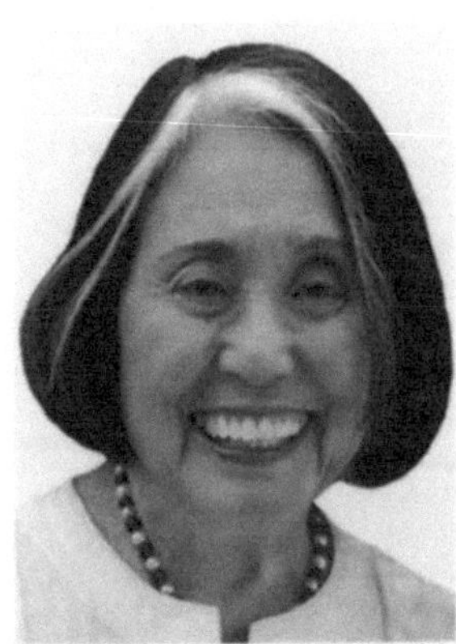

MILL VALLEY, CA, March 1, 2021, Marquis Who's Who, the world's premier publisher of biographical profiles, is proud to honor Jean Shinoda Bolen, MD, with inclusion in Who's Who in the World. An accomplished listee, Dr. Bolen celebrates many years' experience in her professional network, and has been noted for achievements, leadership qualities, and the credentials and successes she has accrued in her field. As in all Marquis Who's Who biographical volumes, individuals profiled are selected on the basis of current reference value. Factors such as position, noteworthy accomplishments, visibility, and prominence in a field are all taken into account during the selection process.

Dr. Bolen is a psychiatrist, Jungian analyst, author, and clinical educator celebrating more than five decades in private practice and teaching, The daughter of Joseph Shinoda, a Pomona College graduate and editor of the college newspaper, who headed a leading firm in the wholesale floral industry, a business started by his father, who immigrated to the United States from Japan, Her mother Megumi Yamaguchi Shinoda, M.D., graduated from Barnard College Phi Beta Kappa and Columbia University Physicians and Surgeons, Alpha Omega Alpha. Her mother was one of four M.D.s in a family of six, whose grandfather Minosuke Yamaguchi, M.D. initially came to the United States to study medicine at Ohio Wesleyan University and settled in New York City. Dr. Bolen was a pre-med and history major while an undergraduate at UCLA, Pomona College, and the University of California, Berkeley, where she graduated in 1958. She received her Medical Degree from the University of California San Francisco, School of Medicine in 1962, took a rotating internship at Los Angeles General Hospital (1962-63) and completed her residency in psychiatry at the Langley Porter Psychiatric Institute, University of California San Francisco Medical Center (1963-66), She became a diplomate of the American Board of Psychiatry and Neurology (1971) and was honored as a Distinguished Life Fellow of the American Psychiatric Association (2006). She entered the analytic training program at C.G. Jung Institute of San Francisco (1966), was certified as an analyst in 1974, and a member of the International Association of Analytical Psychology (IAAP).

In 1967, Dr. Bolen established her private practice in psychiatry and began her teaching career as a member of the clinical faculty at the UCSF Medical Center as s clinical instructor, then assistant clinical professor in 1969, associate clinical professor in 1976, and was appointed as a full professor in 1984, and continued to teach at UCSF until 2010. She is a faculty member and a supervising analyst at the C. G. Jung Institute of San Francisco. She was appointed as a member to the Council of National Affairs of the American Psychiatric Association and became chairperson. With Alexandra Symonds, MD, she co-chaired Psychiatrists for the ERA (Equal Rights Amendment). She then became a board member of the Ms. Foundation for Women. She has served as a NGO representative to the United Nations Commission on the Status of Women, representing Pathways to Peace (USA) and the Women's World Summit Foundation (Geneva). She has been a plenary speaker and honoree at annual Women's Economic Forum conferences in New Delhi and Cairo, and was the leading NGO advocate at the UN for a 5th World Conference on Women (5WCW).

She is the author of 13 books translated into over a hundred foreign editions beginning with the Tao of Psychology, Synchronicity and the Self, Goddesses in Everywoman: Powerful Archetypes in Women's Lives and Gods in Everyman: Archetypes that Shape Men's Lives. Her book The Millionth Circle: How to Change Ourselves and the World led to the formation of the Millionth Circle Initiative (www.millionthcircle.org), its conveners have been active at the UN and at the Parliament of the World's Religions since 2002, More recent books, Like a Tree: How Trees, Women and Tree People can Save the Planet, and Close to the Bone: Life-Threatening Illness as a Soul Journey addresses two current major concerns: global warming and the pandemic. While sheltering in place, Dr. Bolen maintains her private practice virtually, as well as speaking at international conferences and teaching widely on several continents. Her website (www.jeanbolen.com) lists her books, upcoming events, and archived presentations.

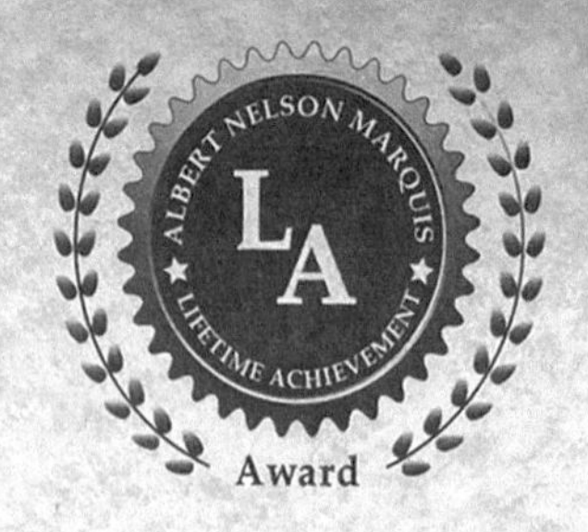

THE MARQUIS WHO'S WHO PUBLICATIONS BOARD

is pleased to recognize

JEAN SHINODA BOLEN, MD

as a recipient of the

Albert Nelson Marquis Lifetime Achievement Award

an honor reserved for Marquis Biographees
who have achieved career longevity
and demonstrated unwavering excellence
in their chosen fields.

Erica Lee
President

2019

A Marquis Who's Who® Publication

Who's Who in Medicine and Healthcare

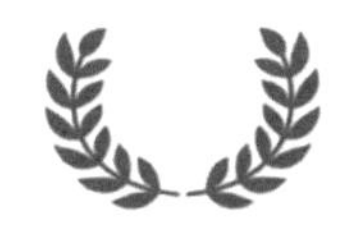

EXECUTIVE SPOTLIGHT

Jean Shinoda Bolen, MD

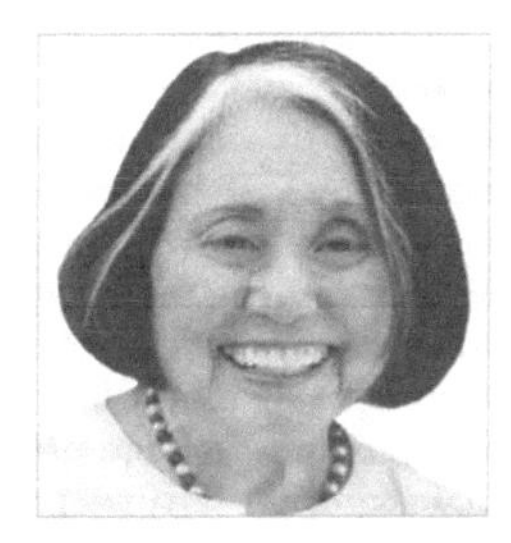

Psychiatrist & Jungian Analyst

Author

MILL VALLEY, CA UNITED STATES

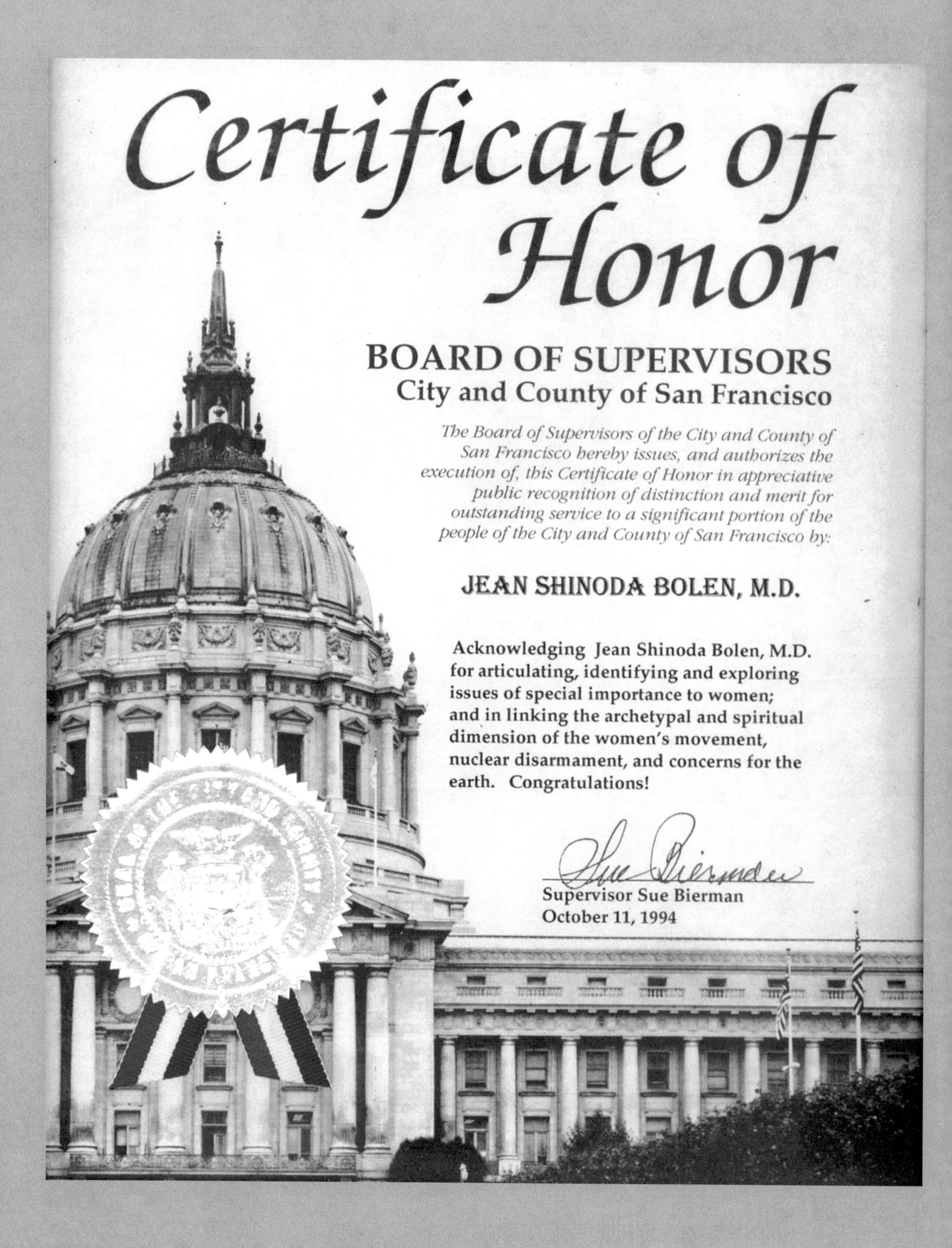

Certificate of Honor

BOARD OF SUPERVISORS
City and County of San Francisco

The Board of Supervisors of the City and County of San Francisco hereby issues, and authorizes the execution of, this Certificate of Honor in appreciative public recognition of distinction and merit for outstanding service to a significant portion of the people of the City and County of San Francisco by:

JEAN SHINODA BOLEN, M.D.

Acknowledging Jean Shinoda Bolen, M.D. for articulating, identifying and exploring issues of special importance to women; and in linking the archetypal and spiritual dimension of the women's movement, nuclear disarmament, and concerns for the earth. Congratulations!

Supervisor Sue Bierman
October 11, 1994

Friends of Langley Porter Institute

Certificate of Appreciation
Presented To

Jean Shinoda Bolen, M.D.

For Encouragement and Support of Mental Health
in the San Francisco Bay Area

Daniel Jenkins
President

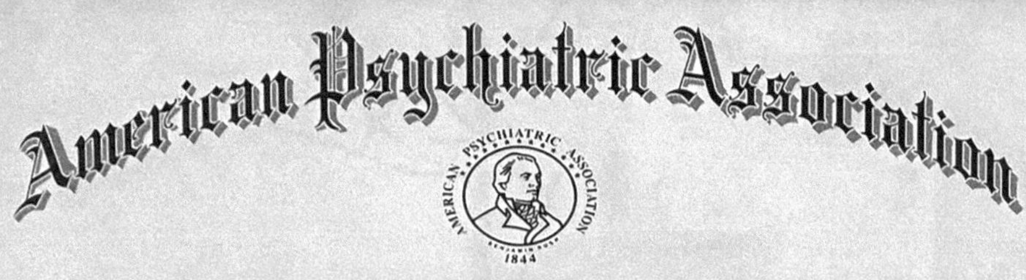

American Psychiatric Association

Be it known to all by these presents that on the recommendation of the Committee on Membership and the approval of the Board of Trustees this Association has elected

Jean Shinoda Bolen, M.D.

to be a

Distinguished Life Fellow

in recognition of significant contributions to Psychiatry. Witness the hand of the President and the Secretary and the seal of the Association this first day of January, 2003.

President

Secretary

The American Board of Psychiatry and Neurology

Incorporated 1934

This is to certify that

Jean Shinoda Bolen, M.D.

has satisfied the requirements of the Board and is hereby certified as qualified to practice the specialty of

Psychiatry

April, 1971

President

Vice-President

Secretary-Treasurer

Certificate No. 11377

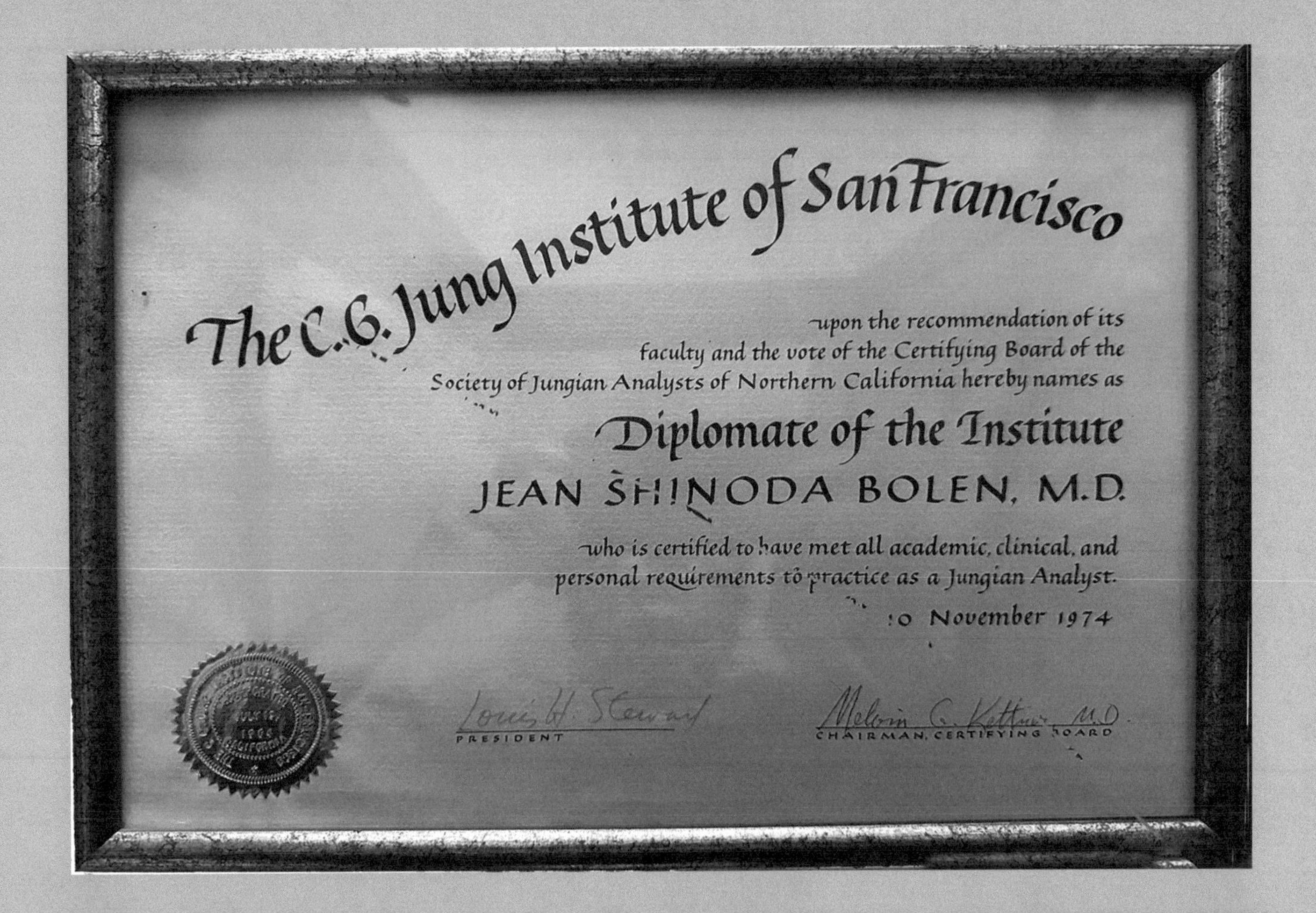

The C.G. Jung Institute of San Francisco

upon the recommendation of its faculty and the vote of the Certifying Board of the Society of Jungian Analysts of Northern California hereby names as

Diplomate of the Institute

JEAN SHINODA BOLEN, M.D.

who is certified to have met all academic, clinical, and personal requirements to practice as a Jungian Analyst.

10 November 1974

Louis H. Stewart
PRESIDENT

Melvin C. Kettner, M.D.
CHAIRMAN, CERTIFYING BOARD

THE REGENTS OF THE UNIVERSITY OF CALIFORNIA

ON THE NOMINATION OF THE FACULTY OF THE SCHOOL OF MEDICINE
HAVE CONFERRED UPON

JEAN MIYE SHINODA

THE DEGREE OF DOCTOR OF MEDICINE
WITH ALL THE RIGHTS AND PRIVILEGES THERETO PERTAINING

GIVEN AT SAN FRANCISCO THIS SEVENTH DAY OF JUNE IN THE YEAR
NINETEEN HUNDRED AND SIXTY-TWO

Edmund G. Brown
GOVERNOR OF CALIFORNIA AND
PRESIDENT OF THE REGENTS

Clark Kerr
PRESIDENT OF THE UNIVERSITY

J.B. deC.M. Saunders
PROVOST AT SAN FRANCISCO MEDICAL CENTER

J.B. deC.M. Saunders
DEAN OF THE SCHOOL

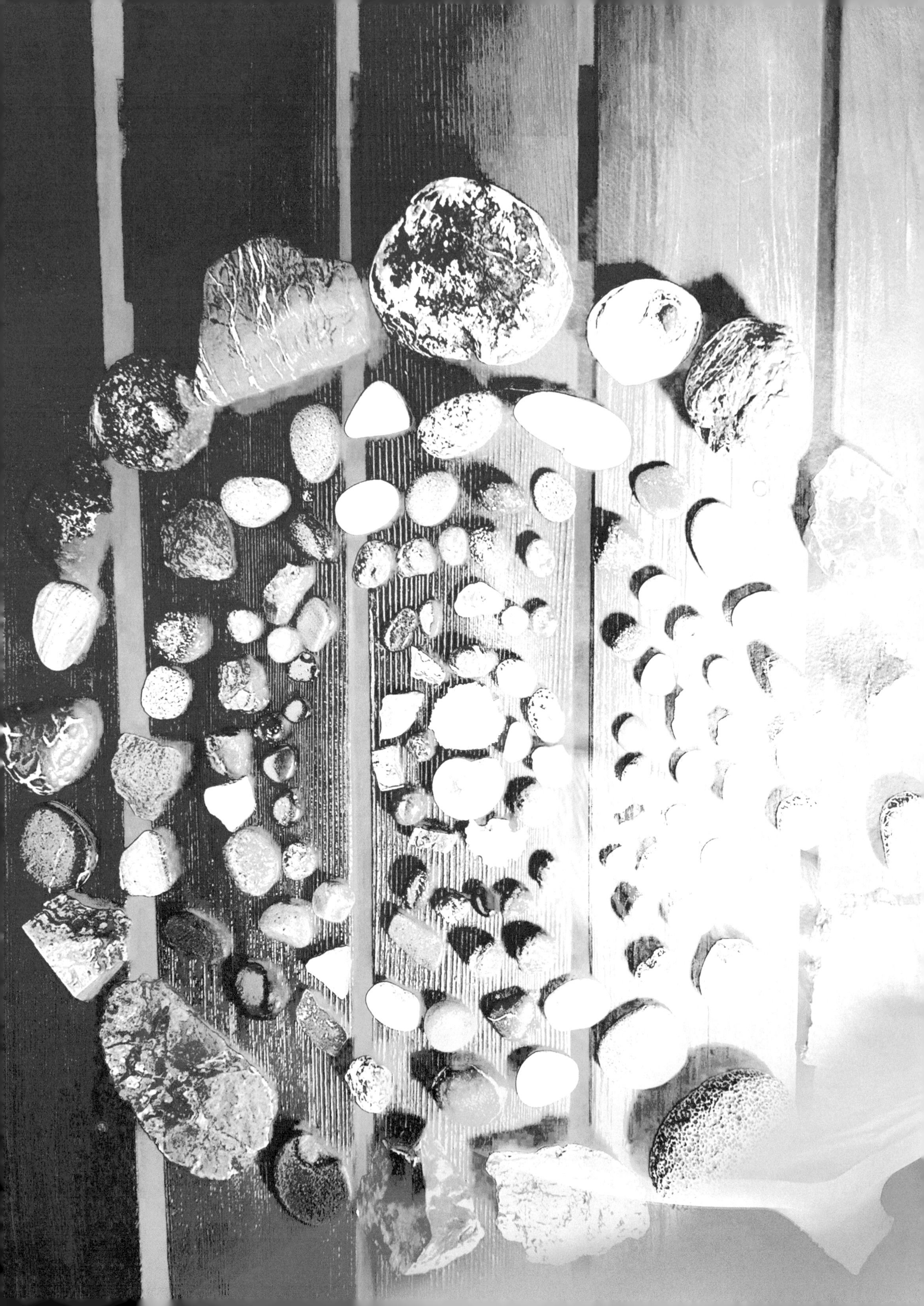

Chapter 33
Wondering: "What Next?". . .

When I returned from Egypt in March 2020 my life became quiet, living up in the hills above Mill Valley in my home surrounded by trees, roads and foot paths, with a panoramic view of the bay and hills and one triangular shaped small mountain directly to the east that I can see when the sky is clear behind Berkeley and Oakland. There also are hills and a ridge behind where I live with a winding descent road to Muir Woods National Park which is between mountain ridges and hills, behind which is the Pacific Ocean.

I am writing the last chapters of this book in a historical time when it is not at all clear what will happen next—to me or to any or all of us. It seems to me that any author of a memoir might end with "to be continued," because of events which may or may not occur after a memoir is written and is in print. An author can't write or type about "when or how I died" or describe what happened "after I died." Yet while we cannot write about such things, we may be able to perceive what happens if we maintain our sense of ourselves, when our physical bodies are no more and yet we still may exist in soul or in spirit and might be seen or heard by people, some in dreams and others who were awake and competent and have even "taken notes." This is what James Bolen did after our son Andre had reviewed his life while paralyzed and had been cheerful in the last months of his life. He awakened me before he took his last breath. Shortly after he was taken to the hospital by ambulance and declared dead, he was seen by his father who went home in grief, until he suddenly could actually see and hear Andy. I learned that for some time afterwards Andy talked to his Dad, who took notes. If he had mistakenly misquoted him, Andy corrected whatever it was he had said. I hope to someday read what Andy had to say.

Whatever we believe in about what happens to soul or spirit when we physically die, we may find out as apparently was the case with our son. Through my own experiences with humans and even some animals, it seems to me that there are numerous people who live out a lifetime as very young souls or immature people, while there are many others who seem to have come into the world and even as youngsters seem to be "old souls," who look around, fascinated at this new situation, and even when physically young, seem to have concern for others. Such individuals often can be very different from their siblings or parents.

Dandelion Effect

I had been traveling for several decades to attend and or speak at conferences or meetings, but once the pandemic began, not traveling led to participating and speaking at more events. I was now accepting invitations to be a speaker on several continents and teaching in seminars while sitting in front of my laptop computer. Many talks were often recorded and then could be seen and heard years later. Or perhaps while I happened to be speaking, a person might tune in and just happen to hear something personally important. I trust what I sometimes call "the dandelion effect" when whatever

I said landed in the heart-mind-soul of a listener who now had words to describe an intuitively felt experience or a dream.

Remember picking the stem of the dandelion flower, and blowing a puff of breath on the light and white airy blossom? Remember seeing that each little seed was attached to its "sail" which if it caught the wind, might land in fertile soil where it could grow? This is a metaphor for what can happen when someone happens to tune in to a talk or interview. A seed of inspiration or a creative idea is a synchronicity when an image or words lands in a creative person's fertile soul. Whenever an idea or image stirs a person's heart, mind, memory, or feeling—it can be like a seed idea or insight that lands in a person's mind or soul. Sometimes it comes through a story in which a listener feels stirred. Once in a while, I do hear about something I said or wrote that mattered, because a heart was receptive or an inspiration was evoked. When I hear about such moments, my heart responds.

The "dandelion effect" is then a mutual experience that neither expected. My talks even when onstage are not written and memorized, though I think up a title or the topic that fits the event and muse on what I may say. Deep in my heart, when I stand in front of the microphone or as now in front of my laptop screen, I don't feel alone and am not afraid that I will embarrass myself now that I am in my mid-to-late eighties and often don't immediately recall names. A "seed" idea is something small that can grow large and beautiful (such is the tiny seed that becomes a redwood tree) and its effect can help a person become who she or he was meant to be.

The Parliament of the World's Religions 2023

It was over three years between my participation in the Women's Economic Forum in Egypt, in 2020, and the Parliament of the World's Religions (PoWR) meeting in Chicago August 14–18, 2023 This PoWR theme was: "A Call to Conscience: Defending Freedom & Human Rights." Held at the largest convention center in North America, McCormick Place near the shore of Lake Michigan in Chicago, over 7,000 attendees from around the world representing more than three hundred religious organizations were there. There were many people who wore religious clothing or covered their heads and hair. Food was generously provided and served by religious organizations in two huge tents filled with tables and chairs. I am grateful for the assistance from Nami Nishiyama, my cousin, who took time off from work and was a real help to me. She accompanied me from the hotel through underground walkways, long corridors, escalators, occasional elevators, and kept track of where each event was to be held.

During the week, every morning before noon, a two- or sometimes three-hour program was held in the huge space called the Community Plenary. Each event was varied, had music and visuals and often cultural dancers on the stage, as well as speakers and chanters or singers, and other individuals. There were thousands of chairs in rows, with walkway space dividing sections. The people on stage could be seen by those who were seated in front of the stage, but everyone who came could see who was speaking, or hearing the music and seeing the dance on three huge screens. Everything was filmed.

I was a very active participant on four panels throughout the week and was honored to be one of fifteen "luminaries" selected to be a Community Plenary speaker on Thursday. For the plenary presentation, as I stood upon a box to be high enough to see and be seen over the stage lectern as my image was projected onto three huge billboard-sized screens during the nine minutes I spoke. I called upon each person in the enormous audience to evolve! I invited every person to recognize we are all an inseparable part of Nature, part of our planet, and of each other. This only requires connecting to our energetic heart for guidance and direction. In this way we individually, and communally, develop into the full potential of whom we are meant to be. It was exhilarating.

Each of the four panels of speakers that I was on included two or three others and a chairperson leading the panel. Each of us usually had different spiritual or religious backgrounds. On Monday, the topic was “The Millionth Circle.” All panel members were conveners of the Millionth Circle who encouraged forming spiritual centered egalitarian circles, with quiet moments at the beginning and end. On Tuesday, the topic was “Healing the Witch Trauma,” referring to the women who were burnt at the stake for healing and helping others, and were considered to have power and often feared. On Wednesday morning, the topic was “A Call to Conscience through Liminality toward a Global Ethic.” On Wednesday afternoon, women spoke in turn on “Evoking, Embodying, and Celebrating the Divine Feminine.” On Thursday in the late afternoon just before dinnertime, the topic I was inspired to name was “The Nun, The Witch, and The Psychiatrist: Shattering Stereotypes, Negative Myths, and Barriers of Separations.”

While this event was exhausting, there were also unexpected encounters that were soul-nourishing. On several occasions, I was stopped by people who approached me in hallways or in the dining areas. They were strangers to me who spoke about how I had helped them and were touched and supported by hearing or reading what had moved them.

For Each of Us: What Next?

Now an elder, a crone, an octogenarian, I observe that may of my contemporaries have contracted and withdrawn from public life. However, I am still here continuing to deepen and grow. I’m not done yet. Loving this life, I am passionate about remaining active, relevant and connected. I hope that my autobiography inspires and educates readers. May the ways I have learned to approach the challenges and joys of life help to inspire and inform others.

The topics that have interested me throughout my life continue to be essential: How do we connect with our soul? Where do we find our true purpose? How can our actions come from a loving heart-sourced place? How can we celebrate our differences and support our common human desires through ever-expanding circles?

While I am well aware of the state of our world-–with the scourge of wars that will affect generations to come; climate catastrophe as a consequence of fossil fuel dependence, decimation of rain forests, pollution, loss of habitat; political unrest with threats to democracy; challenges to women’s and human’s hard-earned rights; and the menace of nuclear annihilation—-I choose to focus on encouraging the power of personal and interpersonal solutions.

I am passionate about continuing my work toward inspiring people, especially women and evolving men, to quietly and actively trust each other to meet regularly together in circles in person or online. Or, if alone, by silently calling on the spirit realm for guidance. In this way I trust the path with heart will reveal the way into the future. Simply tap into the heart chakra in the center of your chest to feel the energy of love and then give it away. It is the one quality in the world that the more you give away, the more love there is in your heart and in the world. Invisible as it may be, it can be felt, and it makes a difference. Each of us is essential and can make a difference in this world we live in together.

May the ways I approach the challenges and joys of my life help to inspire and inform others.

With love, hope, mystical moments, and gratitude,

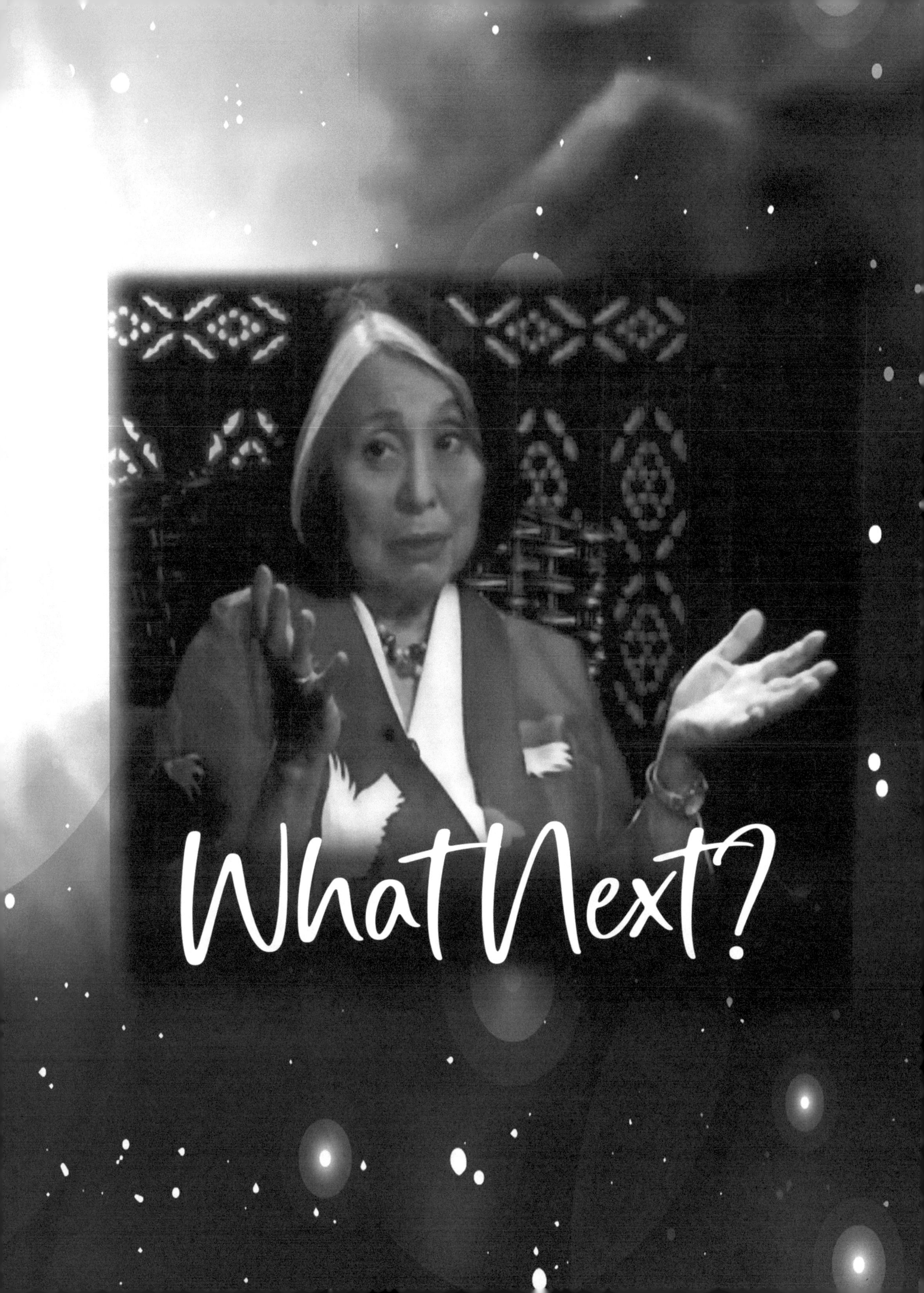

What Next?

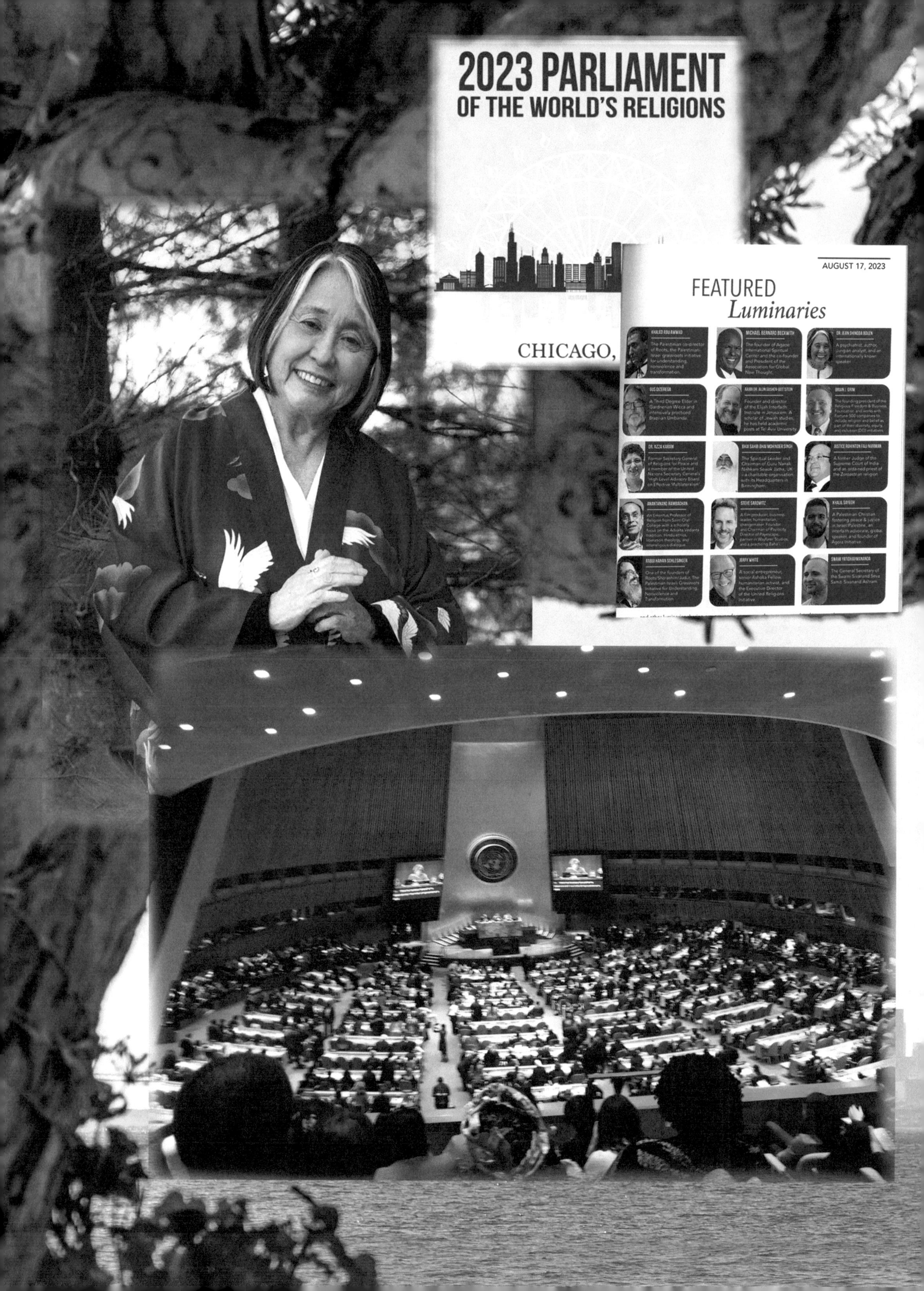
2023 PARLIAMENT
OF THE WORLD'S RELIGIONS
CHICAGO,
AUGUST 17, 2023
FEATURED
Luminaries
KHALED ABU AWWAD
MICHAEL BERNARD BECKWITH
DR. JEAN SHINODA BOLEN
GUS DIZEREGA
BRIAN J. GRIM
DR. AZZA KARAM
JUSTICE ROHINTON FALI NARIMAN
ANANTANAND RAMBACHAN
STEVE SAROWITZ
KHALIL SAYEGH
RABBI HANAN SCHLESINGER
SWAMI YATIDHARMANANDA

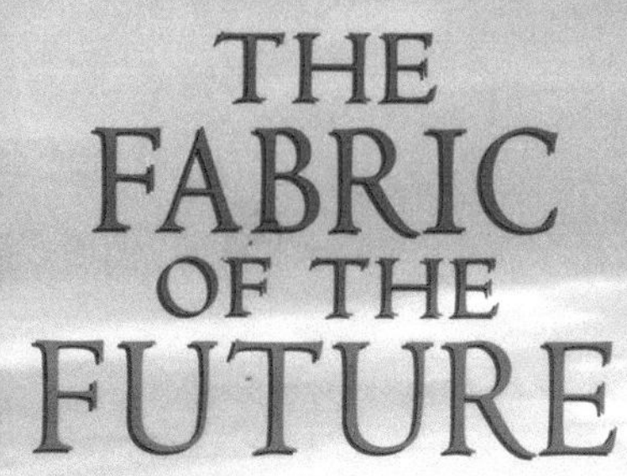

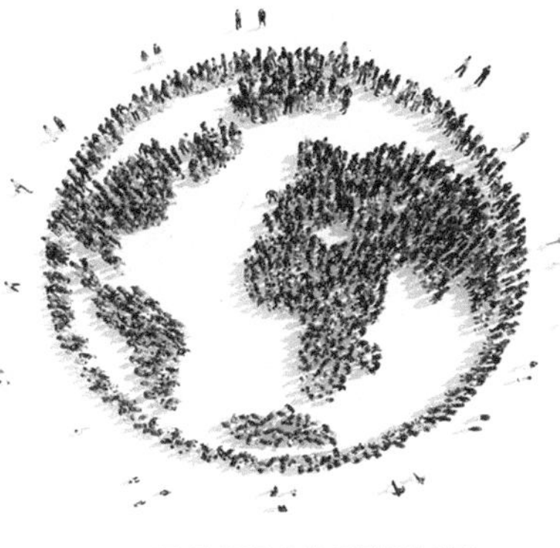

35TH ANNUAL
BIONEERS
REVOLUTION FROM THE HEART OF NATURE
MARCH 28-30, 2024
BERKELEY, CA

Lynda Carré Jean Carole Comeau Beth Baker

Valerie Andrews
Isabel Allende
Jean
Carole Robinson
Pauline Tesler

Millions of Circles

Epilogue

Reflections on Working from Home Finishing my Autobiography

I had been writing my autobiography off and on for over a decade until the pandemic, when I paused to adjust to a new world that kept us sheltered at home and physically separate. I closed my professional office and no longer traveled worldwide as I had been for years. Instead, I met with patients, offered presentations at major world conferences, and provided educational courses—all from the comfort of my Mill Valley home in front my computer.

After the world re-opened to travel, buoyed on my return home with the fresh momentum I experienced with the collective spirit of thousands at Parliament of the World's Religions in Chicago, I completed the final three chapters. Through re-reading my own writing I was able to see, and even re-experience, the earlier life I had written about. In the last chapters I was able to even more fully appreciate my ancestors, supportive family, opportunities, creative spirituality, synchronicities, heart-sourced guidance from those in this world and from beyond, and the never-ending thrill of fully living in this precious, albeit uncertain, world. In the finishing of *Ever Widening Circles & Mystical Moments,* I am grateful for so many people who supported, and collaborated with, me. My friend, Carole Comeau, read through and provided helpful notes in the many versions I sent her in the process of writing this book. I was working with a reliable support person, Carol Hansen Grey, who helped me organize earlier versions of the manuscript for this autobiography and who has managed my personal website for decades (www.jeanshinodabolen.com). As I was finishing writing the last chapters, I became aware that this autobiography was unlike any of my thirteen earlier text-only books. It needed photographs to convey more of my life and the context of the times I have lived through. Then synchronicity happened—I was put in touch with Lynda Carré, a communications professional, graphic design artist, and interfaith chaplain. We reviewed hundreds of personal and historical photos from which she created the evocative photomontages at the end of each chapter and helped me finish writing this book. Lynda also designed the cover of the book incorporating an original artwork I painted. Through my dear friend and author, Valerie Andrews, I was introduced to the wonderful team at Chiron Publications to produce this book. My publicist, Bradley Jones, provided excellent guidance and connections. My former husband and friend, James Bolen, daughter Melody Bolen, son-in-law Amar Tankha, and beloved granddaughter Reiya are in my heart.

I am grateful for these people and many others who are identified within the book. I am also appreciative of the support I rely upon from those in my life who have died and gone "to the other side." I feel their loving presence and trust their guidance.

Having now reached the age of 88, with the expectation of many more years, I expect this book will carry my story for generations to come. I trust it will provide a deeper understanding of my lived experience to those who know me personally as well as those who know me through my work as an activist, author, speaker, psychiatrist, and Jungian analyst.

I invite readers, and listeners to the audiobook, to explore my other books, follow my social media posts on Instagram and Facebook, and visit my website, jeanbolen.com, to see what I am up to.

I hope readers find *Ever Widening Circles & Mystical Moments* to be interesting, inspiring, and helpful in identifying your own authentic soul's purpose, you're your meaningful life path, and realize how essential you are in this precious life. Remember to ask yourself, *Is it meaningful*? *Will it be fun? Is it motivated by love*?

INDEX

Praise for Jean Shinoda Bolen's *Ever Widening Circles & Mystical Moments: Autobiographical, Historical, Spiritual, Psychological & Political*

"Read Doctor Jean Bolen's, Ever Widening Circles and Mystical Moments, *and discover the many and mystical ways that your life and experience are included."*

Gloria Steinem
Feminist Activist, Author Co-Founder Ms. Magazine

"An internationally renowned psychiatrist and a widely respected feminist Jean Shinoda Bolen's Ever Widening Circles & Mystical Moments *is a profoundly inspiring testament to a life lived with courage, purpose, and a deep commitment to humanity. She masterfully weaves her personal journey with universal truths that capture the essence of a life dedicated to transformation, understanding, and the unwavering pursuit of truth. With every page of this autobiography, she offers not just her story, but also an invitation to explore the richness of our own lives and the subtle yet powerful forces that shape them. Her work continues to illuminate pathways for a more compassionate, empathic, inclusive and peace-loving world. A must read for all."*

Ambassador Anwarul K. Chowdhury
Former Under-Secretary-General and High Representative of the United Nations
Founder, Global Movement for The Culture of Peace

"This is the unusual story of an extraordinary woman's life as a Jungian psychiatrist and as a spiritual seeker. In these pages Jean Shinoda Bolen reveals for the first time her private life, including many photographs, and she takes her readers to the realm of the soul as she has done in all her bestselling books. A fascinating memoir for her millions of fans and an open invitation for those who need inspiration in these difficult times."

Isabel Allende
Author

"As she has so generously done throughout her life's journey, Jean Shinoda Bolen offers us - in the form of her memoir - a map to carry readers through the phases of her life's inquiries, challenges and the books she has birthed, that parallel and share insight into the various phases of feminist movements. This is a must read for anyone seeking an archetypal insight into the historical arc of women's evolutionary liberatory movements, discoveries and practices."

Nina Simons
Author, Co-Founder BIONEERS and Chief Relationship Officer

"Jean's autobiographical book, Ever Widening Circles and Mystical Moments, *is a reflective journey, filled with thoughts and insights gained as she engages with her experiences. By being willing to share on a personal level, she encourages the reader to be introspective as well."*

Carole Comeau
LPC (Licensed Professional Counselor)

"Jean Shinoda Bolen is a remarkable changemaker, drawing inspiration from her unique background as a Japanese American who grew up during World War II. Despite the challenges, she succeeded significantly as a medical doctor and psychiatrist in a predominantly male-dominated field. Through her distinguished career as a Jungian analyst, she encourages us to reflect deeply, discover our unique gifts, and offer them to the world with joy and purpose. This volume is a testament to what one person can do to 'bend the arc of history' towards a better world for all."

Justine Willis Toms
Co-founder, Creative Producer, Host New Dimensions Radio
Author of *Small Pleasures: Finding Grace in a Chaotic World*

Made in the USA
Columbia, SC
18 May 2025